HUMAN NEUTROPHILS

The preparation and publication of this study was supported through the Special Foreign Currency Program of the National Library of Medicine, National Institutes of Health, Public Health Service, U.S. Department of Health, Education and Welfare, Bethesda, Maryland, under an agreement with the Coordinating Commission for Polish-American Scientific Collaboration, Scientific Council to the Minister of Health and Social Welfare, Warsaw, Poland.

The study was published pursuant to an agreement with the National Science Foundation, Washington, D.C., by the Foreign Scientific Publications Department of the National Center for Scientific, Technical and Economic Information Warsaw, Poland, 1980

HUMAN NEUTROPHILS

Jerzy Lisiewicz, M.D.

**Associate Professor and Head of Hematological Laboratory,
Division of Hematology, Institute of Internal Medicine,
Academy of Medicine, Cracow, Poland**

THE CHARLES PRESS PUBLISHERS, INC.
BOWIE, MARYLAND

Library of Congress Cataloging in Publication Data

Lisiewicz, Jerzy.
  Human neutrophils.
  Includes index.
  1. Neutrophils.   2. Neutrophils–Diseases.
I. Title.
QP95.8.L57   612′.112   78-74880
ISBN 0-913486-90-6

To My Mother
J.L.

CONTENTS

12

PREFACE

It has recently been strongly suggested that human neutrophils, the phagocytic cells involved in nonspecific resistance to the invasion of microbial agents, play a part in antitumor immunity. A collection and critical evaluation of the data in the literature on this subject seemed appropriate in the light of the extensive advance of knowledge in this field during the past few years. The results of manifold investigations carried out in numerous research centers are discussed, with special attention to the literature of the eastern European countries, which, owing to the language barrier, is less familiar to English-speaking readers. The author decided to omit almost all information on neutrophils of various animal species, including laboratory rodents, and to concentrate solely on neutrophils in man—a subject of primary interest to clinicians.

This monograph has been prepared under a Special Foreign Currency Agreement between the National Library of Medicine, Bethesda, Maryland, and the Coordinating Commission for Polish-American Scientific Collaboration, Scientific Council to the Polish Minister of Health and Social Welfare. The author expresses his gratitude to Dr. Jeanne L. Brand, Chief of International Programs Division, Extramural Programs, National Library of Medicine, for her help in the organization of the preparatory program of the book and for enabling him to visit various American scientific centers in April 1977.

Though the English text of the book has been prepared by the author himself, he is greatly indebted to Dr. Claire Grece Dąbrowska for stylistic corrections, for which he offers his very special thanks.

The numerous electron micrographs included in the book are published by courtesy of Dr. Barbara A. Nichols of the University of California, San Francisco, of Dr. Sylvia Hoffstein of the New York University Medical Center, and of Dr. Li-Tsun Chen of the Johns Hopkins University School of Medicine, Baltimore, to whom the author is extremely grateful. Dr. Jan M. Zgliczyński of the Institute of Medical Biochemistry, Cracow Academy of Medicine, has kindly reviewed the chapters on biochemical aspects of phagocytosis.

In the final preparation of the book, very important help has been given by the author's collaborator, Anna Bodzoń, M.Sc., to whom he is enormously indebted.

The preparation of the book has given an opportunity to present the results of the author's own investigations in the field, which have been carried out in the Division of Hematology of the Institute of Internal Medicine, of which Professor Julian Aleksandrowicz is the Head. During several years of collaboration, Professor Aleksandrowicz has helped the author in many ways, and his initiative has very often given stimulation to new experiments and clinical observations.

The Author

CHAPTER 1

NEUTROPHIL STRUCTURE

The complex structure of neutrophils is related to the unusual locomotional mobility of these cells and their ability to engulf various biologic objects. In light microscope examination the mature neutrophil of the peripheral blood, panoptically stained, represents a rather simple morphologic organization, static in its size and the content of intracellular organelles.

The development of methods enabling the evaluation of the cell structure in conditions resembling the natural, i.e., microkinematography, scanning electron microscopy, phase-contrast microscopy, and transmission electron microscopy, is not yet sufficiently reflected in studies on the human neutrophil. There are no ultrastructural data on the subcellular elements of neutrophils responsible for their locomotion during migration, nor have the morphologic characteristics of the contractile protein molecule, with properties similar to those of actomyosin, in these cells been a subject of numerous studies. Furthermore, the morphologic events accompanying the engulfing of the various particles by neutrophils are not yet well known in detail. In particular, there is a lack of data on the changes in neutrophil surface structure in relation to the type of microorganism phagocytized at the moment when the object to be engulfed is approached. The initial phases of phagocytosis, characterized by intensive surface activity of the cell, are also not known in more detailed form.

NEUTROPHIL FORMATION DURING FETAL LIFE

The embryonic formation of hematopoietic tissue in man has not as yet been studied with the use of a more modern technique. There is an almost complete lack of systematic investigation in this regard, so far as electron microscopic, cytoenzymatic, and biochemical studies are concerned. The morphologic events accompanying hematopoiesis in the bone marrow of the thoracic vertebrae in human fetuses have only recently been clarified. The first stage of formation of the hematopoietic tissue is related to the development of the bone marrow cavity, which represents a unique microenvironment enabling the blood-forming cells to mature and become differentiated. The primary bone marrow development is dependent upon chondrocytic hypertrophy, calcification of the cartilage matrix, and penetration of the blood vessels near the center of the vertebral body (Chen et al., 1975). In a fetus 99 mm in length the cartilage of the central part of the vertebral body is eliminated by chondroclasts, and the subsequent formation of the bone marrow cavity is observed. The cavity is filled with sinuses, primary mononuclear cells containing granules and vacuoles, and mesenchymal cells. The primary site of hematopoiesis is in the extravascular space located between the vascular sinus, the cartilage, and the bone. In a fetus of this size a loosely arranged cellular meshwork and reticular cells are seen. This stage of fetal development is characterized by the absence of recognizable hematopoietic cells.

These cells appear in a fetus 105 mm in length, and are localized in the central part of the bone marrow cavity near the arterioles (Fig. 1). The greater part of the space adjacent to the cartilage and bone, however, does not exhibit hematopoietic cells. In a fetus 120 mm in length, cells with some features of hematopoietic stem cells are much more numerous. The formation of normoblasts takes place during this stage. In a fetus 150 mm in length, numerous developing neutrophils as well as normoblasts, lymphocytes, reticular cells, and megakaryocytes are observed (Fig. 2). During this period well-defined forms of neutrophils in passage through the endothelium occur. In the electron microscope the structural details of neutrophils are visible, i.e., the segmented nucleus and the cytoplasm containing granules of varying size (Fig. 3).

These data are, in general, in accordance with the results of previous studies by other authors indicating that neutrophils appear relatively late during the embryonic development of the hematopoietic tissue. These cells do not occur during the whole mesoblastic period of hematopoiesis, lasting from the second to the eighth week of fetal life. In the peripheral blood the neutrophils appear during the so-called hepatic period of hematopoiesis, i.e., about the 12th week (Mrševič et al., 1972). There is an almost complete lack of data on the ultrastructure of the hematopoietic tissue in the liver and spleen during this period. The ultrastructural differences between the hematopoietic tissue occurring in the bone marrow, on the one hand, and in the liver and spleen, on the other, are especially interesting from the point of view of the microenvironmental characteristics of the various sites of hematopoiesis. A more intensive production of neutrophils is not observed before the myeloid period of hematopoiesis, which begins at the end of the fourth month of fetal life. During the first months of pregnancy, however, the number of neutrophils in the peripheral blood of the fetus is low, ranging from 1000 to 1500/cu mm between the 16th and 24th weeks. The gradual increase in the neutrophil count in the peripheral

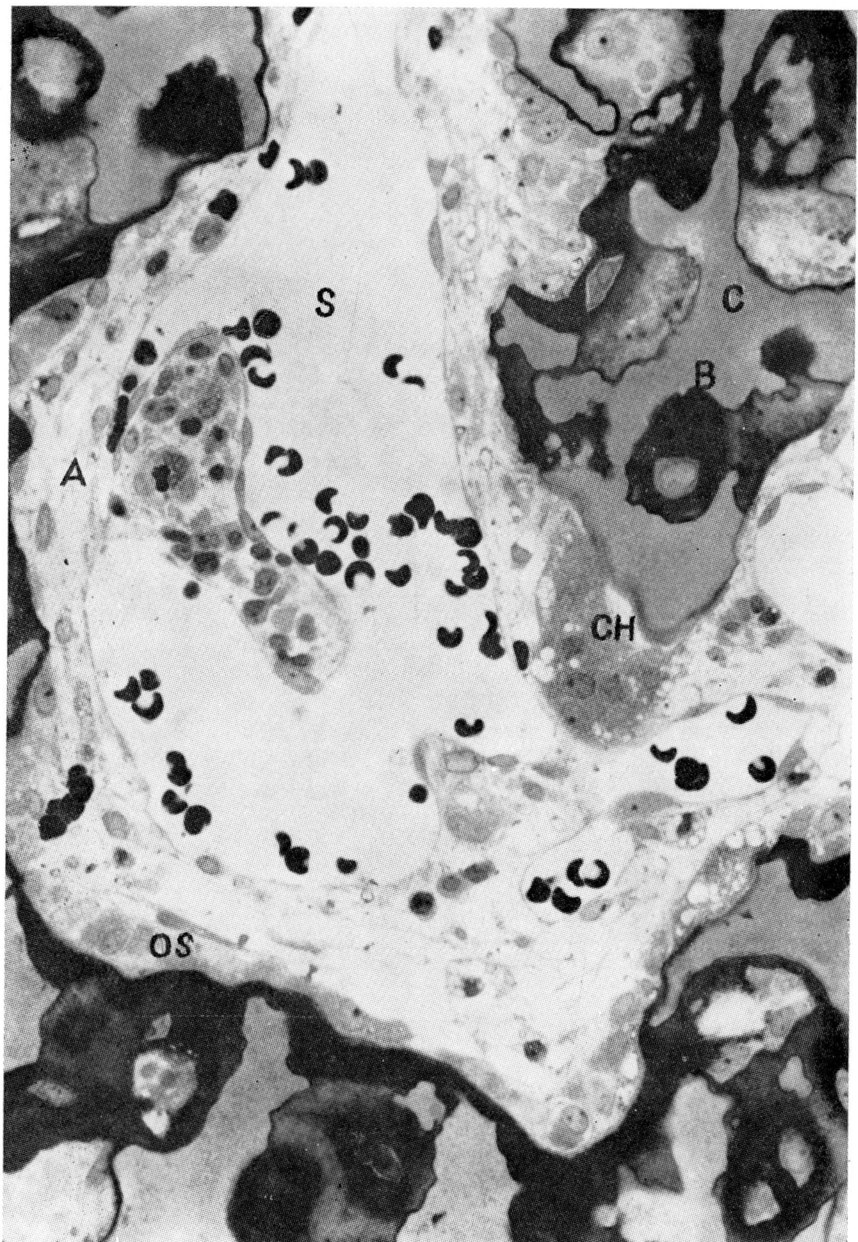

Fig. 1. Fetus, 105 mm in crown-rump length. Within the central marrow cavity the hematopoietic cells begin to appear in the vicinity of an arteriole (A). A few mononuclear cells containing granules or vacuoles are present in the meshwork of the hematopoietic compartment. B, bone; C, cartilage; OS, osteoblast; CH, chondroclast; and S, sinus. $\times$ 500. (Courtesy of Dr. Li-Tsun Chen, Department of Anatomy, The Johns Hopkins University School of Medicine, Baltimore)

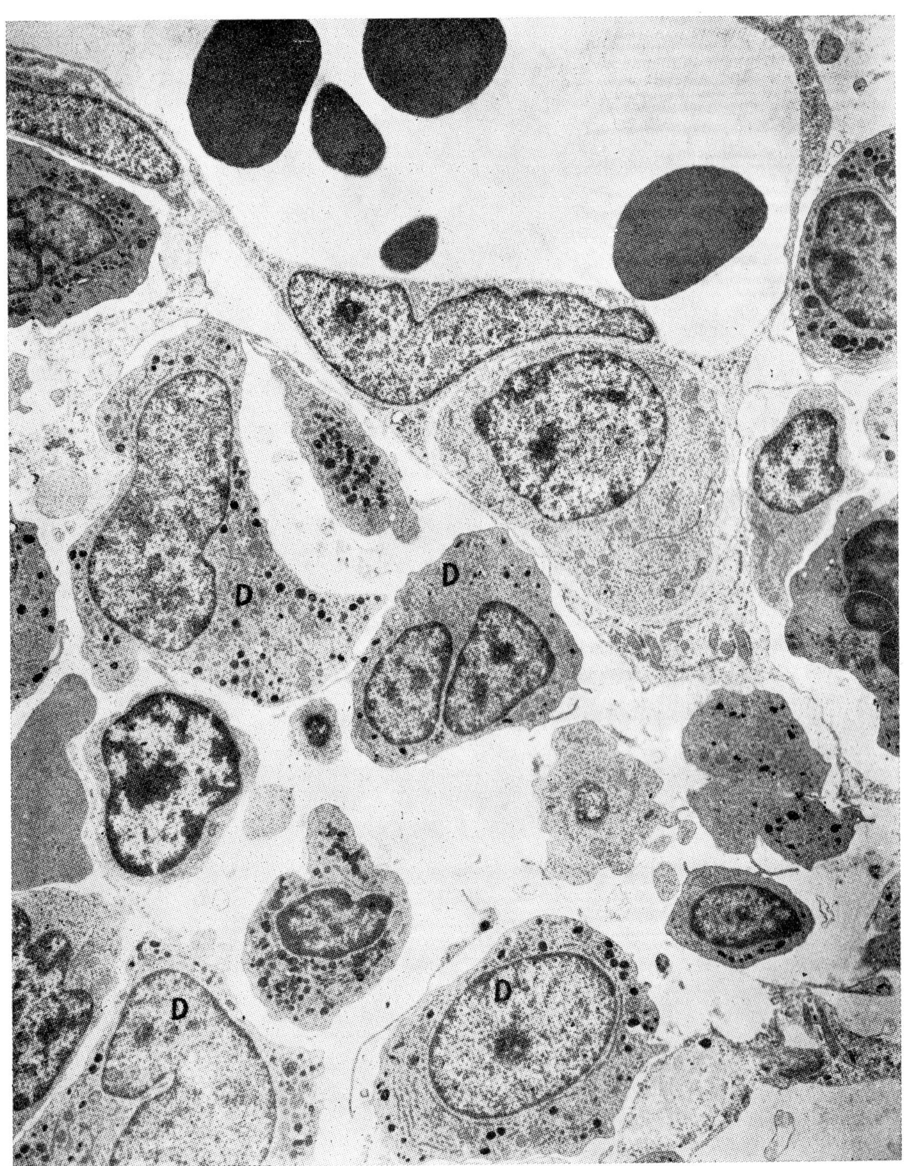

FIG. 2. Fetus, 150 mm in crown-rump length. Developing neutrophils (D) are visible within the central marrow cavity. Various stages of development of the neutrophilic cell series are noted. × 5000. (Courtesy of Dr. Li-Tsun Chen, Department of Anatomy, The Johns Hopkins University School of Medicine, Baltimore)

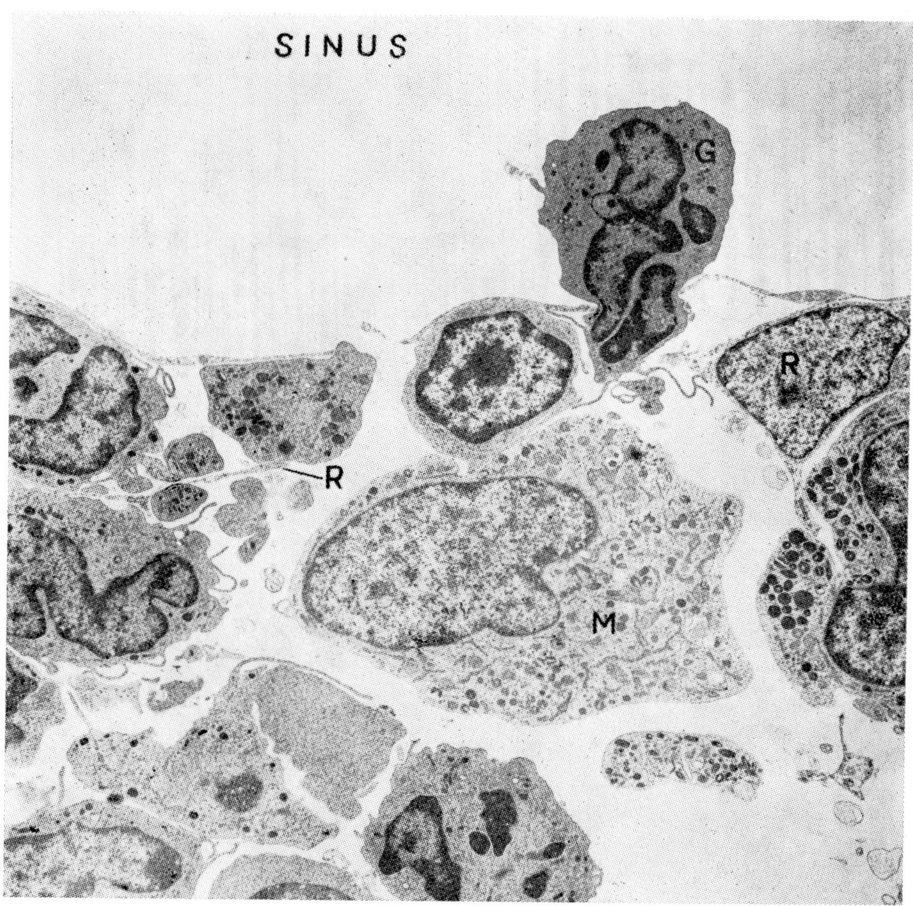

Fig. 3. Fetus, 150 mm in crown-rump length. Detail of the bone marrow cavity. Two neutro-phils are in passage through the endothelium. That on the left (G) is partially revealed. Apertures in the endothelium are observed only when the blood cells migrate through the endothelium. M, developing megakaryocyte; R, reticular cells. × 5000. (Courtesy of Dr. Li-Tsun Chen, Department of Anatomy, The Johns Hopkins University School of Medicine, Baltimore)

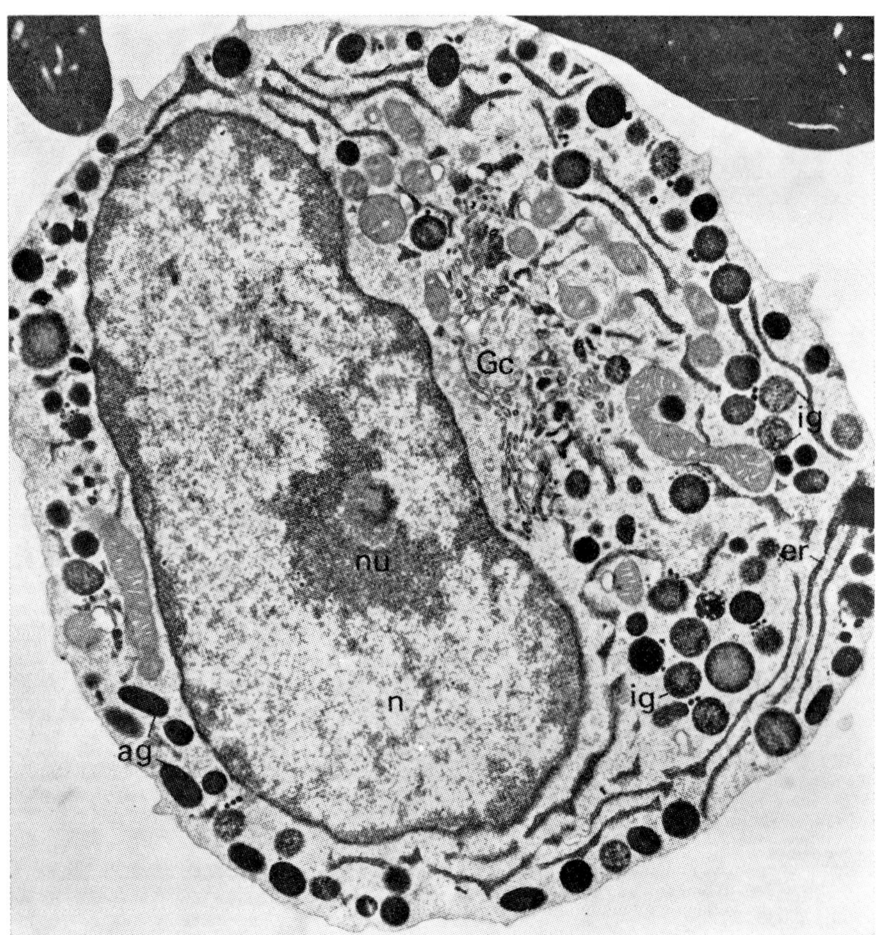

FIG. 4. Neutrophilic promyelocyte. A great part of the cytoplasm is occupied by the immature nucleus (n), which displays a marked lack of chromatin condensation and a large nucleolus (nu). The extensive rough endoplasmic reticulum (er) is filled with a dense peroxidase reaction product, as are the Golgi vesicles and cisternae (Gc), immature (ig) and mature (ag) azurophilic granules. × 12,000. (Courtesy of Dr. Barbara A. Nichols, Francis I. Proctor Foundation for Research in Ophthalmology, San Francisco)

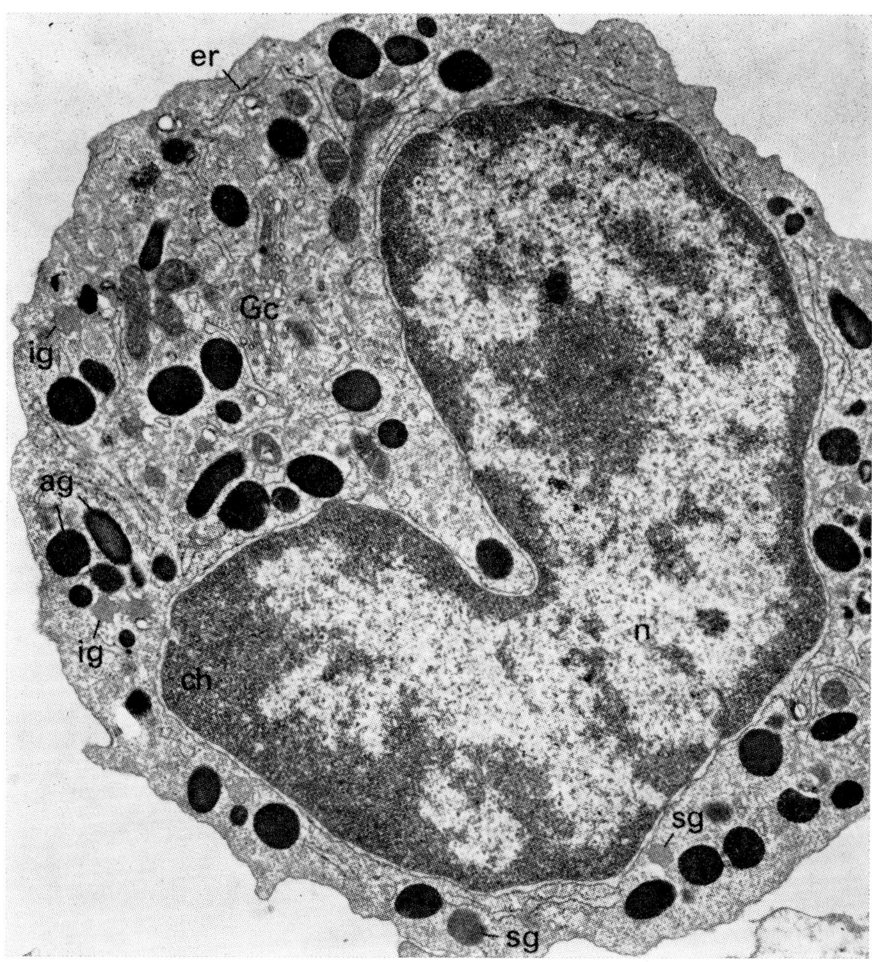

FIG. 5. Neutrophilic myelocyte. With greater maturity, the nucleus (n) reveals increased chromatin (ch) condensation, and sometimes becomes indented. Unlike the promyelocytes, the myelocytes no longer show peroxidase localization in the rough endoplasmic reticulum (er) or Golgi complex (Gc), both of which remain moderately extensive. Besides the peroxidase-containing azurophilic granules (ag) produced earlier during the promyelocyte stage, a few peroxidase-negative specific granules, immature (ig) and mature (sg), are beginning to appear. × 16,200. (Courtesy of Dr. Barbara A. Nichols, Francis I. Proctor Foundation for Research in Ophthalmology, San Francisco)

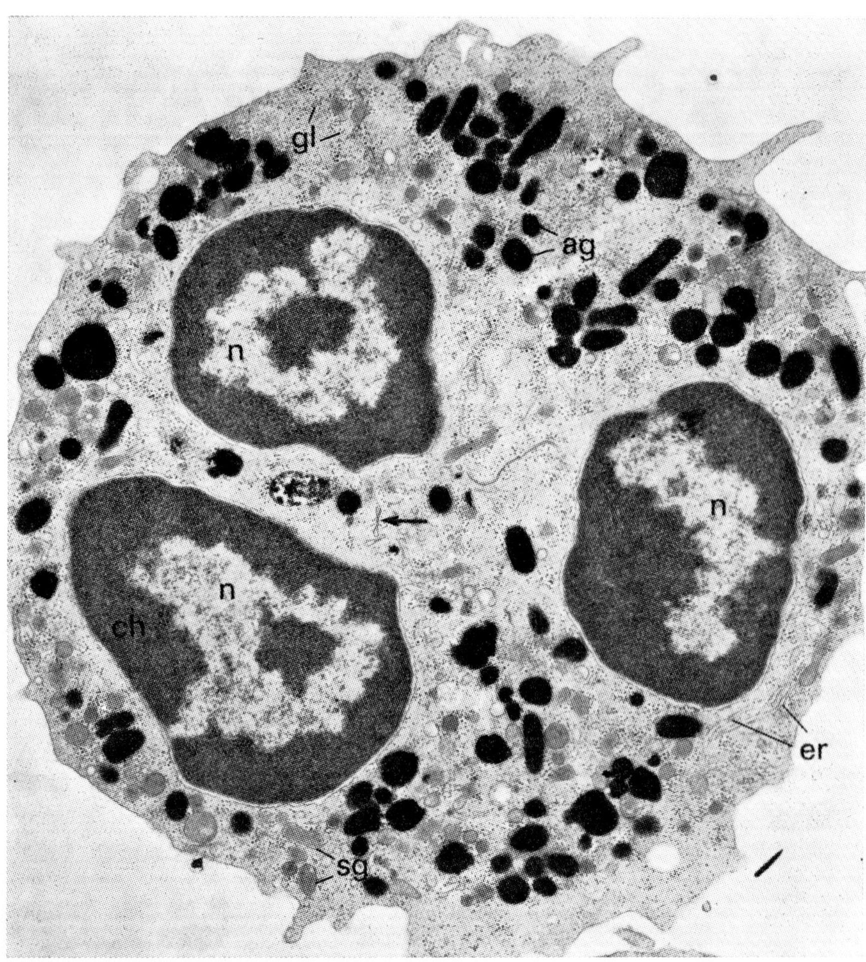

FIG. 6. Mature neutrophil. When fully developed, it has condensed nuclear chromatin (ch) and the nucleus (n) is segmented into lobes (three are visible in this micrograph). The cytoplasm is almost completely filled with granules—peroxidase-positive azurophilic (ag) and smaller peroxidase-negative specific (sg). The peroxidase-negative granules vary considerably in size and shape, and may be very small and elongated (arrow). Most cytoplasmic organelles have disappeared; only a few rough endoplasmic reticulum (er) cisternae remain. Beta particles of glycogen (gl) are liberally distributed throughout the cytoplasm. × 12,500. (Courtesy of Dr. Barbara A. Nichols, Francis I. Proctor Foundation for Research in Ophthalmology, San Francisco)

blood does not occur till the last three months of fetal life (Ławkowicz et al., 1969).

A characteristic feature of neutrophils during the last three months of fetal development is the high alkaline phosphatase activity. Enzyme activity, expressed in score values according to Kaplow, has been observed to exceed 200 in many of the premature infants studied (Bryniak et al., 1975). Simultaneously, high acid phosphatase activity has been noted in the neutrophils of these subjects. The intracellular mechanisms of regulation of the activity of these enzymes during fetal life are not known. Some indirect data indicate that the mechanisms differ from those operating in lymphocytes. It is emphasized that the metabolic activity of resting neutrophils in newborns is similar to that in phagocytizing cells (Park et al., 1970). The resting cells in newborns exhibit increased utilization of oxygen, high activity in the pentose cycle, and increased reduction of NBT.

In the premature infant the state of the neutrophil system may be affected by various diseases and infections. Leukemoid reactions, accompanied by vacuolization of neutrophils and the appearance of immature forms of these cells, are observed in fetuses with congenital syphilis (Aleksandrowicz et al., 1976).

The phagocytic and bactericidal properties of neutrophils in premature and full-term infants are a subject of controversy. On the one hand, there are reports indicating the decreased phagocytic activity of neutrophils in newborns after birth (Miyamoto, 1965; Iwaszko-Krawczuk, 1974), but on the other, normal or even increased phagocytic activity has been noted in analogous groups of subjects (Cocchi et al., 1967; Coen et al., 1969). It has been shown that normal phagocytic activity may be accompanied by a decrease in the ability of cells to kill intracellular bacteria and by a lack of the increase in pentose cycle activity characterizing the phagocytosis process (Coen et al., 1969). The phagocytic activity of neutrophils may be diminished in newborns with severe infections (Ivady et al., 1961).

The changes occurring in the neutrophil system immediately after birth have been the subject of only a few studies. Attention has been called to the fact that the percentage of neutrophils is higher during the first days of life (40%–80%) than between the fifth and the tenth day (30%–40%). These alterations are related to fluctuations in the total leukocyte count, which is high at birth (9000 to 38,000/cu mm) and during the next 10–15 hours decreases gradually. During the first week of life the total leukocytosis count decreases to about 12,000/cu mm. At the end of the first year of life the total leukocyte count is equal to about 12,000, exhibiting fluctuations from 5000 to 21,000/cu mm. A characteristic feature is the occurrence of a significant number of metamyelocytes, reaching 2000/ml of blood, during the first three days of life (Xanthou, 1970).

Neonatal neutrophils are similar to those of the adult so far as ultrastructure and peroxidase localization are concerned (Morris et al., 1975). In the neutrophilic promyelocyte, various stages of the peroxidase-positive azurophilic granule development may be observed (Fig. 4). The localization of these granules changes during the maturation of the neutrophil precursors, and in the myelocyte stage more numerous peroxidase-negative granules are visible (Fig. 5). Details of the mature neutrophil ultrastructure at birth are similar to those in adults (Fig. 6).

NEUTROPHIL PRECURSORS IN THE ADULT

The subsequent stages of neutrophil development in the hematopoietic system of the adult are well known. The details of morphologic characteristics of particular precursors of these cells are also known, and the clinical use of this knowledge, especially so far as the cytologic diagnosis of leukemias is concerned, is well established. The problem of a common stem cell of the various cells in the peripheral blood is, however, still unsolved. No such cell is shown in smears of the normal bone marrow in man. The only precursor cells visible in these smears are related to various cell series—neutrophilic, monocytic, lymphocytic, and others. The only candidates that might be considered pluripotential stem cells able to differentiate into all other bone marrow cell series are found in a small percentage of cells difficult to classify morphologically and characterized by uncertain criteria of their attachment to a given cell clone. Probably these cells represent damaged elements of the lymphoid system, and there is a lack of transitional forms between these poorly classified cells and the early precursors of neutrophils, monocytes, lymphocytes, or erythroblasts.

The Stem Cell Problem

From the very beginning of hematology there has been controversy on whether there is a stem cell for all cells composing the hematopoietic tissue. The concept that all body cells originate from one maternal genetic cell has also affected the approach to the study of hematopoiesis. In the past there have been heated discussions on the origin of particular cell series, in which representatives of the unitarian, dualistic, trialistic, and pluralistic concepts of cytogenesis have been involved. The current discussions of hematologists on this subject are less emotional.

18

It is, however, necessary to emphasize that despite the progress in research on blood cell cytogenesis there is no unequivocal view on the origin of various blood cells. The available facts represent a collection of contradictory or inconsistent information. These data will be briefly summarized:

1. There is a concept that the occurrence of common chromosomal and cell membrane defects in neutrophils, on the one hand, and erythrocytes and platelets, on the other, suggests a common genetic origin of these cell series (Aster et al., 1969; Sandberg et al., 1970). In subjects with the May-Hegglin anomaly, structural defects are noted not only in neutrophils but also in megakaryocytes (Godwin et al., 1974). Some congenital neutrophil defects, e.g., the Chediak-Higashi-Steinbrinck anomaly, however, may also be accompanied by alterations in lymphocytes and monocytes (Page et al., 1962; Kanfer et al., 1968). Such a chromosomal abnormality as the Ph_1 chromosome may occur simultaneously in completely different cell precursors, such as those of neutrophils, erythrocytes, eosinophils, or fibroblasts.

2. The results of studies on human cell cultures indirectly suggest a common origin for neutrophils, monocytes, and eosinophils (Chervenick et al., 1971). These results are thus inconsistent with the data just presented. Furthermore, the occurrence of common congenital defects in both neutrophils and monocytes, such as the myeloperoxidase deficiency, also suggests a common origin for these two cell series (Salmon et al., 1970).

3. There are data indicating the biologic antagonism of the neutrophilic, erythrocytic, and megakaryocytic systems, on the one hand, and the lymphoreticular cell system, to which lymphocytes and plasma cells belong, on the other (Aleksandrowicz et al., 1970). This antagonism consists in different reactions to corticoids and to some cytostatics. Owing to this concept, there is also a lack of data on the occurrence of simultaneous neutrophilic and lymphocytic proliferation of the leukemic type. It seems proper, however, to mention that similar reactions of different cells to a given biologic stimulus do not necessarily indicate the common origin of these cells. Furthermore, casuistic reports on the occurrence of mixed granulocytic and lymphocytic proliferations in patients in whom the only disease previously diagnosed was chronic lymphocytic leukemia are worthy of more discussion (Whang-Peng et al., 1974).

On the whole, the problem of a common stem cell for neutrophilic and other cell series in the hematopoietic system is still a subject of controversy. The hitherto known facts do not permit a clear formulation of the genetic relationship between neutrophils and other cells of the myeloid system such as erythrocytes and megakaryocytes. Furthermore, the existence of defects consisting in a complete lack of development of precursors of both neutrophils and lymphocytes indicates the complex character of the problem of blood cell genesis (De Vaal et al., 1959).

The Myeloblast

Myeloblasts do not occur in the peripheral blood in normal healthy subjects. In the bone marrow these cells represent 1% to 2% of the total marrow cellularity, ranging from 0 to 5%. Myeloblasts are characterized by the presence of a large nucleus, the dispersed nuclear chromatin exhibiting two to five nucleoli. The myeloblast diameter varies from 15 to 20 μm. The number of nucleoli in the myeloblast nuclear chromatin is of basic importance in the differentiation of the myeloblast from the lymphoblast, which usually contains only one nucleolus. The differentiation between these cells is very often helpful in the diagnosis of the cytologic type of acute leukemia and is also used in classifying the leukemoid reactions. This differentiation is more difficult in adults than in children. In an electron micrograph, the myeloblast exhibits numerous mitochondria, the Golgi apparatus, the endoplasmic reticulum, and free ribosomes; frequently polyribosomal structures are visible (Anderson, 1966; Tryfiates et al., 1967; Bessis, 1973). There is still a lack of morphometric study on the nucleoli of myeloblasts which are of significance in evaluation of mesothelial and tumor cells (Valkov et al., 1977).

The presence of azurophilic granules in the myeloblast indicates that further differentiation of the cell will result in the formation of the neutrophilic cell series. At first in young myeloblasts the azurophilic granules are not numerous, but later on their number increases (Bessis, 1973). In the phase-contrast microscope, myeloblasts show a pale, large nucleus containing two or more nucleoli; the differentiation of azurophilic granules from the mitochondria is not easy when using this technique. The myeloblast's ability to perform pseudopodial movements in healthy persons is a subject of controversy (Bessis, 1973; Wintrobe et al., 1975).

The Promyelocyte

Promyelocytes represent the next stage of myeloblast development. The cell nucleus features of these cells are identical with those in the myeloblast (Fig. 4). The promyelocyte cytoplasm, in contrast, is characterized by the appearance of numerous granules varying in number and density. Most of these granules are localized on the cytoplasm periphery. The basophilia of these granules is greater in promyelocytes than in more mature forms of neutrophilic cells. The promyelocyte granules consist of two different subtypes—the first is represented by specific lysosomal granules and the second corresponds to azurophilic granules (Bessis, 1973). Azurophilic granules may undergo transformation into cylindrical inclusions identical with Auer bodies. This transformation is frequently noted in leukemic promyelocytes. The number of mitochondria is lower in promyelocytes than in myeloblasts, in contrast to the endoplasmic reticulum, which is better developed, with ribosomes present along the external surfaces of the endoplasmic reticulum cisternae. The Golgi bodies demonstrate the active formation of both specific and azurophilic granules.

According to numerous authors the azurophilic granules correspond to the so-called primary lysosomes, and the specific granules to the secondary lysosomes. The morphologic precursors of primary granules appear initially as vesicles or vacuoles formed from the lateral terminations of the lamellae associated with the inner aspect of the Golgi region (Davis et al., 1972). During the maturation of these precursors a condensation of electron-dense material takes place, and the crystalline structures appear. The synthesis of the enzymes present in both primary and secondary lysosomes occurs on the ribosomes and within the endoplasmic reticulum. The precursors of the secondary lysosomes are formed from the lateral terminations of the outer aspect of the Golgi region and at the start correspond to vesicles. Electron-dense material appears within the vesicles during the subsequent stages of maturation of these secondary lysosome precursors. The formation of primary lysosomes (azurophilic granules) takes place in the promyelocytes, and that of secondary lysosomes (specific granules) mainly in the myelocytes and metamyelocytes.

Myelocytes, Metamyelocytes, and Stabs

The myelocyte diameter is usually larger than that of the myeloblast and ranges from 16 to 24 μm. In normal conditions the myelocyte is not motile (Bessis, 1973). The nucleoli in this cell are less visible and the nuclear chromatin is more pyknotic (Fig. 5). The cytoplasmic granules are numerous and vary to a lesser degree in cell diameter as compared with that in promyelocytes. Azurophilic granules are larger than specific lysosomal granules. In the myelocyte stage, differentiation in cell basophilia or acidophilia is noted. This is related to further maturation within the cells of the neutrophilic, basophilic, or eosinophilic series. Mitochondria are even less numerous than in the former stage, and the endoplasmic reticulum is transformed into dilated cisternae. Myelocytes are the last cells within the neutrophilic series capable of mitotic division.

Metamyelocytes are characterized by mature neutrophil cytoplasm. This stage of neutrophil maturation exhibits cellular motility (Bessis, 1973). The lysosomal granules undergo diminution and appear as delicate, dark-blue dust dispersed within the cell cytoplasm. The nuclear chromatin becomes more condensed, and the nucleus is horseshoe-shaped. Metamyelocytes are the last developmental stage of neutrophils containing nucleoli within the nuclear chromatin. During neutrophil maturation the number of micronucleoli gradually increases, and the number of dense nucleoli with nucleolonemas diminishes

(Vlastiborova et al., 1972). This is in accordance with the gradual diminution in the size of the nucleoli during neutrophil maturation. The metamyelocyte nucleoli may have a ring- or horseshoe-shaped nucleus (Smetana et al., 1973). They exhibit fibrillar components which probably correspond to synthesized 45 S RNA. In the phase-contrast microscope the metamyelocyte is characterized, in comparison with the mature neutrophil, by the different shape of the nucleus and the presence of a clear centrosomal region (Bessis, 1973). Myelocytes are capable of passing through the capillaries of the bone marrow by diapedesis, similarly to mature neutrophils.

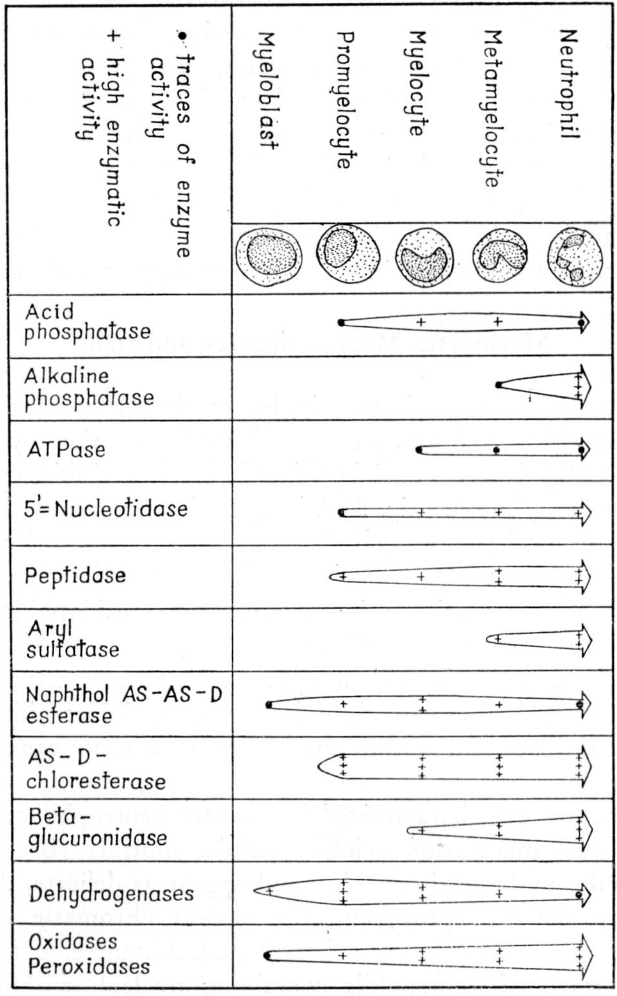

Fig. 7. Scheme presenting the sequence of appearance and activity of various enzymes in precursors of the neutrophil during its maturation. (According to Szmigielski et al., 1965)

Stabs exhibit cytoplasmic features resembling those of mature neutrophils. It has been noted that both stabs and neutrophils present in the bone marrow exhibit lower phagocytic activity than those in the peripheral blood (Altman et al., 1974). This observation suggests a discrepancy between the structural stage of cell development and the phagocytic activity in the bone marrow.

Morphologic evaluation of the neutrophil precursors in clinical practice is based on examination of bone marrow aspirate smears. The percentages of particular types of these precursors, and of mature neutrophils, may change owing to the initial volume of the aspirate. Aspirates in which the volume exceeds 1 ml show higher percentages of neutrophils than those smaller in volume (Dresch et al., 1974). In this way the differences among various authors as regards the evaluation of marrow smears are partially clarified.

Biochemical Components of the Neutrophil Precursors

Knowledge of the biochemical components of the neutrophil precursors is first of all based on cytochemical investigations. In healthy subjects the isolation of appropriate quantities of myeloblasts, promyelocytes, and myelocytes for examination by biochemical methods is in practice impossible. Information on leukemic myeloblasts or promyelocytes isolated from the peripheral blood of patients with acute myeloblastic or acute promyelocytic leukemia cannot be transferred to the corresponding normal cells, since the malignant process affects several metabolic pathways in these precursorlike cells.

During the maturation of cells in the neutrophilic series, some enzymes and biochemical components gradually appear in the cell cytoplasm (Fig. 7). Myeloblasts exhibit the presence of peroxidase, naphthol AS-ASD esterase, dehydrogenases, and oxidase (Szmigielski et al., 1965). The promyelocyte also exhibits acid phosphatase, AS-D-chloresterase, peptidase, and 5'-nucleotidase. Beta-glucuronidase and ATPase appear in myelocytes. Alkaline phosphatase and arylsulfatase are not present before the metamyelocyte stage.

Differential Diagnosis of the Neutrophil Precursors

The differentiation of particular precursors of neutrophils from those of other cells within the blood cell system presents a complex problem, of importance from the clinical and therapeutic points of view. The most important are the differentiations between myeloblasts and lymphoblasts and between promyelocytes and monocytes. The differentiation is based on structural analysis and on cytochemical examination (Table 1).

TABLE 1. Differential characteristics of myeloblasts, lymphoblasts, and monoblasts in patients with corresponding cytologic types of acute leukemia. (According to Hayhoe, 1968; Garg et al., 1972; Ważewska-Czyżewska, 1972; Glick et al., 1974; Schiffer et al., 1975)

Characteristics	Myeloblasts	Lymphoblasts	Monoblasts
Structure			
Nucleoli in the cell nucleus	two or more	one	one to two
Nucleolar membrane	indistinctly outlined	sharp nucleolar border	sharp nucleolar border
Clear zone about the nucleus	present	absent	absent
Nuclear chromatin	fine meshwork	coarse particles	very sparse
Cytochemistry			
Peroxidase	more than 5% of cells positive	negative	positive
PAS reaction	weak or negative	coarse granules in few or many	negative or coarsely positive
Sudanophilia	5% to 90% of cells positive	cells negative or weak	more than 5% of cells positive
Esterase	negative or 0 to 25% of cells positive	negative or weakly positive	more than 50% of cells positive
Other features			
More mature cells associated with	promyelocyte with azure granulations in Wright's stain	prolymphocyte or lymphocytes	promonocytes or monocytes
Phagocytosis of bacteria *in vitro*	positive	negative	positive

MORPHOLOGY OF MATURE NEUTROPHILS

With the light microscope, the characteristic appearance of the cytoplasm and segmented nucleus facilitates recognition of the cell. The light microscope enables the main morphologic features of neutrophils to be evaluated—i.e., their shape, the nuclear structure, and the presence and size of cytoplasmic granules. The mature neutrophil in the human peripheral blood is characterized by a relatively constant diameter of 12 to 15 μm and a uniform shape when examined in a light microscope. The cell nucleus is composed of dense chromatin arranged in separate segments, which vary in number from one to five and are only rarely more numerous. The segments are connected with delicate filaments of chromatin, not easily seen. Sometimes one of the segments may be located on others, and then the whole cell structure may resemble a stab form—the last precursor of the mature neutrophil. Observations made with the phase-contrast microscope indicate that within the living cell particular segments are grouped around the centrosome, which is situated in the center of the cell (Bessis, 1973).

In normal healthy subjects the largest number of neutrophils, that is, 40% to 50%, are cells containing three segments, while smaller percentages of cells have two segments (10% to 30%) or four segments (10% to 20%). The increase in the number of neutrophils with four or more segments, which is also seen in patients with chronic diseases of the liver or kidneys, suggests a vitamin B_{12} or folic acid deficiency. In contrast, an increase in the neutrophil count with a lowered number of segments is noted in patients with infections or in posthemorrhagic states.

A characteristic feature of the mature neutrophil is the presence of numerous granules within the cell cytoplasm. These granules are composed of two different subtypes. The first is represented by specific granules (80% to 90% of all cell granules), and the second by azurophilic granules (10% to 20%). These differences in the granule percentages are due to the fact that the formation of azurophilic granules is stopped at the myelocyte stage during neutrophil development. Further mitotic divisions lead only to a gradual decrease in the number of azurophilic granules, through the subsequent dilutions connected with cell mitosis. Conversely, specific granules are formed during the whole neutrophil life cycle, especially in the myelocyte stage, so that the number of granules gradually increases. In the light microscope specific granules are represented by poorly differentiated dust in the cell cytoplasm. Details of their structure are better seen in the transmission electron miscroscope.

The differences between the specific and azurophilic granules of the neutrophil are presented in Table 2. Morphologically, azurophilic granules in the promyelocyte stage occur in two main subgroups (Bainton, 1977). The first subgroup are spherical, dense, and homogeneous. The second are ellipsoidal or football-shaped, with the presence of crystalline inclusions. The basic differences between the azurophilic and the specific granules are now well established from both the structural and the biochemical standpoints (Bainton, 1977). It seems worth emphasizing, however, that the nomenclature of lysosomal granules

TABLE 2. List of differences between the azurophilic and specific granules of neutrophils. (According to Davis et al., 1972; Ohlsson et al., 1973; Spitznagel et al., 1975)

Characteristics	Azurophilic granules	Specific granules
Presence in cells according to developmental stage	promyelocytes and older cells	mainly myelocytes and older cells
Intracellular formation	lateral terminations of lamellae associated with inner aspect of Golgi region	lateral terminations of lamellae associated with outer aspect of Golgi region
End of granule formation	promyelocytes	all developmental forms and mature neutrophils
Percentage of total number of granules within mature neutrophils	10% to 20%	80% to 90%
Enzymes	myeloperoxidase, elastase, neutral protease, collagenase, antimicrobial basic proteins	lactoferrin, lysozyme, betaglucuronidase, acid beta-glycerophosphatase

within the neutrophil is not uniform in the publications of various authors. The data on some enzyme contents in both azurophilic and specific granules are also controversial. According to some authors beta-glucuronidase belongs to a group of enzymes occurring in specific granules (Spitznagel, 1975), but others are of the opinion that this enzyme is present in azurophilic granules (Davis et al., 1972). Hence the problem of the localization of various enzymes in particular types of neutrophil granules requires further studies.

Supravital staining of neutrophils shows that at a temperature of 37°C these cells are in incessant movement. The neutrophil locomotion is biphasic. The first phase is the primary protrusion of relatively long pseudopodia, consisting solely of cytoplasmic elements, and the second is the translocation of the cell nucleus. These pseudopodia, filled with cytoplasmic fluid, first pull the lysosomal granules and then the nuclear segments from the remaining cytoplasm (Bessis, 1973).

When in the circulating blood, neutrophils have a spherical shape, which does not change before direct contact with surfaces enabling the cells to move actively. These cells can spread over various surfaces, a phenomenon probably similar to ameboid movement. A characteristic feature is the intracytoplasmic movements of the centrosome, which have a specified periodicity lasting 30 sec and an amplitude of about 5 to 10 microns (Bessis, 1973). The neutrophilic granules exhibit several types of movement, including brownian movements, rapid movements in an amplitude ranging from 2 to 3 microns, and the long-distance movements of single granules within a radius of 5 or more microns.

The transmission electron microscope reveals several details of the neutrophil ultrastructure and renders visible the characteristics of the nuclear chromatin structure, the shape and size of the lysosomal granules, the nuclear membrane, and the mitochondria (Fig 6). In the electron micrograph the mature neutrophil of the human peripheral blood presents a segmented nucleus, a small number of mitochondria, and a small but frequently well-formed Golgi apparatus (McCall et al., 1969; Pellegrini, 1974). Other ultrastructural elements of the cell are the rarely visible centriole, dense hyaloplasm with the presence of free ribosomes, and glycogen particles. Single rows of rough endoplasmic reticulum as well as varying numbers of empty vesicles, ranging from 500 to 1000 Å in diameter, are also visible.

The ultrastructure of the lysosomal granules varies greatly in neutrophils. According to several authors, at least three main types of lysosomal granules occur in these cells: 1) ellipsoid granules containing stablike crystalloid structures, 2) spherical electron-dense granules, and 3) small granules varying in size and electron density (Watanabe et al., 1967; Egeberg et al., 1969; Bessis, 1973). The nature of the crystalloid structures present in the large, less dense neutrophilic granules has not been elucidated (Breton-Gorius, 1966). Similarly, the possible relationship between the ultrastructure of the neutrophilic lysosomal granules, on the one hand, and the type of enzyme present within these granules, on the other, has not as yet been established. It is worth mentioning that the characteristic electron density of the lysosomal granules is relative, since it depends on the technique employed and whether lead, uranyl, or combined uranylacetate-lead staining is used (McCall et al., 1969). Granulopoiesis stops in the mature neutrophil stage (Bessis, 1973).

Scanning electron microscopy reveals the neutrophil surface structure. Up to the present there have been only a few studies with regard to this in various diseases and during fetal development. More details are known of the neutrophil spread on glass surfaces (Bessis, 1973).

ABNORMALITIES IN NEUTROPHIL STRUCTURE

Neutrophils may exhibit morphologic abnormalities which are of importance from the clinical point of view. These abnormalities are classified as congenital and acquired. Among congenital abnormalities may be mentioned hereditary hypersegmentation of nuclei; the May-Hegglin, Alder-Reilly, and Pelger-Huët anomalies; bilobed nuclei with alkaline phosphatase deficiency; and the Chediak-Higashi-Steinbrinck anomaly. Among acquired neutrophil abnormalities are Döhle bodies, macropolycytosis, toxic granulation, and other changes occurring in patients with infections, as well as the Philadelphia chromosome. Not much is known about the molecular mechanisms of the genetic alterations leading to the manifestation of these abnormalities. It is striking that in the majority of case reports on congenital defects of the neutrophil structure so far published, no functional or cytoenzymatic findings have been included. Most of the neutrophil abnormalities are associated with various pathologic alterations in the chromosomal system. These alterations are exemplified by the occurrence of such abnormal nuclear structures as pouches, bridges, appendices, and fibrillar bodies in neutrophils from patients with the Down syndrome, which is characterized by the frequent presence of chromosome 21 trisomy (Djaldetti et al., 1974). Abnormal giant granules may appear in both neutrophils and eosinophils in patients with eosinophilic leukemia (Ruzicka et al., 1976).

Hereditary Hypersegmentation of Neutrophil Nuclei

This abnormality may occur in the form of a clinically asymptomatic, autosomal dominant hereditary defect (Undritz et al., 1964; Undritz, 1974). The number of segments in neutrophils in subjects with this defect exceeds four and is usually from six to ten. Nuclear hypersegmentation may be accompanied by the presence of giant neutrophils with a diameter of about 17 microns (Davidson, 1968). The abnormality is dominant and autosomal. In practice, there is sometimes a problem of differentiation between this abnormality and the pseudohypersegmentation associated with a shift to the right in the Arneth-Schilling count. It is essential to establish the hereditary nature of the anomaly before a proper diagnosis can be made. Pseudohypersegmentation occurs in patients with severe infections, chronic renal failure, circulatory insufficiency, and anemias, especially when due to iron deficiency.

May-Hegglin Anomaly

Inclusion bodies in neutrophils from patients with this anomaly are composed of electron-dense fibrils of about 50 Å in longitude (Jordan et al., 1965).

The suggestion that the fibrils are identical with mRNA needs confirmation. The inclusion bodies in the May-Hegglin anomaly correspond to Döhle bodies. They occur not only in neutrophils but also in eosinophils, monocytes, and lymphocytes. The defect is accompanied by leukopenia and giant platelet forms (May, 1909; Hegglin, 1945). In this anomaly the platelets exhibit several functional defects, an increase in the activity of the glycolytic enzymes, and a decrease in the number of granules (Hegglin et al., 1964). The anomaly confirms the common genetic origin of the neutrophil and the platelet systems.

Alder-Reilly Anomaly

This anomaly consists in the occurrence of giant granules in the neutrophils and is accompanied by clinical symptoms of gargoylism (Alder, 1939; Reilly, 1941). The defect varies in its expression and may simultaneously involve neutrophils, monocytes, and lymphocytes, but it may also occur in only one of these cell series (Fricker-Alder, 1958). The differential diagnosis of the anomaly should take into consideration the occurrence of giant granules in neutrophils observed in patients with infections, intoxications, malignancies, the Chediak-Higashi-Steinbrinck anomaly, or basophilic leukemia (Undritz, 1974). There are several subtypes of the Alder-Reilly anomaly, such as the complete, incomplete, or medullar forms. The relationship between this anomaly and Pfaundler-Hurler disease, in which it is frequently noted, is still a subject of discussion.

Pelger-Huët Anomaly

This anomaly consists in the occurrence of bilobed nuclei in neutrophils and the inability to form more numerous segments (Pelger, 1928; Huët, 1932). Genetically the defect is autosomal and dominant. The frequency of this anomaly is equal to 1 per 6000 persons. The anomaly probably does not affect the functional state of the neutrophils. Attention has been called to the fact that in patients with this anomaly and simultaneous infections, nonbilobed nuclei may occur in neutrophils. Sometimes the anomaly has a secondary character and appears in patients with severe infections, leukemias, or disseminated malignancies and then is named pseudo-Pelger-Huët anomaly (Dorr et al., 1959). There are significant differences in the frequency of occurrence of the genes responsible for this anomaly in various countries. Some data (Undritz, 1974) on this problem are presented here per thousand:

Sweden	2.5–6.5	Germany	0.20–0.32
Finland	1.4	England	0.17
Switzerland	1.0	Japan	0.17–0.67

The pseudo-Pelger-Huët anomaly may accompany several diseases differing in etiology (Table 3).

_{TABLE} 3. Occurrence of the pseudo-Pelger-Huët anomaly in patients with various diseases. (According to Undritz, 1974)

Acute myeloblastic leukemia	Lupus erythematosus
Acute lymphocytic leukemia	Agranulocytosis
Chronic lymphocytic leukemia	Fanconi panmyelopathy
Hodgkin's disease	Infectious mononucleosis
Plasma cell myeloma	Malaria
Primary polycythemia	Typhoid fever
Aplastic anemia	Sepsis
Addison-Biermer anemia	Peritonitis
Disseminated malignancies	Uterine cancer
	Cancer of the labium

Bilobed Neutrophil Nuclei with Alkaline Phosphatase Deficiency

A neutrophil anomaly has been described which consists in the presence of a bilobed nucleus, the complete absence of alkaline phosphatase, and a significantly diminished number of specific granules with a small diameter in the cell cytoplasm (Strauss et al., 1974). This anomaly was observed as a congenital defect in a boy with recurrent infections. In contrast to the Pelger-Huët anomaly, the defect was characterized by loosely aggregated nuclear chromatin, the deficiency of alkaline phosphatase, and no familial occurrence. The changes observed were solely related to specific granules. The azurophilic and the glycogen-containing granules exhibited no detectable alterations. In this patient an abnormal phagolysosome formation and disturbed bactericidal activity in the neutrophils against *Staphylococcus aureus* were also demonstrated. Recently, a genetic disorder characterized by the occurrence of monolobed neutrophils and deformed thumbs and great toes, dislocation of hips, limitation of motion of the joints of the lower extremities has been reported (Plum et al., 1978).

Chediak-Higashi-Steinbrinck Anomaly

This anomaly consists in the occurrence of abnormal giant granules within the neutrophils (Steinbrinck, 1948; Chediak, 1952; Higashi, 1954). Clinically the anomaly is associated with albinism, occurs in both sexes, and is autosomal and recessive. The abnormal granules appear in mature neutrophils, myelocytes, and myeloblasts, as well as in the cells of the eosinophilic and basophilic series. They resemble Döhle bodies, are from 2 to 5 microns in diameter, and are peroxidase-positive (Page et al., 1962). The granules may also be noted in lymphocytes and monocytes. The surface granularity of the membranes surrounding these giant cellular inclusions differs in its ultrastructure from that of normal granule membranes (White, 1973). Electron microscopic studies have also shown that in neutrophils from patients with this anomaly two separate types of giant granule exist. It has been suggested that the first type of granule represents enlarged but not actually altered lysosomal granules, and the second develops as a result of the constant fusion of small giant granules during neutrophil maturation. The two types of abnormal granule probably originate from the azurophilic granules, and their differentiation takes place during the maturation of the neutrophilic cell series. The association between the morphologic changes accompanying the anomaly and the azurophilic granules is expressed in a diminution of the peroxidase activity within the neutrophils of patients (Davis et al., 1972). The activity of beta-glucuronidase, which is an enzyme belonging to the specific granule enzymes, however, is also simultaneously diminished in the cells.

Attention has been called in various publications to the fact that in patients with this anomaly infections are strikingly frequent (Kanfer et al., 1968). It has been shown that it is related to decreased bactericidal function in the neutrophils (Wolff et al., 1972). One of the intracellular causes of this phenomenon is a lack of ability in the giant granules to fuse and form phagocytic vacuoles (Padgett et al., 1967). Disturbances in chemotaxis and phagocytosis are other examples of the biologic insufficiency of abnormal neutrophils (Clark et al., 1971; Stossel et al., 1972, 1974). On the other hand, there have been reports that phagocytic properties, migratory capabilities, and the appearance in the Rebuck skin window are not affected in these neutrophils.

There are suggestions that the main defect of neutrophils in the Chediak-Higashi-Steinbrinck anomaly consists in disturbed intracellular cyclic nucleotide metabolism. In favor of this concept there is an observation that the addition of cholinergic agents and cyclic 3',5'-guanosine monophosphate improves abnormal degranulation and normalizes the bactericidal capacity of neutrophils from patients with this anomaly (Boxer et al., 1977). There are also data suggesting that it may be possible to correct the microtubule defect of these cells by an agent increasing cyclic GMP generation (Oliver, 1976). It has been observed that after treatment of the cells with ascorbate their bactericidal activity is enhanced (Boxer et al., 1976).

Jordans' Anomaly

Neutrophils in patients with this anomaly exhibit abnormal vacuolization (Jordans, 1953). Abnormal vacuoles are observed in almost 100% of the neutrophils. The vacuoles are pale structures differing in size and exhibiting lipids when stained with Sudan III. The anomaly is inherited recessively and may be accompanied by muscular dystrophy and fatty degeneration of the liver. A characteristic feature of the anomaly is the occurrence of pathologic vacuolization not only in neutrophils but also in monocytes, eosinophils, basophils, and lymphocytes. There have been reports on the occurrence of the anomaly solely in neutrophils without the simultaneous involvement of other cells, but the classification of these cases is difficult (Rosenszajn et al., 1966).

Alius-Grignaschi Anomaly

This anomaly consists in a total peroxidase deficiency in the neutrophils (Grignaschi et al., 1963; Undritz, 1966). In addition, neither neutrophils nor monocytes exhibit positive reactions for oxidases and lipids. The anomaly has been observed in both sexes, but its mode of inheritance has not been sufficiently elucidated in the cases so far published (Undritz, 1974). Autosomal recessive inheritance has most frequently been noted. The relationship of the anomaly to the myeloperoxidase deficiency described in the section on phagocytosis defects is not clear.

Döhle Bodies

Döhle bodies are pale blue cystic inclusions, usually localized on the neutrophil cytoplasm periphery. In the original Döhle publication the bodies were observed in patients with diphtheria (Döhle, 1911). The bodies, however, are also observed in patients with various infections, malignancies, pregnancy, traumatic lesions, or burns. They are distinctly demarcated from the surrounding cytoplasm (Wilson's staining) and may occur in varying numbers. Usually, the occurrence of Döhle bodies is accompanied by other changes in neutrophils, such as a decrease in the nucleus/cytoplasm ratio and the appearance of more dense granules (Itoga et al., 1962).

Macropolycytosis

This anomaly consists in the occurrence of abnormally large neutrophils and their precursors. The neutrophils in patients with this anomaly are from 15 to 25 μm in diameter (normal values are within the range of 12 to 15 μm). The abnormality is observed in subjects with folic acid deficiency and involves the cells of the erythroblastic and megakaryocytic series, and also the cells of the jejunal mucosa, bladder, and vagina. Macropolycytosis may also be noted in patients with infections or myeloproliferative syndromes treated with antimetabolites. In some cases, the abnormality is a hereditary trait (Davidson et al., 1960).

Abnormalities Associated with Infections

It has long been known that infections differing in etiology may be accompanied by morphologic alterations in the neutrophils (Aleksandrowicz et al., 1976). In severe infections these alterations are manifested to a greater degree. They have been seen in patients with bacterial endocarditis, tuberculosis, rheumatic fever, or typhoid fever (Aleksandrowicz et al., 1976). Moreover, various structural changes in neutrophils have also been seen in patients with variola, leprosy, tonsillitis, pneumoconiosis, intoxications with chemical agents, schizophrenia, or puerperal complications. Toxic granulations appear in neutrophils from patients with Hodgkin's disease or a neutrophil nucleus anomaly of the Pelger-Huët type. They are frequently seen in fibrinoid pneumonia as well as in patients after X-ray therapy (Rudyk, 1966). The granulations are of irregular size and reddish violet or dark brownish red in color. The most intensive staining of these granulations takes place in an environment of pH 5.4, in contrast to normal dusty granulations, which stain most intensively in a pH of 6.0 to 7.0.

There have been suggestions in the past that toxic granulations are formed under the influence of various infections and toxic agents, especially of the local inflammation type, or that they are surviving promyelocyte granulations. On the other hand, these granulations have been considered to be a result of increased neutrophil phagocytic activity against bacteria or the protein components of various microbial agents.

Electron microscopic studies have indicated that toxic granulations may occur as large homogeneous granules exhibiting low electron density or as large granules containing crystalloid inclusions (Egeberg et al., 1969). These changes are probably due to an accumulation of lysosomal enzymes. It has been demonstrated that neutrophils containing toxic granulations exhibit decreased concentration of these enzymes, which indirectly favors the concept that the granulations represent nothing else but lysosomes (Koszewsky et al., 1967).

It has, however, been noted that the content of lysosomal enzymes in neutrophils varies greatly and is dependent on the enzyme type (McCall et al., 1969). The intracellular distribution of lysosomal enzymes has not been studied as yet in regard to the presence or absence of toxic granulations.

From the clinical standpoint it is of importance that toxic granulations are an expression of a severe inflammatory process or deep metabolic disturbances. A decrease in the number of granulations or their disappearance from the cells is usually accompanied by amelioration of the patient's state and remission of the pathologic process. The significance of the occurrence of toxic granulations in the differential diagnosis of various diseases has been emphasized. The shift to the left of the Arneth-Schilling neutrophil count and the appearance of toxic granulations may suggest a diagnosis of a leukemoid reaction and not of leukemia, though the granulations may accompany secondary infections in the course of leukemias (Williams et al., 1977; Wintrobe et al., 1975).

It is worth mentioning that a neutrophil with toxic granulations may exhibit several other structural alterations as compared with normal cells. Among these alterations the following may be mentioned:

1. The occurrence of rough endoplasmic reticulum lamellae in one or more focuses of the cell cytoplasm.

2. The presence of a prominent Golgi apparatus.

3. The appearance of a greater number of large granules (McCall et al., 1969).

There is an opinion that the presence of aggregates of rough endoplasmic reticulum (Döhle bodies) and azurophilia in some of the granules within neutrophils with toxic granulations may reflect immaturity of the cytoplasm due to the precocious release of cells from the bone marrow.

The Philadelphia Chromosome (Ph$_1$)

Chromosome Ph$_1$ was first described in 1960 in neutrophils from patients with chronic granulocytic leukemia (Nowell et al., 1960). This chromosome was small and noted in 80% to 90% of patients. It is easier to detect in the bone marrow than in the peripheral blood cells. Chromosome Ph$_1$ has also been observed in eosinophils (Kauer et al., 1964), normoblasts, and megakaryocytes (Whang et al., 1963). This chromosome belongs to the G-chromosome group and is numerically designated as chromosome 22 (O'Riordan, 1971). The small size of the chromosome is due to the loss of part of the long arm. There are data indicating that this loss is due to translocation to chromosome 9 rather than to any other mechanism (Rowley, 1973). In some cases the presence of chromosome Ph$_1$ is accompanied by a loss of chromosome Y. If chromosome Ph$_1$ occurs in a given patient it may be detected in almost all the cells of the bone marrow. These data are related to the problem of the congenital or acquired character of the occurrence of chromosome Ph$_1$. The observation that this chromosomal defect does not occur in the healthy member of a twin pair of which one contracts chronic granulocytic leukemia argues against the concept that it is congenital (Goh, 1967).

The existence of chromosome Ph$_1$ indicates the clonal nature of proliferation in this disease. The conditions for the appearance of abnormal cell clones are not known. The presence of chromosome Ph$_1$ was found in patients in whom leukemia developed after irradiation (Engel, 1964). Initially it was supposed that studies on chromosome Ph_1 would clarify the etiopathogenesis of chronic granulocytic leukemia. Later, however, it was shown that small abnormal chromosomes of the G group also occurred in irradiated subjects in whom this disease did not develop (Ishiwara et al., 1967). The familial incidence of the chromosome has been reported (Wiener, 1965). The question of the familial incidence of both chromosome Ph_1 and chronic granulocytic leukemia has not been solved, since in some families leukemia occurred in more than one member and the presence of the pathologic chromosome was not detected. Data on the prevalence of chromosome Ph_1 in patients with acute myeloblastic leukemia, erythroleukemia, myelofibrosis, primary thrombocythemia, and primary polycythemia argue against its pathognomonic role (Sandberg, 1971). In the course of chronic granulocytic leukemia a second chromosome Ph_1 may appear (Canellos et al., 1976). The significance of this phenomenon is not clear. Probably it is related to the action of previously used cytostatics, which may induce chromosomal aberrations, or to the formation of a new cell clone. On the other hand, it is not certain whether the disappearance of chromosome Ph_1 may not be due to the treatment applied. In the majority of cases the chromosome is found to be present despite symptoms of hematologic remission of the disease.

Recently a cell clone with chromosome Ph_1 was obtained in a culture from the cells of the pleural exudate of a patient in the terminal phase of chronic granulocytic leukemia (Lozzio et al., 1975). In addition to the presence of this chromosome, the cultured cell line was characterized by other abnormalities of the karyotype, such as the long acrocentric marker associated with translocation of chromosome 17 and the long arm of chromosome 15. The cell line obtained is an unusually valuable subject for various experimental studies. Cells of this line transplanted into a nude mouse strain preserve the chromosomal aberrations mentioned and undergo a malignant growth in the form of solid vascularized tumors (Lozzio et al., 1976). The spleen cells of patients with chronic granulocytic leukemia were also the subject of an interesting cytogenetic study (Spiers et al., 1975), in which it was shown that chromosome Ph_1 occurs more frequently in those with a myeloblastic exacerbation of the disease. The Philadelphia chromosome was recently the subject of an extensive review (Lawler, 1977).

SEX CHROMATIN

In neutrophils from healthy females a chromatin body 1.5 microns in diameter occurs. It is attached to one of the nuclear lobes by a fine chromatin filament. This chromatin body is morphologically described as a "drumstick" or "badminton racket" (Parameshwaran, 1971). The body occurs in 1% to 10% of neutrophils. In a group of 107 adults the mean percentage of chromatin body occurrence was equal to 4% and ranged from 2% to 8% (Parameshwaran, 1971). Sex chromatin is present exclusively in the neutrophils of women and does not occur in men. The chromatin is visible to a lesser degree in eosinophils and basophils than in neutrophils. The drumstick is regarded as a homolog of the sex chromatin (Barr bodies) observed in epithelioid cells and associated with the condensed, nonactive chromosome X (Davidson et al., 1954). The incidence of sex chromatin in the neutrophil drumstick, on the one hand, and in various cells, on the other, is not parallel. For instance, in a normal adult woman sex chromatin (Barr bodies) may occur in 25% of the epithelioid cells and in only 0.5% of the neutrophils. In some cases an inverse situation may occur: drumsticks are present in 1% to 2% of the neutrophils and sex chromatin is not detectable in the other cells. In 107 women studied in this regard, sex chromatin (Barr bodies) was noted in 16% to 34% of the epithelioid cells, and drumsticks were observed in 2% to 8% of the neutrophils (Parameshwaran, 1971). It was demonstrated that the number of drumsticks in the neutrophil nucleoli of a given woman is constant in subsequent examinations (Kapustin, 1974). This may serve in the identification of persons in forensic medicine. Drumsticks may also be detected in men with the Klinefelter syndrome, as may Barr bodies. This phenomenon is related to the presence of chromosome 47 (XXY), which is a characteristic feature of the syndrome. In patients with various diseases conditioned genetically, including those characterized by the occurrence of 4 chromosomes X (XXXX or XXXXY), the number of Barr bodies and of drumsticks is equal to the number of chromosomes X less one. A constitutional defect consisting in an increased number of drumsticks in the neutrophils has been reported (Undritz, 1974). In chromatin-negative women with the Turner syndrome, drumsticks do not occur. A decrease in the number of drumsticks has been reported in patients with chronic granulocytic leukemia in which low alkaline phosphatase activity in the neutrophils was noted (Tomonaga, 1961). Double drumsticks are rarely observed.

LE CELLS

The term LE cell refers to a neutrophil that has phagocytized the nucleus of another cell. LE cells exhibit a large phagosome, take Giemsa stain, and show a positive Feulgen reaction. These cells are demonstrable in the majority of patients with lupus erythematosus and related diseases. The cells are not pathognomonic, however, since they have been found in patients with myasthenia, hemocytopathies, chronic arthritis, or allergic syndromes.

During the first phase of LE cell formation after exposure to the patient's serum the homogenization of the neutrophil nucleus takes place, the nuclear chromatin loses its normal appearance, the cell segments undergo fusion, and the nucleus volume increases (Robineaux et al., 1956). During the second phase the damaged neutrophil is surrounded by other neutrophils. This period lasts from 10 to 60 min. Next the LE cell is formed; the damaged cell with the homogenized nucleus is phagocytized by one of the undamaged neutrophils. This phagocytosis is selective, since it includes the cell nucleus and not the cytoplasmic debris. The whole phenomenon is a result of the presence of anti-nuclear antibodies in the patient's serum (Hargraves, 1969).

CHAPTER 2

BIOCHEMISTRY OF NEUTROPHILS

The biochemical composition of neutrophils corresponds to the complex antimicrobial functions of these cells and reflects, as in other body cells, the presence of various metabolic pathways associated with energy production, glycogen utilization, and nucleic acid, lipid, and protein metabolism. Progress in research on neutrophil biochemistry is closely related to the development of methods of neutrophil separation from blood cells, and of biochemical methods, especially those used in the isolation of particular enzymes and other cell components.

In the past, several studies have been made using neutrophil samples contaminated with other blood cells. These are first of all studies on patients with congenital metabolic defects and leukemias. It is known that a suspension of white blood cells from patients with chronic granulocytic leukemia contains cells of the neutrophilic series in varying stages of maturation as well as many other cells, including eosinophils, basophils, and lymphocytes. The results of investigations on such cell suspensions are of limited value as far as knowledge of the neutrophil is concerned.

A number of investigations on neutrophils have been carried out on animals, but in many cases the results of these studies are useless for a knowledge of humans. Recently, numerous fresh data indicate that the extrapolation of research results from animals to man, at least from the hematologic point of view, should be very cautious.

It is also obvious that the results of studies on the composition of many enzymes, biologically active polypeptides, and other substances, as far as the amino acid sequence and other structural details are concerned, cannot be related to man without criticism. It has recently been shown that the sequence of amino acids in the fibrinogen fibrinopeptides varies in various species of mammal. This may be of significance in the evaluation of results of various studies on fibrinogen and the fibrinogen derivative contents in neutrophils, the fate of the derivatives and the mechanism of their enzymatic degradation within these cells, etc. Hence, as in other parts of this book, we shall summarize only the results of studies on man, and details relating to animals will be omitted.

NUCLEIC ACIDS AND PROTEIN SYNTHESIS

DNA and RNA

Information on the structure, content, and metabolism of DNA and RNA in neutrophils and their precursors in healthy subjects is very scanty. DNA is synthesized by the polymerization of deoxyribonucleotides catalyzed by DNA polymerase. The DNA polymerase activity diminishes during the subsequent stages of neutrophil maturation, and in the mature cell only traces of the enzyme are detectable. In leukemic cells of the neutrophilic series in patients with chronic granulocytic leukemia the enzyme activity is significantly higher as compared with that in subjects exhibiting reactive inflammatory neutrophilia (Ove et al., 1968). The increase in enzyme activity in leukemic cells exceeds the values that may be expected, owing to cell immaturity.

Experimental studies have shown that the last cell of the neutrophilic series, incorporating ^{3}H-thymidine, is the myelocyte. This cell is also the last capable of mitotic divisions and DNA synthesis. There is very little information of the intracellular regulation of this synthesis in neutrophils. More recent clinical observations suggest that specific chalones inhibit the proliferation of both leukemic and normal cells in the neutrophilic series (Rytömaa et al., 1976). Hence it may be supposed that the neutrophilic chalones, which are endogenous regulators of cell proliferation, may change or inhibit the metabolism of these cells, especially in regard to DNA or RNA metabolism.

As in other body cells, RNA synthesis in neutrophils is controlled by DNA (Silber et al., 1968). There are several data confirming this concept—the RNA synthesis is inhibited by actinomycin D and the neutrophilic RNA is susceptible to the action of ribonuclease. RNA, which is synthesized independently of DNA, is resistant to this enzyme.

As compared with normal cells in the neutrophilic series, cells from patients with chronic granulocytic leukemia or acute myeloblastic leukemia, when at a similar stage of maturation, exhibit increased DNA synthesis (Silber et al., 1968). The nature of this increase in not as yet known.

There is an almost total lack of information on DNA and RNA synthesis in the neutrophils of healthy subjects in relation to the biologic cycles, age, sex, and other physiologic conditions. The available data on the cyclic occurrence of some neutrophilic functions such as phagocytosis or the production of neutrophils indicate that the biologic cycles may also affect nucleic acid synthesis.

Protein Synthesis

Information on protein synthesis in normal neutrophils is scanty. It is known that the incorporation of radioactive amino acids is more intensive in leukemic cells in the neutrophilic series than in normal cells (Weisberger et al., 1954; Nadler et al., 1961).

Nucleotide Synthesis

Not much is known about the polymerization of deoxyribonucleotides and ribonucleotides into DNA and RNA in the neutrophils of healthy patients. Polymerization is associated with the *de novo* synthesis of the purine and pyrimidine nucleotides. In normal conditions neutrophils contain numerous enzymes catalyzing pyrimidine synthesis. These enzymes include carbamyl aspartyl transferase, dihydroorotase, dihydroorotic dehydrogenase, and orotidyl decarboxylase (Smith et al., 1959). In patients with leukemias involving the neutrophilic cell series, the activity of these enzymes is more intensive in less mature cells (Smith et al., 1960). It is not known whether an analogous phenomenon occurs in normal cells. From the standpoint of general biology, however, such a phenomenon might well be expected.

Several studies have been made on the synthesis of nucleotides in normal and leukemic neutrophils with reference to the mature of leukemic proliferation (Marsh at al., 1964; Silber et al., 1968). The results of these studies will be discussed extensively in the chapter on neutrophils in leukemias. It is worth mentioning here that normal neutrophils are capable of synthesizing pyrimidine deoxynucleotides but are incapable of performing the early stages of purine synthesis (Gallo et al., 1968). The site of the synthesis of the early precursors of purines—adenine and guanine, compounds necessary for the further steps of purine synthesis in neutrophils—is not known. It may be assumed that these cells utilize the total body pool of these early precursors, synthesized in the liver.

The mutual interconversions of the pyrimidine deoxyribonucleotides are complex. It is generally accepted that despite synthesis *de novo* these nucleotides may be synthesized via the salvage pathway through the kinase-catalyzed interaction of ATP with nucleosides and deoxynucleosides. Among the enzymes of the pyrimidine deoxyribonucleotides in the cells of the neutrophilic series thymidine kinase, dTMP kinase, pyrimidine deoxyribosyl transferase, thy-

midylate synthetase, deoxycytidylic deaminase, and ribonucleotide reductase
may be mentioned.

The intracellular regulation of these enzymes as well as that of the ribonucleotides and deoxyribonucleotides in normal neutrophils and their precursors
has not as yet been finally elucidated. The role of chalones in this regard is not
yet clear (Rytömaa et al., 1976). The fact that gold therapy in patients with
rheumatoid arthritis may inhibit the synthesis *de novo* of pyrimidine nucleotides
and cause neutropenia is a complication of this therapy (Westwick et al., 1974).

VITAMIN B_{12}, FOLIC ACID, OTHER VITAMINS

Neutrophils contain an $alpha_1$-B_{12}-binding protein, transcobalamin I (Simons et al., 1966). According to some authors these cells perform secretory
functions in regard to this protein. This concept is favored by data indicating
that the transcobalamin level in the blood is proportional to the neutrophil
mass. High levels of transcobalamin are noted in patients with leukemic proliferation of the neutrophil system, whereas low levels are seen in patients with
leukopenias. There are also data indicating that neutrophils produce transcobalamin III. An increase in the total serum B_{12}-binding capacity (TBBC) related
to an increase in the transcobalamin I and III levels exhibits a positive correlation with the neutrophil count in the blood (Kane et al., 1974). The metabolism
of vitamin B_{12} and of folic acid is of importance in understanding the nucleic
acid synthesis pathways in neutrophils. Coenzymes of folic acid take part in the
thymidine and purine syntheses. In neutrophils several enzymes of folic acid
metabolism are present, among which serine hydroxymethylase, tetrahydrofo-
lic methylene N^5,N^{10}-dehydrogenase, and the formate-activating enzymes may
be mentioned (Bertino et al., 1963). Several studies have been made on dihydrofolic reductase in neutrophils; in normal cells only traces of the activity of this
enzyme occur, whereas in leukemic cells of the neutrophilic series the activity
of this enzyme is higher. Despite the fact that the activity of dihydrofolic reductase increases during treatment with folic acid antagonists, it seems that this
enzyme represents the target enzyme of these antagonists.

Investigations on the metabolism of DNA, RNA, vitamin B_{12}, folic acid,
and proteins in neutrophils have not revealed all the regulators, feedback mechanisms and inhibitors of particular reactions in these cells. Relatively few
studies have been devoted to the intracellular factors controlling cell proliferation, such as chalones. Similarly, only a few studies refer to vitamin C, ribo-
flavin, and vitamin B_6 in neutrophils. Most studies on this subject have been
made using neutrophil samples contaminated with other white blood cells. It

is known that in patients with deficiencies of these vitamins their intracellular content is diminished. In experiments *in vitro* the addition of ascorbic acid to a neutrophil suspension activates the pentose cycle (DeChatelet et al., 1972). It is suggested that this mechanism may represent an alternative mode of hydrogen peroxide production in neutrophils which is independent of myeloperoxidase.

ENERGY METABOLISM

The neutrophil is a cell that utilizes large quantities of energy, especially during phagocytosis. Glycolysis is the main mode of producing energy in these cells. All normal cells of the body, except neutrophils, exhibit a diminished production of lactate via glycolysis in the presence of oxygen. This phenomenon is known as the Pasteur effect. Neutrophils are able to perform a normal degree of glycolysis in the presence of oxygen. Attention has been called to the fact that in some tumor cells the Pasteur effect does not occur. This striking similarity between neutrophils, on the one hand, and tumor cells, on the other, has not yet found any clear explanation. Comparative studies on normal neutrophils and neutrophils from the blood of patients with chronic granulocytic leukemia have shown that normal cells produce much more lactic acid than leukemic cells (Beck, 1958). This phenomenon is associated with differences between normal leukemic cells as far as the enzymes involved in regulation of lactate production are concerned. In leukemic neutrophils the contents of hexokinase, phosphofructokinase, glycero-3-phosphate dehydrogenase, pyruvic kinase, and lactic acid dehydrogenase are lowered as compared with these in normal cells (Beck, 1958; Sznajd et al., 1971). Moreover, the content of some enzymes in the pentose cycle, such as glucose-6-phosphate dehydrogenase or 6-phosphate-gluconate dehydrogenase, is also low in leukemic cells, though the level of phosphopentose isomerase in these cells is normal. A comparison of the main alterations in the activity of various enzymes involved in glycolysis and the glycogen synthesis of normal and leukemic neutrophils indicates a frequent decrease in the activity of these enzymes in patients with chronic granulocytic leukemia (Table 4). The results of these studies throw a new light on the energy metabolism of neutrophils, though the nature of the difference between normal and leukemic cells remains obscure.

The main source of the glucose metabolized in glycolysis and the pentose cycle in neutrophils is glycogen. These cells contain the largest amount of glycogen among all leukocytes (Gibb et al., 1949). The amount of mucopolysaccharide is also high in neutrophils (Kerby, 1955). During neutrophil maturation the glycogen content varies in subsequent stages of development in cells of the neutrophilic series. In myeloblasts, glycogen does not occur at all or only in traces. Myelocytes exhibit larger amount of glycogen (Wagner, 1947). In mature

TABLE 4. Comparison of the enzyme content of neutrophils from the peripheral blood of healthy subjects and patients with chronic granulocytic leukemia. (According to Sznajd et al., 1971)

Increase in enzyme content in leukemic neutrophils	Decrease in enzyme content in leukemic neutrophils
Amylo-1,6-glucosidase	Hexokinase
Glycogentransglucosidase	Phosphofructokinase
Dihydroorotase	Lactic acid dehydrogenase
Orotic acid dehydrogenase	Pyruvic acid kinase
Dihydrofolic dehydrogenase	Thymidylate phosphorylase
DNA polymerase	Alkaline phosphatase
Thymidylate synthetase	UDPG-phosphorylase
Acid phosphatase	Phosphoglucomutase
Muramidase (lysozyme)	Glycogen UDPG-synthetase
Histidine decarboxylase	
Total proteolytic activity	

neutrophils the amount of glycogen is higher than in immature cells. The absence of glycogen in myeloblasts is a feature differentiating these cells from lymphoblasts, which contain large amounts of glycogen. Neutrophils from patients with chronic granulocytic leukemia exhibit low amounts of glycogen; in contrast, cells from patients with primary polycythemia, inflammatory leukocytosis, or bone marrow metaplasia contain relatively high amounts of this polysaccharide (Wachstein, 1949; Valentine et al., 1953; Gahrton, 1966).

LIPID METABOLISM

Neutrophils from healthy subjects contain lipids represented by 10% in the form of cholesterol and 35% phospholipids (Gottfried, 1967). Among the phospholipids present in neutrophils phosphatidyl ethanolamine, ethanolamine glycerophosphates, sphingomyelin, phosphatidyl serine, and phosphatidyl inositol may be mentioned. The presence of free cholesterol and triglycerides was found in the neutral lipid fraction, which contained only small amounts of esterified cholesterol. Triglycerides represent the main portion of the inclusions formed within the cell cytoplasm in resting neutrophils *in vivo* (Lutas et al., 1977). These inclusions are probably the storage form of the free fatty acids which may participate in membrane synthesis during phagocytosis.

Immature forms of the neutrophilic series isolated from the blood of patients with chronic granulocytic leukemia contain smaller amounts of lipids and cholesterol and have a lower cholesterol/lipid phosphorus ratio than normal neutrophils (Gottfried, 1967). The metabolic basis of these differences is not known (Gigante et al., 1962). Furthermore, in additon to the components mentioned, the presence of oleinic, palmitinic, and linolenic acids has been shown in cells of the neutrophilic series (Chiaroni et al., 1966).

The degree of lipid synthesis is greater in the neutrophilic cell series of patients with chronic granulocytic leukemia or acute myeloblastic leukemia than in normal cells (Kidson, 1961, 1962). Neutrophils from patients with primary polycythemia exhibit no differences in lipid synthesis as compared with cells from healthy subjects. In subjects exposed to the action of industrial toxins the neutrophil lipid content is lowered (Andarzhanov et al., 1974).

Mature neutrophils are capable of enlargement of the fatty acid chains (Majerus et al., 1967). The mechanism of this phenomenon is not known. It has only been found that mature neutrophils do not contain acetyl CoA carboxylase, which occurs solely in blasts, the youngest neutrophil precursors. The enzyme is of fundamental importance in the synthesis of long-chain fatty acids.

*

Studies on the lipid metabolism in neutrophils, employing ^{14}C-acetate, have indicated that radioactivity is collected mainly in neutral lipids, and only a small portion is found in the phospholipids (Marks et al., 1960). In patient with chronic granulocytic leukemia, ^{32}P applied therapeutically is quickly incorporated into leucine, phosphatidyl ethanolamine, phosphatidyl serine, inositol phosphate, and sphingomyelin (Firkin et al., 1961).

It seems worth mentioning that ^{14}C-acetate incorporation into leukemic neutrophils refers mainly to phospholipids. In normal neutrophils this incorporation is observed first of all in regard to glycerides, free fatty acids, cholesterol, and its esters, while phospholipids are involved to a much lesser degree.

TRACE METALS AND OTHER ELEMENTS

A decrease in the supply of trace elements in the diet may cause a decrease in the immune system reactivity and alter the functional state of neutrophils (Aleksandrowicz et al., 1976). This decreased supply, according to some authors, is due to the development of industrial civilization, which introduces artificial soil fertilization and alters the natural composition of food. The greater frequency of infections in animals fed a diet deficient in trace elements confirms this concept. It has also been suggested that a diminished supply of certain trace elements may lead to a greater susceptibility of cancer and leukemias (Aleksandrowicz, 1975). The role of environmental factors in human immunity as related to the neutrophil system has only recently become a subject of interest. It has been noted that in children living in an area occupied by petrochemical industry the neutrophil count is lowered (Andarzhanov et al., 1974). The peroxidase, glycogen, and lipid contents of these cells is also diminished. These data indicate a need for the preservation of the natural environment, proper town-planning projects, and hygiene, in a broad sense, of the habitable environment of man.

Lithium

Experimental studies *in vitro* have demonstrated that LiCl stimulates the production of neutrophils in bone marrow (Harker et al., 1975, 1977). The mechanism of lithium action has not yet been fully clarified, but it has been shown that LiCl increases colony-stimulating activity by lung tissue. This effect is inhibited by puromycin. In patients with manic-depressive syndromes, lithium increases neutrophilic leukocytosis (Shopsin et al., 1971). After cessation of lithium therapy the leukocytosis abates within a week. It has also been shown that lithium carbonate increases the neutrophil count in healthy subjects but does not induce this effect in patients with malignancies of the hematopoietic tissue (Tisman et al., 1976). Our observations on the action of lithium carbonate upon the neutrophil system in patients with chronic neutropenia indicate that this antidepressant agent increases not only the neutrophil count but also the neutrophil acid phosphatase activity.* Clinical trials of the use of lithium carbonate in the treatment of patients with neutropenia deserve to be continued (Gupta et al., 1975). Our observations on the action of lithium carbonate on the neutrophil count in the peripheral blood of patients with bone marrow hypoplasia have indicated that the neutrophil system is stimulated by this agent. There are, however, reports on agranulocytosis after lithium therapy.

Copper

There are only scanty data on the effects of copper on the neutrophilic system. In children in whom the serum copper level is higher than normal, the neutrophils exhibit an increased ability to reduce NBT (Jankowski et al., 1975). There is a lack of data on neutrophil function in patients with copper deficiency.

---

* Blicharski J. et al.: Acta Haematol. Pol., 1980, 1, 17–23.

Selenium

The role of selenium excess or deficiency in the diet in the etiology of malignant tumors and leukemias has been a subject of numerous studies in recent years (Ermakov et al., 1974). There is a theoretical possibility that selenium deficiency may disturb the antimicrobial and antitumor functions of neutrophils.

In preliminary observations we have stated that in patients with chronic lymphocytic leukemia treated with small doses of sodium selenate, the absolute neutrophil count diminishes and neutrophil alkaline phosphatase activity does not change. These facts are in accordance with the observation that infectious bacterial complications in these patients are frequent.

Zinc

Experimental deficiency of zinc in the diet induces a decrease in neutrophil acid phosphatase activity in mice (Lisiewicz et al., 1977). The absolute neutrophil count is also diminished (Fig. 8). The decrease affects both enzyme-positive and enzyme-negative cells. These observations have shown that zinc is of importance in maintaining the normal state of the lysosomal apparatus in neutrophils. The mechanisms involved in the regulation of enzyme activities within the neutrophil by zinc are not clear. It has been observed that zinc neutralizes the histidine and cysteine effects by diminishing neutrophil alkaline phosphatase activity (DeChatelet et al., 1971).

Magnesium

In personal investigations we have observed that magnesium salts (Delbiase) cause a transient increase in the neutrophil count in the peripheral blood of patients with chronic lymphocytic leukemia (Aleksandrowicz et al., 1970). Magnesium has an important effect on the normal course of neutrophil degranulation, and also alters the chemotactic properties of these cells (Estensen et al., 1976). The molecular mechanism of this action of magnesium is not known. In experimental conditions mangesium deficiency in mice causes an increase in the absolute neutrophil count associated with an increase in acid phosphatase-positive cells (Lisiewicz et al., 1977), though the general indices of enzyme activity remain unchanged. This indicates a difference between the magnesium and zinc deficiencies in regard to lysosomal acid phosphatase and the lysosomal apparatus as a whole in neutrophils.

Calcium

Calcium alters the chemotactic properties of neutrophils (Estensen et al., 1976). The mechanism of action of bivalent ions on these properties of neutro-

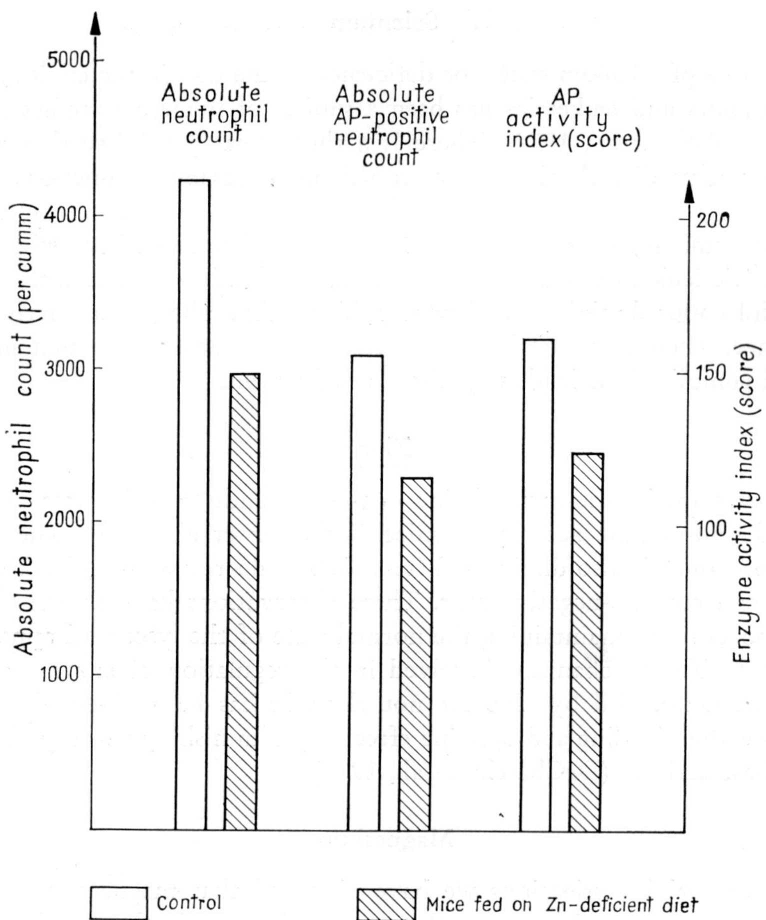

FIG. 8. Effect of zinc deficiency on acid phosphatase (AP) activity in mouse neutrophils. (According to Lisiewicz et al., 1977)

phils has not been fully elucidated (Gallin et al., 1974). In experimental conditions calcium may induce the excretion of lysozyme from neutrophils (Goldstein et al., 1974).

Iron

There is a lack of systematic studies on the iron effect on neutrophil functions. The content of this element within neutrophils has not been studied in various physiologic and pathologic conditions. In healthy subjects the iron content in neutrophils is low (Koszewsky et al., 1967). It has been suggested that toxic granulations present in these cells in patient with various infections contain hemosiderin as the result of an active uptake of iron.

NEUTROPHIL ANTIMICROBIAL INTRACELLULAR SYSTEMS

A characteristic feature of neutrophils is a biochemical component enabling biologic attack on a given microbial agent by means of several intracellular antimicrobial systems. The first group of these systems acts by means of oxygen and the intracellular production of hydrogen peroxide; the second group acts independently of cellular oxygen. The oxygen-dependent systems induce a direct oxidative effect, inhibiting a number of microbial enzymes and destroying the homeostasis of microbial oxidoreductive processes. The suggestion that the action of the oxygen-dependent systems is prior to the slower action of the oxygen-independent systems needs further study, since there are data indicating that the start of phagocytosis is accompanied by the release of enzymes from specific and azurophilic granules (Bainton, 1973). The oxygen-independent systems degrade particular components of microbial agents through enzymatic digestion and so cause a decrease in the pH, diminishing their chance of surviving within the neutrophils. The antimicrobial cationic proteins are an important component of these systems. The main biologic properties of neutrophils are their ability to produce energy despite a lack of oxygen and to degrade anaerobically glucose despite the presence of oxygen. This indicates the adaptation of these cells for the synthesis of hydrogen peroxide solution in regions situated deep in the tissues without a sufficient supply of blood and oxygen.

OXYGEN-DEPENDENT SYSTEMS

Among the oxygen-dependent systems of the neutrophils hydrogen peroxide, superoxide anions, singlet oxygen, and myeloperoxidase should be mentioned. Particular components of the oxygen-dependent systems may act independently or their actions may be related to one another. The myeloperoxidase-hydrogen peroxide system induces a much stronger bactericidal effect than myeloperoxidase or hydrogen peroxide alone (McRipley et al., 1967; Klebanoff et al., 1972; Klebanoff, 1975). Real progress in this field was made by the demonstration that myeloperoxidase isolated from neutrophils catalyzed the chlorination reaction (Zgliczyński et al., 1975). The formation of Cl^+ ions enables the spontaneous chlorination of the amino compounds which are components of the microbial agents. In the light of these studies it may be accepted that the main element of the oxygen-dependent antimicrobial systems in neutrophils is the myeloperoxidase–H_2O_2–Cl^+ system.

The Myeloperoxidase–H_2O_2–Halide System

The system composed of myeloperoxidase (MPO), hydrogen peroxide, and halide is probably the strongest antimicrobial system in the neutrophil. The biologic significance of this system has been learned only recently (Zgliczyński et al., 1975; Sbarra et al., 1976). In this system the halide component may be represented by Cl^-, J^-, or Br^- ions. Iodine may be replaced by iodine-containing thyroid hormones such as triiodothyronine or thyroxine. The source of hydrogen peroxide in the system may be in the group of enzymes producing it (e.g., glucose and glucose oxidase) or in bacteria producing this compound (pneumococci, streptococci, lactic bacteria). Hydrogen peroxide alone may induce antimicrobial action. In certain conditions, however, the amount of this substance may be insufficient to kill phagocytized bacteria. During phagocytosis the intracellular production of hydrogen peroxide increases. The reaction of hydrogen peroxide, myeloperoxidase, and one of the halides mentioned leads to the formation of an antimicrobial system exhibiting an unusually strong action. Neutrophil myeloperoxidase in man is able to catalyze the decarboxylation and deamination of amino acids in the presence of hydrogen peroxide. The MPO–H_2O_2–Cl^- system may also chlorinate amino acids and subsequently lead to the formation of amino acid chloramines (Fig. 9). The oxidation of Cl^- by H_2O_2 induces conversion of Cl^- into Cl^+. The antimicrobial system in question functions independently of the intracellular pH. The mechanism of breakage of the peptide bonds for decarboxylation of the amino acids through the MPO–H_2O_2–Cl^- system is not known. This system interacts with the free amino acids, leading to the formation of amino acid chloramines. These chloramines are unstable and undergo decomposition in the presence of water into aldehydes, CO_2, and NH_4Cl. Another biologically important property of the MPO–H_2O_2–Cl^- system is its ability to form singlet oxygen in the presence of chloride ions. Singlet oxygen induces a separate antimicrobial effect. It has recently been shown that the biologic role of the MPO–H_2O_2–Cl^- system does not lie only in antimicrobial action. The system may induce a cytotoxic effect on mammalian tumor cells (Clark et al., 1975).

Two main components of the MPO–H_2O_2–Cl^- system, MPO and H_2O_2, deserve more extensive discussion. H_2O_2 induces a strong antimicrobial effect and is produced intracellulary in neutrophils. During phagocytosis an increase in H_2O_2 production is noted (McRipley et al., 1967). The mechanism of this production is not clear in detail. Probably H_2O_2 is formed in the course of NADP regeneration with the participation of $NADPH_2$ oxidase (Iyer et al., 1961). There are data indicating that the toxicity of H_2O_2 against microbial agents increases in the presence of iodines and ascorbic acid; the role of this phenomenon in man has not been fully elucidated. It is also not clear whether the neutrophil has an intracellular mechanism of defense against H_2O_2 produced during phagocytosis; it cannot be excluded that the mechanism is associated with the presence of the sulfhydryl group within the cell (Mandell, 1972).

The antimicrobial action of MPO may be demonstrated in the absence of H_2O_2, but the action is weaker than that in the presence of H_2O_2 (McRipley et al., 1967; Klebanoff et al., 1972). The mechanism of activation of the

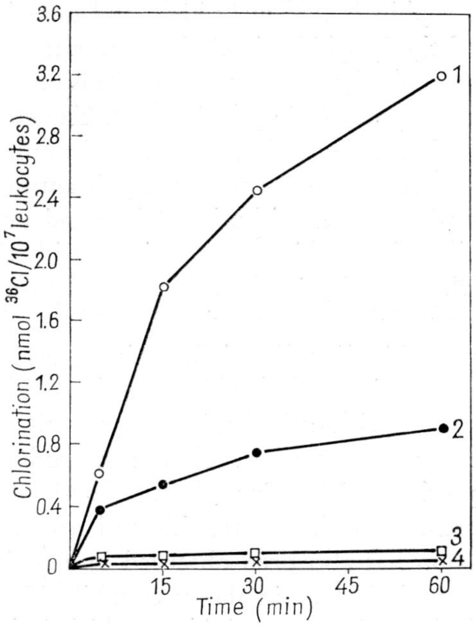

FIG. 9. The time course of the chlorination process in leukocytes (predominantly neutrophils). The composition of the samples was as follows: *1*—leukocytes + bacteria; *2*—leukocytes + bacteria in the presence of 1 mM NaN_3; *3*—leukocytes only; *4*—bacteria only. Chlorination depends on the presence of bacteria; it is not due to the metabolic processes in bacterial cells, since the control sample with bacteria, but without leukocytes, does not exhibit ^{36}Cl incorporation. (Courtesy of Dr. J. M. Zgliczyński, Institute of Medical Biochemistry, Cracow Academy of Medicine)

$MPO-H_2O_2$ system is not known in detail. It is only known that activation is accompanied by the decrease in the intracellular pH, the activation of $NADPH_2$ oxidase, and the release of myeloperoxidase from the lysosomal granules. Some inhibitors of this system, such as NAN_3, KCN, and aminotriazol, are also known.

The antimicrobial action of the $MPO-H_2O_2$ system against viruses (Belding et al., 1970), bacteria (McRipley et al., 1967; Klebanoff, 1968; Mandell, 1974), *Mycoplasma* (Jacobs et al., 1972), and fungi such as *Candida albicans*, *Aspergillus niger*, or *A. fumigatus* (Lehrer, 1969) has been demonstrated. The ability of

^{4*}

neutrophils to kill *Candida albicans* is inhibited by theophylline and prostaglandin E_1 (Bourne et al., 1971).

Myeloperoxidase occurs in the large azurophilic granules and is regarded as a marker of these granules (Bainton et al., 1971). This enzyme has been obtained in highly purified form (Schultz et al., 1964; Rohrer et al., 1966), and has also been isolated from the peripheral blood leukocytic mass of patients with chronic granulocytic leukemia (Zgliczyński et al., 1968). The myeloperoxidase content in neutrophils is extremely high, and in cells from healthy subjects may reach 5% of the lyophilized cellular material (Schultz et al., 1962). The ability of MPO to act in a broad spectrum of pH is of significance for bactericidal function of this enzyme (Zgliczyński, 1979). The enzyme occurs within the neutrophils in two forms depending on the environmental pH. It reflects the basic role of the enzyme among the neutrophil antimicrobial systems. In some studies the general activities of both catalase and peroxidase have been estimated in neutrophils. Neutrophils from patients with chronic granulocytic leukemia exhibit a higher activity in these enzymes than normal subjects (Żupańska, 1970). In patients with myeloperoxidase deficiency the iodination defect and a decreased ability to kill *E. coli* and *C. albicans* has been observed (Stendahl et al., 1976). Abnormal intracellular killing of bacteria has also been noted in neutrophils from patients with defective H_2O_2 synthesis, though this defect is observed only after engulfing bacteria which do not produce H_2O_2 themselves. In contrast, bacteria producing H_2O_2 introduce the deficient component of the cell antimicrobial system into the neutrophil and are killed to the normal degree. This phenomenon has also been observed in a patient with glucose-6-phosphate dehydrogenase deficiency in the neutrophils (Owusu, 1973). It may also be mentioned that bacterial neuraminidase, which induces the removal of neutrophil membrane sialic acids, impairs the stimulation of O_2^- production while it has no effect on phagocytosis and the phagocytosis-associated burst of the hexose monophosphate shunt (Tsan et al., 1977).

Superoxide Anions

Superoxide anions are radicals exhibiting high reactivity in the course of oxygen reduction. These anions may act as both oxidative and reductive agents (O_2^-). There is an opinion that superoxide anions are intermediate factors in H_2O_2 formation. The formation of singlet oxygen from superoxide anions is expressed in the formula for the reaction

$$O_2^- + O_2 + 2H^+ = O_2 + H_2O_2$$

The formation of oxygen from these anions is catalyzed by superoxide dismutase; hence this enzyme inhibits reactions depending on the presence of superoxide anions. It has been demonstrated that superoxide anions are intermediate products of H_2O_2 formation (Klebanoff, 1975). This concept is based on the fact that cytochrome C inhibits H_2O_2 formation through the mechanism of the reaction between cytochrome C and the superoxide anion. In the presence of superoxide dismutase this inhibitory effect of cytochrome C is not observed, since the enzyme prevents the occurrence of this reaction and causes O_2 formation. It has also been shown that the presence of the enzyme protects microbial agents from the toxic effects of superoxide anions (Gregory et al., 1973). This phenomenon is due to the fact that the rapid formation of O_2 from these anions causes their removal from the environment of the microbial agents, and O_2 is utilized in the metabolic processes.

There are some data indicating that human neutrophils are able to form superoxide anions. These cells reduce ferricytochrome C, and the addition of superoxide dismutase inhibits this reduction (Babior et al., 1973). In these experiments it was also shown that the intracellular production of superoxide anions increases during phagocytosis. The demonstration that the content of these anions is lower in the neutrophils of subjects with chronic granulomatous disease than in healthy persons indicates their clinical significance (Curnutte et al., 1974).

Singlet Oxygen

The term singlet molecular oxygen refers to the electronically activated state of oxygen exhibiting chemiluminescence during return to the triplet ground state. This phenomenon is observed during the incubation of bacterial particles and their phagocytosis by normal human neutrophils (Allen et al., 1972). In patients with chronic granulomatous disease this phenomenon has not been observed (Stjernholm et al., 1973). The intracellular sources of singlet molecular oxygen are not known in detail. One of its sources is probably the MPO-mediated antimicrobial system, and another is the dismutation process of superoxide anions (Kasha et al., 1970; Allen et al., 1973). The mechanism of the antimicrobial action of molecular singlet oxygen has not been fully elucidated. It has been suggested that the oxygen may react with certain chemical groups, especially with those having double bonds, and form dioxetans, in this way inducing a toxic effect on microbial agents (Allen et al., 1972). Molecular singlet oxygen would then be responsible, to a certain degree, for the bactericidal effect of the myeloperoxidase system. The possiblity that singlet oxygen acts upon microbial agents through photodynamic reactions seems to be of special interest. The toxic effect of eosin on *E. coli* increases significantly in the simultaneous presence of both light and oxygen (Klebanoff, 1975).

It has already been mentioned that one of the most striking features of neutrophils is their ability to degrade glucose and to produce intracellular energy, in anaerobic conditions, so the possibility that neutrophils maintain their antimicrobial properties in anaerobic conditions is *a priori* suggestive. There are several methodologic difficulties in studying the oxygen-independent antimicrobial systems in these cells in the complete absence of oxygen, since there are no available methods for the total elimination of oxygen from a cell, and so there is always a possibility that traces of oxygen persist within the neutrophil. Among the neutrophil oxygen-independent systems lysosomal enzymes, lysozyme, lactoferrin, antibacterial cationic proteins, and hydrogen ions should be mentioned.

Lysosomal Enzymes

Lysosomal enzymes in neutrophils cause the biochemical degradation of various components of the microbial agent engulfed within the inner space of the phagocytic vacuole. The possible role of these enzymes in the mechanisms of mitotic division (Seelich, 1975), and in the hydrolysis of intracellular materials (Davis et al., 1972) has also been discussed. Lysosomal enzymes occur in lysosomal granules, which are characterized by structural polymorphism. One group of these granules is represented by primary lysosomes, corresponding to azurophilic granules, and the other is composed of "specific" granules. During neutrophil maturation in the bone marrow, azurophilic are formed prior to specific granules (Bainton et al., 1971). Azurophilic granules are composed of two structural subpopulations. The first is round-shaped, the second is ellipsoid. The ellipsoid forms are characterized by the frequent presence of crystalloid structures. Azurophilic granules contain myeloperoxidase, arylsulfatase, and beta-glycerophosphatase (Bainton et al., 1969; Ullyot et al., 1970). Specific lysosomal granules represent another group in the lysosomal apparatus. They appear later than azurophilic granules during the development and maturation of neutrophils and are seen in the myelocyte stage. Characteristic features of specific granules are the pale, homogeneous matrix and spherical shape.

There are numerous unsolved problems as regards lysosomal enzymes. It is not known whether a single lysosomal granule may contain one or more enzymes. The mechanism of activation of lysosomal enzymes during lysosome fusion and the formation of the phagocytic vacuole is also unknown. The relationship between the intracellular content of these enzymes and neutrophil antimicrobial activity has not been well established. In other words, the lowest intracellular level of lysosomal enzymes that does not significantly alter neutrophil bactericidal activity is not yet known. It is not known whether the presence of all the lysosomal enzymes is necessary to maintain the normal bactericidal functions of these cells. Only a few cases of congenital defects in intracellular bacteriolysis associated with deficiencies of the lysosomal enzymes are known.

The neutrophil lysosomes contain large amounts of various hydrolases which enable the degradation of most of the components of phagocytized bacteria. Only a few of these hydrolyses have been extensively studied in man. The majority of biochemical studies have been on the isolation of these enzymes, their localization in cell subfractions, and their general biochemical properties. There is a striking lack of studies on the intracellular mechanisms of enzyme activation and the composition of various lysosomal enzymes as far as the content and sequence of the amino acids are concerned. In many instances the biologic role of a particular lysosomal enzyme is not clear. Attention has been called to the possible participation of neutrophil lysosomal proteases in the activation of the kinin system and in the release of kinin from kininogen (Movat et al., 1973). The possible part played by neutrophils in the activation of vasoactive peptides and in alterations in blood vessel permeability deserves further study.

Several enzymes belong to the lysosomal enzyme group. Among them acid phosphatase (Clarke, 1965), lysozyme (Welsh et al., 1971), alpha-glucosidase, beta-glucosidase, and beta-glucuronidase (Clarke, 1965; Hirschhorn et al., 1965) should be mentioned. N-acetyl-beta-glucosaminidase has been the subject of more recent studies (Lisiewicz et al., 1976). Alpha-amylase, laminarinase, dextranase, and alpha-mannosidase represent other enzymes in this group (Clarke, 1965). A separate subgroup of lysosomal enzymes is represented by peptidases such as leucinaminopeptidase, carboxypeptidase, prolidase, iminodipeptidase, acid proteinase, and neutral proteinase (Haschen et al., 1966). Elastase (Janoff et al., 1971), collagenase (Lazarus et al., 1968), and lipase (Braunsteiner et al., 1965) also belong to the group of lysosomal enzymes. Some proteases are localized extralysosomally and are closely associated with the cell membrane fraction (Wintroub et al., 1974). The neutrophil neutral proteases have various tissue substrates as well as a substrate circulating in the blood (Table 5). This reflects the manifold biologic functions of these proteases. These enzymes take part in the degradation of numerous components of the joint membranes and activate the complement components, plasminogen, kininogen, and fibrinolysis (Goldstein, 1976; Johnson et al., 1976). It has been found that elastase and cathepsin G, isolated from the azurophilic granules in neutrophils, stimulate B lymphocytes and increase the incorporation of ^{3}H-thymidine into these cells (Bretz et al., 1976). These data suggest that neutrophil enzymes released into an inflammatory environment may affect the functional state of the lymphocytes and enhance the reactions of antigen recognition and production of specific antibodies. The source of neutral proteases in an inflammation area may, however, be in cells other than neutrophils.

The list of neutrophil lysosomal enzymes includes enzymes capable of the hydrolytic degradation of such microbial components as nucleic acids, protein, carbohydrates, lipids, and monosaccharides. Among neutrophil lysosomal enzymes nucleotidases, nucleosidases, ribonucleases, deoxyribonucleases, alkaline

TABLE 5. Biologic substrates of the neutrophil neutral proteases. (According to Goldstein, 1976)

Tissue substrates	Blood substrates
Cartilage glycosaminoglycan	Kininogen
Lung connective tissue	Plasminogen
Vascular basal membrane	Fibrin
Elastine	C_5
Collagen	C_{1s}
Basal membrane of kidney glomeruli	

proteases like chymotrypsin and cathepsin, as well as other enzymes such as arylsulfatase, acid phosphatase, esterases of fatty acids, and lipases may also be mentioned. The localization of 5-nucleotidase in neutrophils has not as yet been established. The content of this enzyme in human neutrophils is very low, and the enzyme occurs in the membrane fraction (Szmigielski et al., 1967; Strauss et al., 1975). A relatively high activity of arylsulfatase is noted in promyelocytes, myelocytes, metamyelocytes, and mature neutrophils. In cytochemical studies this enzyme has been demonstrated in small granules, and no diffuse reaction has been noted (Szmigielski et al., 1974).

Only a few neutrophil lysosomal enzymes have been studied in detail in patients with various diseases. The majority of these studies have been on acid phosphatase, collagenase, catalase, and the esterases. Extracts of neutrophilic granules hydrolize hemoglobin, fibrinogen, albumin, and casein (Asghar et al., 1976).This hydrolysis is enhanced by the addition of urea. The mechanism of this phenomenon is not clear. It has been found that human serum containing alpha$_1$-antitrypsin strongly inhibits this hydrolysis (Asghar et al., 1976).

The mechanism of enzyme release from the lysosomal granules are not well known. Probably a certain role in this is played by the complement component C_{5a}, which selectively releases the neutrophil lysosomal enzymes (Lewis, 1974). C_{5a} activity may be generated by the incubation of isolated C_5 with lysates of neutrophil lysosomes, probably owing to the action of neutral proteases. A nonenzymatic mechanism of this generation by the activation of the serum complement may also be involved. C_{5a} also affects the surface charge of neutrophils and changes the chemotactic properties of these cells. Neutrophil

TABLE 6. Effect of thymus extract (TFX) on lysosomal acid phosphatase (AP) activity in mouse neutrophils.
(According to Lisiewicz et al., 1976)

	Day after TFX injection		Absolute neutrophil count (per cu mm)	Absolute AP-negative neutrophil count (per cu mm)	Absolute AP-positive neutrophil count (per cu mm)	AP-activity index (score)
Control group		$\overline{X}$	2827.4	728.6	2098.8	142.0
		SD	1350.6	839.5	1146.9	73.1
Group studied	8	$\overline{X}$	1981.8	199.1*	1829.7	205.8*
		SD	999.8	178.6	880.6	37.0
	15	$\overline{X}$	2364.8	278.0*	2086.8	198.5*
		SD	1937.6	278.8	1916.6	46.4

* Statistically significant differences.

lysosomal enzymes may also be released by aggregated IgA from patients with plasmocytoma (Spiegelberg et al., 1974).

Acid Phosphatase

Acid phosphatase (AP) is one of the better known neutrophil lysosomal enzymes. In the course of fetal development the enzyme appears in fetuses aged 12 to 14 weeks, as in lymphocytes (Lisiewicz, 1976). In personal observations we have found a high activity of lysosomal AP in neutrophils from premature infants. The significance of this fact is not clear; in contrast, the activity of this enzyme in the lymphocytes is low (Lisiewicz, 1976). We have also demonstrated that AP activity is increased in neutrophils from patients with cancer of the larynx (Gierek et al., 1977; Lisiewicz et al., 1977). This increase may be related to the mobilization of neutrophils caused by the inflammatory changes in the tissues surrounding the tumor or may reflect the neutrophil system reaction against the tumor components.

The hormonal control of AP activity in human neutrophils has not been a subject of more systematic studies. In mice we have ascertained that calf thymus extract (TFX, thymus factor X), a well-known stimulator of the lymphocyte system, induces a significant increase in the AP activity indices in peripheral blood neutrophils (Lisiewicz et al., 1976). This increase was accompanied by a decrease in the absolute neutrophil count (Table 6). The intracellular mechanism of the increase in AP activity was not elucidated in our studies. It is of interest, however, that a similar increase in enzyme activity is also noted in lymphocytes after the application of TFX. These observations support the concept that thymus extract nonspecifically stimulates the lysosomal apparatus in both neutrophils and lymphocytes.

In other studies we have shown that irradiation with 450 r induces a slight increase in AP activity in mouse neutrophils (Aleksandrowicz et al., 1976). This increase may be due to the reaction of neutrophils against the tissue components released after damage from irradiation (Fig. 10).

Characteristic changes in AP activity occur in the neutrophils of pregnant women. The activity of the enzyme increases during the consecutive months of pregnancy and is parallel to the total neutrophil count (Lisiewicz et al., 1977). In pregnant women with Rh-incompatibility similar alterations in enzyme activity have been observed.

AP activity in the neutrophils also increases in patients with chronic granulocytic leukemia, aplastic anemias, certain tumors, or myocardial infarction, and in a certain percentage of patients with primary polycythemia (Aleksandrowicz, 1969). In patients after surgery an increase in AP activity is noted for a week or more, and the dynamics of its changes differ from

58

those of alkaline phosphatase (Bogusz et al., 1967; Cichocki et al., 1968) AP activity is lowered in patients with acute myeloblastic leukemia and chronic lymphocytic leukemia. In children with acute lymphoblastic leukemia, AP activity in the neutrophils is not altered as compared with healthy subjects.

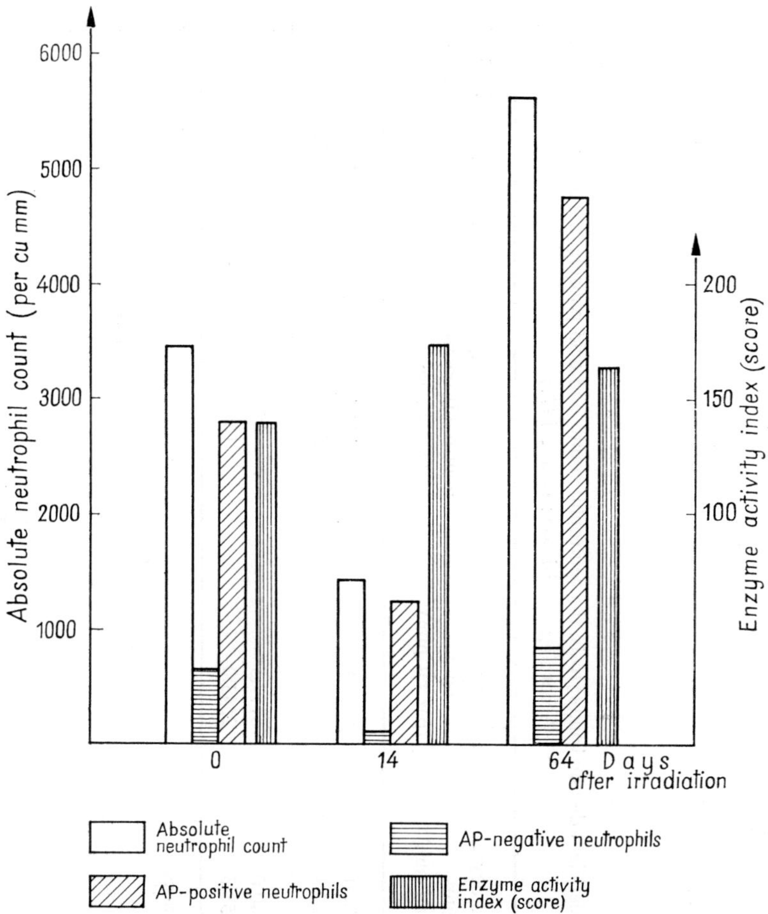

Fig. 10. Effect of calf thymus extract on the neutrophil count and lysosomal acid phosphatase activity in mice irradiated with 450 r. A transient decrease in numbers of the enzyme-positive cells is noted on the 14th day after irradiation. (According to Aleksandrowicz et al., 1976)

A magnesium-deficient diet in mice induces an increase in the absolute AP-positive neutrophil count accompanied by a decrease in the enzyme-negative cell count (Table 7) (Lisiewicz et al., 1977). At the same time, the enzyme activity index does not change significantly. A zinc-deficient diet, conversely, induces a decrease in both the absolute AP-positive neutrophil count and the enzyme activity index.

TABLE 7. Effect of magnesium-deficient diet on leukocytosis, the neutrophil count, and acid phosphatase activity in mouse neutrophils. (According to Lisiewicz et al., 1977)

		Leukocyte count (per cu mm)	Absolute neutrophil count (per cu mm)	Absolute AP-negative neutrophil count (per cu mm)	Absolute AP-positive neutrophil count (per cu mm)	AP-activity index (score)
Control group	$\overline{X}$	11,010.0	4238.4	1135.1	3103.4	158.1
	SD	2023.1	959.7	371.6	927.0	26.5
Group studied	$\overline{X}$	9540.0	6777.5*	85.3*	6692.3*	165.8
	SD	2958.3	2543.0	168.0	2568.9	33.4

* Statistically significant differences

Collagenase

Recently collagenase has been isolated from a homogenate containing mainly neutrophils from the blood of healthy donors. The molecular weight of the enzyme is equal to about 61,000 (Wojtecka-Łukasik et al., 1974). It has been shown that the optimum pH of the enzyme is about 7.8, which differentiates this enzyme from the acid lysosomal hydrolases. It has been suggested that collagenase plays a part in the local resorption of collagen. There are data showing that collagen is degraded in two different phases. During the first phase the large collagen molecule (TC) undergoes a breakdown into two smaller parts. TC^A and TC^B, which during the second phase are degraded into small peptides by neutral protease. Recently this protease has been isolated from a leukocytic mass (Sopata et al., 1974).

Catalase

Catalase is an enzyme easily detected cytochemically with the use of 3,3-diaminobenzidine tetrahydrochloride (DAB). It was previously suggested that the enzyme is localized in specific granules differing from those containing myeloperoxidase (Szmigielski, 1972). Investigations made by a complex technique involving histochemistry and electron microscopy seem to indicate, however, that the enzyme is localized in the azurophilic granules, that is, in the primary lysosomes (Nishimura et al., 1976). It is not known whether a single lysosomal granule may contain simultaneously both catalase and myeloperoxidase. In personal studies we have found that catalase present in chronic granulocytic leukemia neutrophils may induce an antiheparin effect (Sznajd et al., 1969). Cationic proteins and enzymes such as myeloperoxidase as well as ribonuclease isolated from neutrophils, however, also have antiheparin properties.

A characteristic feature of acatalasemia is the total lack of catalase in the neutrophils in the peripheral blood. Up to the time of writing the so-called Swiss and Japanase types of acatalasemia have been described (Nishimura et al., 1976).

Esterases

A characteristic feature of neutrophils in various stages of maturation consists in the positive cytochemical reactions to esterolytic activity. Especially numerous studies have been made on this subject with the use of naphthol AS-D-chloroacetate (NASDCA). Biochemical studies have shown that the esterase activity is localized in the granular fraction of human neutrophils and exhibits maximal activity at pH 7.4 (Rindler et al., 1973). Esterase heterogeneity has been demonstrated by means of acrylamide gel (Rindler et al., 1971, 1973). There have been suggestions that the esterase activity is localized in the azurophilic granules (Schmalzl et al., 1971; Rindler et al., 1973). Attention has been called to the fact that the highest esterase activity is noted in the promyelocyte stage, and in more mature forms a gradual decrease in enzyme activity occurs (Schmalzl et al., 1971). This phenomenon is parallel to a decrease in the number of the azurophilic granules during subsequent mitotic divisions (Bainton et al., 1971). NASDCA esterase activity is higher in cells from patients with acute myelocytic leukemia than in those from patients with acute lymphoblastic leukemia (Morimoto, 1975). The diagnostic significance of this difference is of clinical value.

The esterolytic activity of human neutrophils depends on the proteases and esterases present in the lysosomal granules. NASDCA may be hydrolyzed by chymotrypsin, trypsin, and elastase. There are data indicating that the main esterolytic activity in neutrophils is due to a specific esterase activity and not to a chymotrypsinlike protease (Rindler et al., 1974). It is of interest that fractions having esterolytic and proteolytic activity are difficult to separate from one another and that fractions exhibiting no proteolytic activity have also no esterolytic activity. Neutrophil esterase is associated with cationic proteins and lysozyme. Electrophoresis with acrylamide gel showed that the mobility of esterase differs from that of acid phosphatase, beta-glucuronidase, betagalactosidase, and arylsulfatase (Rindler et al., 1973). The esterolytic activity of human neutrophils is higher than that of rabbit neutrophils (Dewald et al., 1975). Cytochemical studies of esterases enable the differentiation of various cells in the blood and bone marrow, especially in regard to promyelocytes and promonocytes (Table 8).

Oligosaccharases

Most of the data available refer to beta-glucuronidase and N-acetyl-betaglucosaminidase. Neutrophil beta-glucuronidase activity increases in patients after surgery (Cichocki et al., 1968). This increase is less evident than that in the acid phosphatase. In patients with cancer of the larynx we have observed a characteristic lowering of the beta-glucuronidase activity index in neutrophils; the N-acetyl-beta-glucosaminidase activity was significantly decreased in subjects with precancerous state of the larynx (Lisiewicz et al., 1977; Gierek et al., 1979).

Factors Activating the Lysosomal Apparatus of Neutrophils

Activation of the neutrophil lysosomal apparatus includes the formation of new lysosomal granules, the formation of abnormal lysosomal granules such as toxic granulations, and the release of the lysosomal granule content. Little is

TABLE 8. Cytochemistry of the esterases in circulating blood and bone marrow cells in man*.

Substrate / Cells	Alpha-naphthyl acetate	AS-naphthyl acetate		Chlor-AS-D naphthol acetate
		with NaF 1.5 mg/ml	without NaF	
Myeloblast	1	1	1	0
Promyelocyte	1–2	1–3	2–3	2–5
Myelocyte	1–2	2	2	3–5
Neutrophil	0–1	1–2	1–2	3–4
Eosinophil	0 or trace	0–1	1	0
Promonocyte	2–4	0 or trace	1–4	0–1
Monocyte	3–5	0 or trace	3–5	0–1
Erythroblast	1	0 or trace	0 or trace	0
Erythrocyte	0 or trace	0 or trace	0 or trace	0–1
Megakaryocyte	2–5	1–3	2–5	0
Thrombocyte	2–3	1	1	0
Plasma cell	2	1–2	2	0
Reticulocyte	3–4	3–4	3–4	0
Lymphoblast	1	1	1	0
Lymphocyte	1–2	1	1	0

* The numerical data refer to the number of esterase-positive granules within a single cell.

known of the factors affecting this last phenomenon. The release of lysosomal enzymes from neutrophils occurs, e.g., after the exposure of these cells to immune complexes (Weissmann et al., 1971). Factors increasing the intracellular content of cAMP, like theophylline, diminish this effect. The release of lysosomal enzyme from neutrophils also depends on the calcium concentration (Goldstein et al., 1975). There is a complex interaction between calcium, C_{5a}, and some release-activating agents such as cytochalasin B in regard to discharge of enzymes from lysosomal granules.

Concanavalin A

Concanavalin A is a substance capable of binding with the glycoproteins on the cell membrane surface of neutrophils. It has been shown that this binding is associated with the intercanalization of the cell membrane and depends on the state of the microtubular apparatus (Smith et al., 1972; Ryan et al., 1974). It has been suggested that concanavalin A acts solely upon the specific lysosomal granules and releases, e.g., lysozyme, but has no effect on the azurophilic granules containing peroxidase (Hoffstein et al., 1976). There have been suggestions that microtubule assembly is related to the concanavalin A-influenced cell surface.

It has been shown that this agent significantly increases lysozyme release from neutrophils (Hoffstein et al., 1976). The action of cytochalasin B alone is weaker than that of concanavalin A. The mechanism of cytochalasin B action has not been fully elucidated (Zurier et al., 1973). Some observations also indicate that cytochalasin B enhances the release from the lysosomal granules of the enzyme that converts kininogen into kinin (Movat et al., 1973).

Phorbol Myristate Acetate

Phorbol myristate acetate releases enzymes from the specific lysosomal granules of neutrophils but does not affect the azurophilic granules (Goldstein et al., 1975). In cells stimulated by cytochalasin B, the release involves the azurophilic granules, and not only lysozyme but also beta-glucuronidase are released in these conditions. In phorbol myristate acetate-treated neutrophils the number of visible cytoplasmic microtubules increases.

*

The mechanisms of enzyme release from the lysosomal granules of neutrophils are not well known in detail. There is a relationship between the number of microtubules in the neutrophils and the degree of lysozyme release from these cells (Hoffstein et al., 1976). After stimulation with concanavalin A, the number of microtubules increases in the pericentriolar region and in the peripheral areas of the cytoplasm. Since a number of these microtubules are associated with the internal cell membrane at the sites of concanavalin A binding, the suggestion has been formulated that the microtubules play a role in releasing the lysosome content of the cells into the surrounding areas. Another view is that concanavalin A increases lysozyme release from the neutrophils. Alphamethyl-mannoside inhibited the lysozyme release induced by concanavalin A, and cytochalasin B enhanced this release. It seems possible that the biologic trigger mechanism is different for specific and for azurophilic granules. The observation that concanavalin A releases solely enzymatic material from the specific granules and does not change the state of the azurophilic granules favors this concept.

The hormonal control of lysosomal enzyme release from neutrophils has been the subject of only a few studies. Epinephrine, isoproterenol, and cyclic AMP inhibit beta-glucuronidase release from lysosomes; in contrast, acetylcholine and cyclic GMP enhance this release (Ignarro et al., 1974). Hence it has been suggested that the immunologic release of lysosomal enzymes from human neutrophils is regulated by the autonomic neurohormones. On the other hand, it has been shown that the protein factor present in the poorly purified thyroid-stimulating hormone and in the luteinizing hormone causes an increase in the cyclic AMP concentration and iodine accumulation in neutrophils (Stolc, 1975). Little is known of the interactions in these cells between the hormones, on the one hand, and the enzymes and metabolic pathways, on the other. It is known that catecholamines, epinephrine, norepinephrine, and DOPA induce *in vitro* an increase in neutrophil oxygen utilization and stimulate the hexose monophosphate shunt (Qualliotine et al., 1972). The stimulation of the pentose cycle in these experiments seemed to be independent of cyclic AMP. It has been suggested that the mechanism of these changes consists in epinephrine oxidation to adrenochrome, which reacts with NADPH to produce NADP; this concept, however, needs confirmation.

Lysozyme (Muramidase)

The bacteriolytic activity of lysozyme (muramidase) has been known since the time of Fleming (Fleming, 1922). The main source of this enzyme in blood and inflammatory exudates is in neutrophils (Senn et al., 1970), but monocytes also exhibit its presence (Perillie et al., 1968). In the course of neutrophil maturation the content of this enzyme within the cells increases. There is a correlation between the degree of leukocytosis and the serum lysozyme concentration. The enzyme in the blood is heterogeneous (Söder et al., 1970).

In inflammatory exudate, the intracellular lysozyme content decreases during 8 to 24 hourse and its concentration in the extracellular environment increases, especially after neutrophil lysis. The increase in enzyme activity in the serum of patients with monocytic leukemia probably depends on an increase in the number of the monocytes producing the enzyme (Sternberger et al., 1970). The content of the enzyme in neutrophils from patients with chronic granulocytic leukemia is low, and the enzyme is absent from these cells in patients with acute myeloblastic or chronic lymphocytic leukemia (Asamer et al., 1969).

Recently, an important advance in our knowledge of the metabolism, transfer, turnover, and renal filtration of lysozyme has been made (Hansen, 1974; Hankiewicz et al., 1976). It has been demonstrated that lysozyme occurs in leukemic blasts but is not detectable in normal blastic cells. In patients with leukemias during remission the neutrophil lysozyme content is lowered. The enzyme concentration in the serum of patients with neutropenias is low, but in those with neutrophilia it is high.

Lactoferrin

Lactoferrin is a protein characterized by the ability to bind the iron present in neutrophilic granules (Masson et al., 1969; Baggiolini et al., 1970).

The mechanism of the antibacterial activity of lactoferrin may be associated with its chelating properties against iron utilization during the growth of bacteria. It is generally accepted that lactoferrin occurs in specific neutrophilic granules. The antimicrobial effect of the lowered iron levels in the blood of patients with various infections has been the subject of a recent review (Aleksandrowicz et al., 1976).

Antimicrobial Cationic Proteins

These proteins were isolated from animal neutrophils with the use of diluted acid. It is not known, however, whether human neutrophils contain these proteins. The substances known as phagocytin (Hirsch, 1956) and leukins (Skarnes et al., 1956) isolated from neutrophils are included in the group of these antimicrobial proteins. Their composition, properties, and mechanism of action are now well known (Zeya et al., 1966). The proteins occur in the lysosomal fraction of guinea-pig neutrophils (Zeya et al., 1966). Large amounts of arginine have been found in these proteins.

Antibacterial action against gram-negative and gram-positive bacteria and *Candida albicans* has been observed in these proteins. This action is blocked by anionic substances like heparin, the nucleic acids, and endotoxin. An excess of iron ions has a similar effect (Gladstone et al., 1970). The presence of antibacterial proteins within phagocytic vacuoles has been demonstrated cytochemically (Spitznagel et al., 1963).

Three different cationic proteins have been isolated from human neutrophils by means of affinity chromatography on sepharose-4-phenylbutylamine (Rindler et al., 1975). These proteins correspond to the neutral proteases and differ from elastase and collagenase. The proteases hydrolyse casein and the chymotrypsin substrate, i.e., N-acetyl-L-thyrosine ethyl ester. The specific inhibitor of chymotrypsin, N-tosyl-L-phenylalanylchlormethane, and the natural inhibitor of alpha-antichymotrypsin, alpha-1-antitrypsin, inhibit the neutral proteases. Chymotrypsins isolated from soybeans and lima beans also exhibit an inhibitory effect against the proteases. A chymotrypsinlike protease, purified with sepharose-4-phenylbutylamine, is a cationic protein with an electrophoretic mobility similar to that of lysozyme (Rindler et al., 1974).

The results of these studies indicate that the so-called neutral proteolytic activity of human neutrophils depends not only on elastase and collagenase but also on at least three other enzymes with a chymotrypsinlike activity. The investigations cited have been made on the general antimicrobial mechanisms operating in neutrophils. Enzymes belonging to the cationic protein fraction of these cells probably hydrolyze peptide bonds in proteins which are components of the bacterial cell membranes.

<h1 style="text-align:center">Hydrogen Ions</h1>

Changes in the hydrogen ion concentration and a decrease in pH within the phagocytic vacuoles represent elements involved in the antibacterial action of neutrophils. It has been demonstrated in rats that in the course of phagocytosis the pH may be lowered down to 4.0 in 7 to 15 min. In man, a similar decrease in pH is within the range of 6.0 to 6.5 (Mandell, 1970). These alterations, of course, depend on the experimental conditions and the properties of the phagocytized material. It may be stated, however, that the pH values in phagocytic vacuoles induce a bacteriostatic or bactericidal effect in particular micro-organisms. The pH values are significant in the action of some enzymes, e.g., acid phosphatase.

*

In general, it may be said that the neutrophil has at its command several antimicrobial systems inducing instant or more distant effects. This explains the biologic effectiveness of the cell systems operating in various conditions, both aerobic and anaerobic. The sequence of intracellular events related to the actions of particular antimicrobial systems, as well as several feedback-conditioned interactions between the systems and single enzymes, on the one hand, and the components of microbial objects, on the other, still requires further studies.

NEUTROPHIL CYTOCHEMICAL TESTS OF SPECIAL CLINICAL IMPORTANCE

Nitroblue Tetrazolium Reduction

Nitroblue tetrazolium reduction (NBT) has become a cytochemical test widely used in studying neutrophils. The cytochemical reaction consists in the formation of red insoluble diformazane precipitate during reduction with nitroblue tetrazolium. The intracellular conditions in the normal course of this reaction have not been unequivocally explained. It is known that the presence of $NADH + H^+$ and of oxidase within the cell is critical for the occurrence of the reaction. The extent of NBT reduction is expressed in terms of the percentage of NBT-positive neutrophils (Park et al., 1968). The stimulated NBT test is even more widely used. The percentage of NBT-positive neutrophils in healthy subjects ranges from 3% to 10% (the mean value equals 8%). In children the percentage is a little higher (Kobielowa et al., 1973). High NBT test values are seen in neonates during the first months of life. Low test values are a characteristic feature in patients with chronic granulomatous disease. The results of the NBT test may be modified by factors present in the serum or within the neutrophils (Nydegger et al., 1973; De la Vega et al., 1973).

An increase in the NBT test values in neutrophils is noted in patients with infections of the upper respiratory tract, bacterial meningitis, and sepsis due to infection with *Candida albicans* (Park et al., 1968; Kobielowa et al., 1973). A similar increase in NBT reduction is observed in patients with endocarditis, miliary tuberculosis, variola, malaria, and parasitic infections. The NBT test exhibits values higher than normal in 10% of patients with cystic fibrosis (Sullivan et al., 1973). The addition of serum from patients with this disease and exhibiting the presence of antibodies against *Pseudomonas aeruginosa* to a suspension of normal neutrophils results in an increase in the NBT test values (Koch et al., 1973). Increased values of the test have also been noted in patients with Hodkin's disease or various lymphomas and in children with acute lymphoblastic leukemia during remissions (Soonattrakul et al., 1973; Pituch 1977). The test is of value in the differentiation of bacterial and nonbacterial infections (Matsuda, 1975). In children with viral infections the NBT test shows lowered values (Kolanowska et al., 1976). It has also been found that peroral contraceptives composed of progesterone and estrogens may elevate the test values (Arrowsmith et al., 1973). The increase of the NBT reduction has also been noted in women being in the puerperal period (Sułowicz et al., 1977). Though NBT reduction does not show changes due to circadian rhythm, in subjects after physical exercise the reduction increases (Żaboklicki et al., 1976).

The mechanism of the increase in NBT values in patients with inflammatory or infectious conditions is not well understood. In many conditions such as primary lung tuberculosis, rheumatic fever, or disseminated lupus erythematosus, the test values are not changed (Park et al., 1968; Ng et al., 1972). In experiments *in vitro* an increase in NBT reduction has been observed after the exposure of neutrophils to adenoviruses of types 4 and 7 (Rosenbaum et al., 1974). Methylene blue, an agent stimulating oxidative metabolism associated with the hexose monophosphate shunt, has a similar effect (Humbert et al., 1973). Probably methylene blue acts as a transfer factor for electrons between NBT and the 2-pyridine nucleotides, which are of importance in the oxidative pathway of neutrophils. There have been reports on an increase in NBT-positive cells in patients after kidney transplantation treated with prednisone (Matula et al., 1971). Transient functional defect associated with a decrease in NBT reduction has been observed in a patient with ataxia-telangiectasia (Kretschmer et al., 1972). In newborns the reduction of NBT is physiologically lowered (Merkiel et al., 1977). The effect of heparin on NBT reduction has been the subject of controversial reports.

Neutrophil Alkaline Phosphatase

Most of the information on neutrophil alkaline phosphatase (NAP) originates from cytochemical investigations. The majority of these studies were made by means of Kaplow's method (Kaplow, 1955, 1963). NAP estimation has found practical application in the differentiation of elevated leukocytosis in patients with chronic granulocytic leukemia, leukemoid reactions, or inflammatory conditions.

The intracellular localization of NAP has been a subject of controversy. On the one hand, the enzyme has been found in the microsomal and cell membrane fractions (West et al., 1972), but, on the other, NAP has been said to be present in the perinuclear cisternae, the Golgi apparatus, or the cytoplasmic lysosomal granules (Geddes et al., 1975). During neutrophil maturation NAP activity appears first in the myelocyte stage and gradually increase in more mature forms until it reaches the highest values in the mature neutrophil.

NAP activity depends on the stage of ontogenetic development, sex, and hormonal effects. In the premature infant the activity of the enzyme is very high (Bryniak et al., 1975). The purpose of this phenomenon is not clear. It seems probable, however, that it may be related to the hormonal influence of the mother, in whom NAP activity also significantly increases (Cardinali et al., 1970; Lisiewicz et al., 1974). In children aged 1 to 15 years the activity of the enzyme is higher as compared with that in adults (Mehta et al., 1974).

Several hormones alter NAP activity. The activity of the enzyme is higher in men than in women (Polishuk et al., 1970; Mehta et al., 1974). This probably depends on the activating action of estrogens. Stilbestrol also significantly increases NAP activity (Moszczyński, 1976). It has also been observed that the activity of the enzyme increases during the second half of the menstrual cycle (Radwańska et al., 1971). In women with anovulatory cycles this phenomenon does not occur. Testosterone also has an activating effect on NAP. This is of importance in patients with various internal diseases treated with this hormone, since an increase in NAP activity may be regarded as a sign that inflammation is present (Lisiewicz et al., 1975). Similar effects of testosterone have been observed in animals (Ebadi et al., 1966). In patients with the Cushing syndrome, NAP activity is also elevated (Szathári et al., 1971). A correlation between the enzyme activity and the 17-OH-corticoid level in the serum has been observed in these patients.

The significance of hormonal factors in the regulation of NAP has also been demonstrated in our studies on patients with postpuerperal hypothalamosis, juvenile hypothalamosis, or ovarian insufficiency of hypothalamic origin (Bacz et al., 1974). In women with the latter entity the NAP values were lower than in the other groups studied. Treatment with extracts of the posterior lobe of the pituitary gland induced, in all groups studied, an increase in NAP activity (Table 9).

NAP activity may serve as a very sensitive index of a discrete inflammatory state which is not reflected in the physical examination results or in leukocytosis. We have observed that in the asymptomatic period of lung tuberculosis the NAP acivity index increases to a detectable extent (Lisiewicz et al., 1972). Delicate inflammatory states of the uterine endothelium provoked by intrauterine mechanical contraceptives are also reflected in an increase in NAP activity (Urrego et al., 1971).

TABLE 9. Neutrophil alkaline phosphatase activity in women with postpregnancy hypothalamosis, juvenile hypothalamosis, or ovarian hypofunction of hypothalamic origin treated with posterior pituitary lobe extract.* (According to Bacz et al., 1974)

Group studied	Neutrophil alkaline phosphatase activity index (score) (according to Kaplow's method)		
	before treatment	during treatment	
		day 2	4	6
Postpregnancy hypothalamosis	55.2	64.6	70.0	70.6
Juvenile hypothalamosis	56.7	59.2	69.2	70.7
Ovarian hypofunction of hypothalamic origin	79.9	83.7	84.2	85.3

* The figures in the table represent the mean values of neutrophil alkaline phosphatase activity in a total group of 37 women with these clinical entities.

Alterations in NAP activity in patients with diseases of the blood and hematopoietic organs present separate problems. The most important use of the NAP activity test is in the differential diagnosis of leukemoid reactions of the neutrophilic system and chronic granulocytic leukemia. The leukemoid reactions are characterized by high and the leukemia by low NAP activity. In certain conditions, however, neutrophils from patients with chronic granulocytic leukemia may exhibit a high activity of the enzyme. A high activity of NAP in these patients is observed during such complications of the disease as pneumonia, colitis, or other local inflammatory states. Treatment with ACTH, corticoids (Mdzewski, 1963) or testosterone (Janicki et al., 1977) results in an elevation of NAP activity. Only few patients treated with cyclophosphamid exhibit a moderate increase of the enzyme activity (Moszczyński, 1976). Low

NAP activity values in patients with acute myelocytic leukemia may be accompanied by chromosomal translocation of the C-G type or the absence of chromosome Y (Kamada et al., 1976). The mean survival time of patients with low activity of this enzyme is longer in comparison with those with normal or high NAP activity. The significance of this observation requires further studies.

Relatively high NAP activity is observed in patients with acute lymphoblastic leukemia, whereas patients with acute myeloblastic leukemia usually exhibit a low activity of this enzyme (Hayhoe, 1968). High NAP activity is also noted in patients with erythroleukemia (Mdzewski, 1963; Garg et al., 1972) or primary polycythemia (Szczepkowska et al., 1973). In patients with this last entity, treatment with myleran does not change the NAP activity. The characteristic increase in the activity of this enzyme in patients with myelosclerosis facilitates the differentiation of this disease from chronic granulocytic leukemia.

Alterations in NAP activity are also observed in patients with infectious diseases, inflammations, trauma, or several diseases of the blood (Table 10). In some states NAP activity exhibits a characteristic evolution depending on the particular stage of the disease and the treatment employed. In patients with reactive neutrophilic leukocytosis after surgery, the increase in the activity of this enzyme is parallel to the degree of leukocytosis and exhibits its maximum on the third or fourth day after operation (Bogusz et al., 1967). A similar association between the degree of neutrophilia and the enzyme activity is noted in women during the puerperal period (Fig. 11); we have observed the maximal increase in NAP activity in these women on the second day after delivery (Lisiewicz et al., 1974). Posthemorrhagic increase in leukocytosis may be accompanied by an increase in the activity of this enzyme (Diamant et al., 1970). Recently, an increase in the enzyme activity has been observed in patients intoxicated with carbon monoxide (Moszczyński et al., 1977).

In patients with infectious diseases, the relationship between NAP activity and the degree of neutrophilic leukocytosis varies, depending on the causative agent. In patients with streptococcal pneumonia, high values of this enzyme's activity are noted from the onset of illness (Mirecka et al., 1970). The gradual decrease in leukocytosis in these patients is accompanied by a lowering of the enzyme activity. In patients with tetanus, the maximal values of NAP are observed from the fifth to the seventh day of hospitalization (Caban et al., 1970). In patients in whom the disease takes a severe course, the mean values of the enzyme activity index are higher than when the course is milder. Hence NAP activity may be regarded as one of the few objective laboratory indices of the severity of tetanus. Alterations in NAP activity depending on the stage of the disease are also observed in patients with tularemia, Q fever, or pappataci fever (Beisel, 1966). After the injection of pyrogen, leukocytosis and NAP activ-

TABLE 10. Neutrophil alkaline phosphatase in various normal and pathologic conditions. (Accord. ing to Mdzewski, 1963; Beisel, 1966; Sznajd et al., 1971; Aleksandrowicz et al., 1976)

<table>
<tr><td colspan="2" align="center">Increase in enzyme activity</td></tr>
<tr><td>

Physiologic states
  the premature infant
  the full-term infant
  women in the second half of
    the menstrual cycle
  pregnant women
  women in the puerperal period

Infectious diseases
  lung tuberculosis
  streptococcal pneumonia
  streptococcal tonsillitis
  tularemia
  Q fever
  pappataci fever
  tetanus
  bacterial meningitis

Diseases of the blood
  erythroleukemia
  primary polycythemia
  leukemic reactions
  chronic lymphocytic leukemia
  Hodgkin's disease
  myelosclerosis
  pancytopenia (some cases)

</td><td>

Other diseases
  postsurgery states
  myocardial infarction
  diabetes mellitus
  trauma
  hemorrhage
  cancer of the larynx
  carbon monoxide intoxication
  cirrhosis of the liver
  mechanical jaundice
  peptic ulcer
  inflammatory states
  Down's syndrome

Drugs
  ACTH
  corticosteroids
  testosterone
  pyrogen
  estrogens
  intrauterine contraceptives

</td></tr>
<tr><td colspan="2" align="center">Decrease in enzyme activity</td></tr>
<tr><td>

Infectious diseases
  viral hepatitis
  infectious mononucleosis
Diseases of the blood
  chronic granulocytic leukemia
  preleukemic states
  lymphosarcoma
  reticulosarcoma

</td><td>

children born from mothers with leukemias
subjects exposed to irradiation
congenital spherocytosis
symptomatic polyglobulia
paroxysmal nocturnal hemoglobinuria
Addison-Biermer anemia
pancytopenia (some cases)
acute or chronic monocytic leukemia

</td></tr>
</table>

ity decrease within the first hour, and a subsequent increase in these indices is then observed (Ban et al., 1966).

Decreased NAP activity is seen above all in patients with chronic granulocytic leukemia. About 90% of these patients exhibit a low activity of this enzyme (DeChatelet, 1970). The intracellular mechanism by which the enzyme activity is lowered has not been clarified as yet. Initially it was suggested that low NAP activity is related to the presence of the pathologic chromosome Ph_1, but later studies revealed that NAP activity may be lowered in patients either with or without the chromosome (Sandberg et al., 1970; Gralnick, 1971). Subsequently, the data on the absence of any relationship between chromosome Ph_1

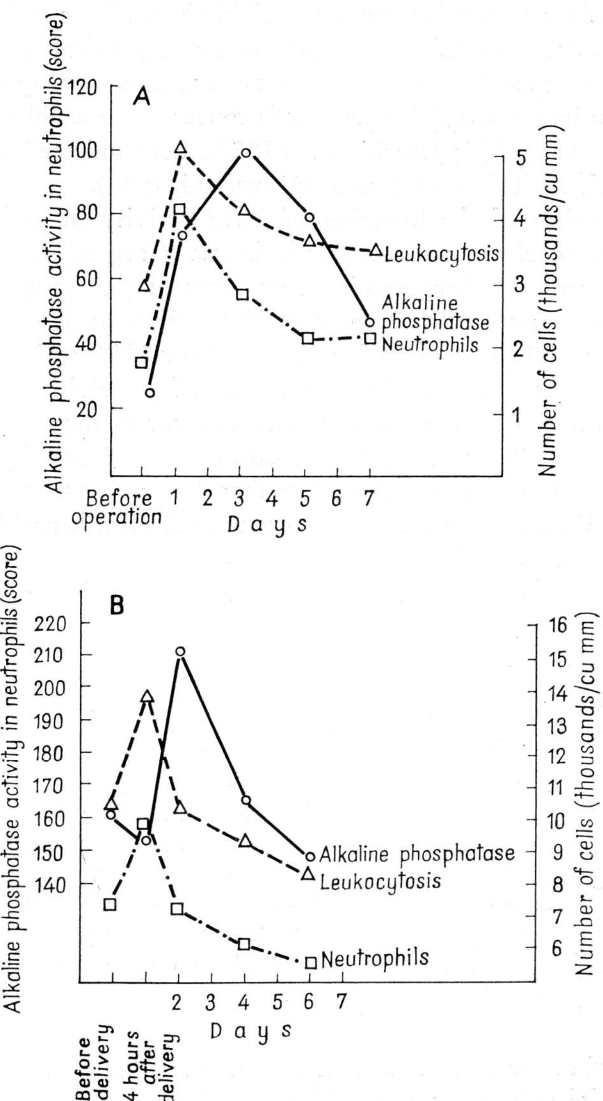

FIG. 11. Changes in neutrophil alkaline phosphatase activity in patients with reactive inflammatory leukocytosis after surgical operations (*A*) and in women during the puerperal period (*B*). Maximal increase in the enzyme activity occurred after maximal increase in the neutrophil absolute count. (According to Bogusz et al., 1967 and Lisiewicz et al., 1974)

and low NAP activity received additional confirmation (Chikkappa et al., 1973). The preliminary suggestions on the biochemical differences between NAP in patients with chronic granulocytic leukemia and NAP in normal subjects (Bottomley, 1969) were not confirmed, and it was also demonstrated that the lowering of NAP activity in these patients is not related to the molecularly abnormal enzyme synthesis in leukemic cells (Rosenblum et al., 1975). It seems probable that the intracellular apparatus of NAP synthesis in leukemic cells is not disturbed, since in certain conditions the activity of this enzyme increases. We have demonstrated that the response of leukemic neutrophils to testosterone, as far as an increase in NAP activity is concerned, resembles that of normal cells (Lisiewicz et al., 1975; Janicki et al., 1977). Leukemic cells also respond to stimulation with ACTH or corticoids (Mdzewski, 1963).

The mechanism of the lowering of NAP activity in patients with such diseases as acute or chronic monocytic leukemia (Garg et al., 1972), preleukemic states, congenital spherocytosis, some cases of pancytopenia (Mdzewski, 1963), infectious mononucleosis, hemolytic anemias, or idiopathic thrombocytopenia (Garg et al., 1972) remains obscure. Low NAP activity has also been observed in patients with nocturnal paroxysmal hemoglobinuria (Lewis et al., 1967); it is of interest that in patients with this entity the acetylcholinesterase activity is also low (Ross et al., 1964). Lowered NAP activity has also been noted in children born from leukemic mothers, in subjects exposed to irradiation or industrial carcinogens, and in patients with viral hepatitis (Aleksandrowicz et al., 1976).

CHAPTER 3

PRODUCTION, KINETICS, AND FATE OF NEUTROPHILS

The production, kinetics, and fate of neutrophils are parts of the general mechanism maintaining the homeostasis of the whole neutrophilic cell system. In contrast to the erythrocyte and the erythron, our konwledge of the neutrophil, as far as its kinetics and fate are concerned, is still rather scanty. The majority of studies on the production, fate and distribution of neutrophils have hitherto been made on experimental animals. The results obtained, however, have not given any satisfactory insight into neutrophil production in man. Quantitative determinations of the total content of neutrophils and their precursors in human beings are posible only with great approximations. The significance of these determinations from the clinical point of view has not yet been well established.

The production of neutrophils in the adult is regulated by biologic cycles and hormonal effects. The agents of importance in the regulation are chalones. The cybernetic character of the mechanisms controlling neutrophil production has been known for a long time (Wheldon et al., 1974). The positive and negative feedback loops are known in this respect. The main site of neutrophil production is in the bone marrow, which is the basic reservoir of these cells and their precursors. Neutrophil production may take place during fetal development and in some pathologic conditions in extramedullary spaces such as the liver and the spleen. Human cord-blood contains numerous colony-forming cells (Knudtzon, 1974).

The term kinetics of neutrophils refers not just to data on the survival time of these cells in the blood, and their movement within the vascular system. The whole system of cells in the neutrophilic series, like other cell systems in the hematopoietic tissues, goes through an incessant cycle of alterations, including the production of neutrophils in the bone marrow, release of these cells into the circulating blood, passage through the vascular walls into the tissues, grouping at sites of sequestration, and finally death and disintegration.

The subtle regulation of the neutrophil count in the peripheral blood depends on the effective action of a number of hormonal factors, feedback loops, and other agents inhibiting the release of these cells from the bone mar-

row and their rate of proliferation. The main external agents affecting neutrophil kinetics are bacterial derivatives such as endotoxin. The bacteria, after
penetrating the body, may enter the circulating blood either directly or via
their derivatives, and induce rapid changes in the neutrophil count through the
ejection of the cells from the marrow, the alteration in the proportion of particular pools of neutrophils, and the collection of these cells in some anatomic
regions, e.g., in the lungs. The mobilization of neutrophils in the blood in conditions of microbial invasion displays the biologic efficiency of the kinetic
mechanisms. Leukergy also exemplifies the alterations in neutrophil kinetics
conditioned by several agents of microbial origin.

Progress in research on neutrophil kinetics in man has mainly been due to
advances in various methods enabling the fate of these cells in the body to be
traced. Some of these methods will now be discussed, in the first place those
that are of clinical use.

METHODS OF INVESTIGATION OF NEUTROPHIL PRODUCTION
AND KINETICS

Among the various techniques for the evaluation of neutrophil kinetics
the following will be briefly presented: radioisotopic techniques using cells
labeled by means of ^{51}Cr, DF-^{32}P, ^{3}HTdR, or ^{35}PO$_4$; techniques employing antineutrophilic serum, endotoxin, or etiocholanolone; the leukopheresis technique;
and total bone marow mass evaluation.

Evaluation of the Total Bone Marrow Mass

In conditions *in vivo* the evaluation of the bone marrow volume in man
is impossible in practice. Studies on totally exsanguinated subjects have shown
that the bone marrow represents 3.4% to 5.9% of the total body weight (Mechank, 1926). Indirect calculations involving the mean size of the neutrophil
precursors, the mature cells, and other cells, have enabled the determination of
the total mass of nucleated cells within the human bone marrow (Wilbur, 1966).
Comparative studies on the mean size of nucleated cells in various mammals
have revealed that it, as compared with that in man, is greater in monkeys
and smaller in rabbits and rats (Donohue et al., 1958). The highest values of the
neutrophil cell series per kilogram of body weight were found in monkeys; in
man and the other animals mentioned these values were lower.

76

<h1 style="text-align:center">Leukopheresis</h1>

In literature the terms leukocytopheresis, leukopheresis and leukapheresis are used to indicate the same process. Leukopheresis refers to the elimination of leukocytes from the circulating blood to a degree causing a decrease in the total pool of these cells in the body. For a long time it has been known that the main body of circulating neutrophils within the capillary lumen is localized near the capillary endothelium (Bierman et al., 1961, 1963). The mass of these cells is termed the marginal pool of neutrophils. The technique of leukopheresis has enabled deeper insight into the capabilities of neutrophil production in healthy donors, the evaluation of changes in the neutrophil system in donors after numerous repeated leukophereses, and the evaluation of their clinical results in patients with leukemias. A more detailed presentation of these problems will be found in Chapter 5 on the immunologic properties of neutrophils.

<h1 style="text-align:center">Endotoxin</h1>

The acute stages of sepsis in clinical conditions resemble, to a certain degree, the phenomena observed after the experimental injection of endotoxin. Endotoxins from gram-negative bacteria induce fluctuating changes in the neutrophil count consisting of an initial phase of neutropenia and subsequent neutrophilia in the blood. Leukopenia after an injection of endotoxin occurs within a few minutes and lasts from 30 to 60 minutes. A gradual increase in the neutrophil count, reaching its maximum after 4 to 8 minutes, is subsequently noted. Those observations have been used in evaluating the marrow pool of neutrophils (Craddock et al., 1960; Fink et al., 1962; Marsh et al., 1964). The extent of neutrophil mobilization in the peripheral blood reflects to a certain degree the bone marrow efficiency with regard to the production of these cells and the antibacterial activity of the whole neutrophil system. Evaluation of the mobilization capacity of neutrophils after the injection of endotoxin is of practical importance in patients with malignancies in whom chemotherapy provokes neutropenia. The effects of endotoxin on neutrophils may be inhibited by some antibiotics, auch as polymyxin B sulfate (Corrigan et al., 1974).

<h1 style="text-align:center">Etiocholanolone</h1>

Etiocholanolone (delta-4-androsten-3,17-dion) induces an increase in the neutrophil count starting after a latent phase lasting from 6 to 8 hours which is preceded by a leukopenic phase (Vogel et al., 1967). This shows the difference between the actions of endotoxin and etiocholanolone.

It should be emphasized, however, that the evaluation of differences between the actions of various agents inducing neutrophil mobilization is not simple in every case. A comparison of the actions of the *Salmonella abortus equi* endotoxin (Lipexal) etiocholanolone, hydrocortisone, and prednisone has not revealed any major differences (Dale et al., 1975).

Antineutrophilic Serum

Antineutrophilic serum causes neutropenia unaccompanied by the destruction of the immature neutrophil precursors in the bone marrow; hence, it has been suggested that the antigenic detertminants reacting with the serum do not appear before the mature cells. There is a lack of data on the composition and properties of antineutrophilic serum analogous to the data on antilymphocytic serum.

Radioactive Orthophosphate

The use of labeled DNA in studies on neutrophil kinetics is based on the fact that the mature neutrophil does not undergo mitotic divisions. Hence, labeled DNA is a relatively stable marker which does not leave the cell during its life. Methodologic difficulties arise from the fact that after cell death the labeled DNA is reutilized.

The mean survival time of neutrophils in healthy subjects determined by means of $^{32}PO_4$ is from 8 to 9 days (Ottesen, 1954). It has been established by means of these methods that neutrophils which have left the vessel lumen and passed into the extravascular spaces do not return to the circulating blood. These data contradict the previous opinion that there is a constant recirculation of mature neutrophils between the blood and tissues. It has also been found that neutrophils containing ^{32}P incorporated into DNA do not appear, after the marker application in the blood, before 5 days. This period corresponds to the time taken by neutrophils to mature in the bone marrow. During these 5 days the following events should take place: the incorporation of ^{32}P into neutrophil precursor DNA, total DNA synthesis, a subsequent series of mitoses in the myeloblasts and myelocytes, and the process of neutrophil maturation.

Labeled Thymidine

The use of labeled thymidine has given an insight into the course of particular phases of the cell cycle. The cell cycle consists of the following phases: 1) phase G_1 (postmitotic rest period); 2) phase S (phase of DNA synthesis, during which the replication of chromosomes from the diploidal to the tetra-ploidal number occurs); 3) phase G_2 (premitotic rest); and 4) phase M (mitosis). The term generation time refers to the interval between one mitosis and another. The appearance in and disappearance from the blood of neutrophils labeled with ^{3}HTdR may be useful in evaluating the kinetics of these cells in various pathologic conditions. Abnormal regulation of neutrophil kinetics has been found *inter alia* in patients with the Chediak-Higashi-Steinbrinck anomaly (Blume et al., 1968).

Other Markers

Several investigations on neutrophil kinetics have been made with the use of ^{51}Cr. These investigations concerned the survival time of cells *in vivo* in various conditions (McCall et al., 1955; McMillan et al., 1966), and the kinetics of local cellular exudates in patients with acute leukemias (Perillie et al., 1964). Similar studies have been carried out with the use of DF-^{32}P (Athens et al., 1961; Boggs, 1960; Boggs et al., 1964) and of ^{3}H-DFP (Meuret et al., 1973). The last technique is particularly useful in the evaluation of neutrophilia induced by cortisol and enables measurements to be made of the cell flow rate in and out of the circulating pool of neutrophils; this technique is also applicable in studying patients with severe neutropenia (Rothstein et al., 1971).

BIOLOGIC SITES OF NEUTROPHIL PRODUCTION

The formation of mature neutrophils and their precursors needs special microenvironmental conditions. The microenvironment of the bone marrow presents particular conditions enabling neutrophils and other blood cells to be formed. Vascularization of the bone marrow cavity is only one of these conditions. Others are not well known. There is an almost complete lack of information on the differences between the microenvironmental conditions in the bone marrow cavity and the other extramedullary sites of hematopoiesis.

Bone Marrow

In bone marrow smears, all forms of neutrophil precursors—myeloblasts, promyelocytes, myelocytes, metamyelocytes, and stabs—are visible. These cells exhibit particular morphologic features which enable particular cellular forms to be differentiated. The majority of quantitative studies of the neutrophil system in the bone marrow have been based on the evaluation of the percentages of given cell lines. The diagnostic value of such an evaluation is well known, but quantitative studies by means of this method are possible only with great approximations. In the first place, there are several difficulties in establishing the exact time of mitoses and the mitotic index of the neutrophil precursors. Data on the neutrophil precursor content in bone marrow obtained by various authors differ on account of differences in age, race, diurnal variations, geographic factors, etc. The comparison of the data obtained by various authors is given in Table 11. The differences among authors are

TABLE 11. Differential count of cells of the neutrophilic series in the bone marrow. (According to Wintrobe et al., 1975; Williams et al., 1977; Miale, 1972)

Cells \ Author	Wintrobe (1975)	Miale (1972)	Osgood, Seaman (1944)	Vaughan, Brockmyre (1947)	Berman (1949)	Glaser et al. (1950)
Myeloblast	0.9	1.3	0.4	1.3	3.0	1.2
Promyelocyte	3.3	3.4	1.4	—	9.0	1.8
Myelocyte	12.7	7.9	4.2	8.9	6.0	16.5
Metamyelocyte	15.9	10.1	6.5	8.9	9.0	23.0
Stab	12.4	18.0	24.0	23.9	31.0	—
Mature neutrophil	7.4	15.0	15.0	18.5	17.0	12.9
Cells of neutrophilic series (total)	53.6	55.7	51.5	51.4	55.0	65.4

more pronounced when the differential count of cells belonging to the neutrophilic series is presented as a percentage of the total number of cells in the bone marrow (Table 12). It is emphasized that some differences among the data from various studies may be due to the fact that the volumes of marrow aspirates are not the same. Marrow samples containing more than 1 ml exhibit a greater percentage of mature neutrophils than smaller samples, owing to the admixture of peripheral blood (Dresch et al., 1974).

The controversy on the pluripotential hematopoietic cell should be mentioned here. In the bone marrow of the adult there are no cells corresponding to candidade of such a cell. The only period when hematopoietic pluripotential cells, which may be regarded as the common precursors of all blood cells, are visible in the bone marrow cavity is during the first stages of fetal development of hematopoietic tissue (Chen et al., 1975). Hence neutrophil production during fetal life and in the adult should be considered separately. Not much is yet known on the factors conditioning the differentiation of primitive stem cells into more mature and more differentiated cell forms in fetuses.

80

TABLE 12. Differential count of cells of the neutrophilic series in the bone marrow (expressed as a percentage of the total marrow cell count). (According to Dresch et al., 1974)

Author Cells	Wintrobe (1967)	Flandrin (1971)	Donohue (1958)	Harrison (1962)	Doll (1970)	Cronkite (1971)	Uchida (1971)	Kurnick (1971)	Northup (1972)
Myeloblasts	3.3	5	0.5	2.9	4.9	0.4	3.3	3.1	
Promyelocytes	8.2	10.8	1.3	2.7	13	1.2	6.9	6.2	45
Myelocytes	19.7	19.4	22.4	22.3	25.5	19.5	9.2	10.2	
Metamyelocytes	36.1	26.8	23.3	48.7	15.2	15.7	80.6	80.5	55
Mature neutrophils	32.7	38.0	52.5	23.4	41.4	63.2			

The production of neutrophils is closely related to the distribution and fate of these cells. The three main anatomic areas in which neutrophils function are the bone marrow, the peripheral blood, and the tissues.

Within the bone marrow there occur three basic pools of neutrophil precursors—the mitotic, the maturation, and the storage pools. The mitotic pool includes myeloblasts, myelocytes, and promyelocytes. These cells are able to undergo mitotic division (Boll et al., 1965). There are from five to seven mitoses between the myeloblast and the mature neutrophil (Warner et al., 1964). The maturation pool includes all cells from promyelocytes to stabs. The storage pool consists of mature neutrophils, stabs, and metamyelocytes which do not undergo mitotic divisions, and the morphologic differences between them correspond to the maturation stage.

During mitotic divisions, processes of simultaneous maturation take place, shown in the formation of azurophilic and specific lysosomal granules. The cells in the storage pool do not synthesize DNA or incorporate tritiated thymidine. The intracellular mechanisms leading to division of the cell nucleus into segments and the mechanisms of changes related to maturation noted in the cell cytoplasm are not well understood.

There is an evident gap between the mitotic compartment and the maturation compartment. Information on the mitotic divisions within the mitotic compartment is relatively plentiful. Analysis of the percentages of particular precursors of neutrophils in the bone marrow suggests that during the whole process of normal proliferation of the neutrophil system, starting from the myeloblast, four or five mitotic divisions take place (Warner et al., 1964). Data obtained by means of DF-^{32}P marker indicate that the myelocyte undergoes at least three mitoses (Warner et al., 1964).

Despite attempts at a mathematical approach to the problems of the frequency and course of mitotic divisions in the neutrophil system, our understanding of events in this regard is not sufficient. A mathematical formula cannot take into consideration the simple fact that not all myelocytes must undergo mitoses; neither is it known whether a given myelocyte will undergo another mitosis or not. It is always possible that a given cell may represent the last form in a mitotic cycle, and in a short time will mature to the stage of a nondividing metamyelocyte; neither can it be omitted that the variations in calculations of the mitotic index for nucleated cells in the bone marrow are very great, depending on the authors and the methods used. The differences are striking in many cases (Japa, 1942; Killman et al., 1962). The circadian rhythms of cell mitotic activity may also be of importance in evaluating the differences among the calculations of various authors (Mauer, 1965). Attention should also be drawn to the fact that so far the available methods do not permit the quantitative determination of particular precursors of neutrophils in the bone marrow as a whole. Other difficulties stem from the fact that labeled material is reutilized and eluted and that the radioactivity of this material may affect the course of mitoses.

Similar problems arise when tritiated thymidine is used as a label in the evaluation of the mitotic index of neutrophil precursors. In man, the labeling indices for the myeloblast, promyelocyte and myelocyte are 0.85, 0.65, and 0.33, respectively (Cronkite et al., 1964), but these data are also disputable owing to various possible errors.

The evaluation of neutrophil production by calculating the labeled metamyelocytes appearing after injection of ^{3}HTdR is also not free from errors. Since metamyelocytes do not undergo mitoses or incorporate ^{3}HTdR, the appearance of labeled metamyelocytes may be considered as a result of their efflux from the mitotic compartment of myelocytes. In man, a 3-hour interval is observed between the injection of ^{3}HTdR and the appearance of labeled metamyelocytes (Cronkite, 1969). This time interval corresponds to the subsequent phases, i.e., the uptake of the marker by the myelocytes, the transition through the G_2 and M phases, and the formation of metamyelocytes.

After passing from the bone marrow into the blood, neutrophils form a total neutrophil pool, which consists of two subpopulations: the first, in movement, is called the circulating neutrophil pool (CNP), and the second, adhering to the walls of the small vessels, is called the marginal neutrophil pool (MNP). Little is known of the equilibrium between these pools in man. MNP represents a large reserve of cells which may be mobilized, e.g., during local inflammations, and may migrate from the blood to the tissues without a simultaneous increase in the neutrophil count in the circulating blood. This means that the initial phases of inflammation may not be indicated by detectable changes in leukocytosis. The half-survival-time of neutrophils in the blood is, according to various authors, from 6 to 7 hours (Cartwright et al., 1964; Galbraith et al., 1965).

It may be supposed that there should exist a steady state of equilibrium between the production of neutrophils and their content in various compartments, on the one hand, and the extent of their elimination from the blood and disruption in tissues, on the other. The efflux of cells from one pool (K_{out}) should be equal to the influx of cells into this pool (K_{in}) plus all the cells produced within a given pool, designated as K_b (born).

$$K_{out} = K_{in} + K_b$$

It seems, however, that owing to various technical difficulties the precise determination of the size of a particular pool in a single patient will not be possible for a long time yet. The data so far obtained are merely approximations.

Very scanty data refer to the fate of neutrophils in the tissues. It is generally accepted that the survival time of these cells after passing from the blood into the tissues is about 4 to 5 days. After this period the cells undergo death and disintegration, and their remnants are reutilized by various cells of the body.

Interesting data on the production of neutrophils have been obtained in studies on the blood neutrophil turnover rate (NTR) by means of labeling with DF-^{32}P. This method enables the determination of the total blood neutrophil pool (TBNP) and of the extent of disappearance of labeled cells from the blood. It has been calculated by this method that the daily production of neutrophils in man is from 62 to 400 $\times$ 10^7 cells per kg (Bishop, 1971). Other data from these studies are presented in Table 13.

TABLE 13. Blood neutrophil kinetic parameters in 71 normal subjects.
(According to Bishop, 1971)

	Mean	95% limits
TBNP (cells $\times$ 10^7/kg)	61	27–128
CNP (cells $\times$ 10^7/kg)	31	13–49
MNP (cells $\times$ 10^7/kg)	29	8–115
T 1/2 (hours)	6.3	4–10
NTR (cells $\times$ 10^7/kg/day)	160	62–400

TBNP = total blood neutrophil pool
CNP = circulating neutrophil pool
MNP = marginal neutrophil pool
T = total
NTR = neutrophil turnover rate

It is obvious that the relationships among the parameters presented in Table 13 undergo constant fluctuations under the influence of various factors. A shift between CNP and MNP is observed after the injection of endotoxin. During the first period after injection, TBNP does not change significantly and its increase is noted only after some hours. The extent of the passage of neutrophils between the blood and tissues corresponds to NTR and in healthy subjects is 160 $\times$ 10^7/kg/day (Bishop, 1971). It has already been mentioned that as a rule neutrophils that reach the tissues do not reenter the blood.

Spleen, Liver, and Lymph Nodes

The formation and production of neutrophils in the spleen take place during the fetal period of hematopoiesis. Little is known about this period of neutrophil production. There is more information on neutrophil formation in the spleen of adults with myeloid metaplasia. Our knowledge on the formation of neutrophils in the liver is also only scanty. Very few data relate to the hepatosplenic period of hematopoiesis in the fetus and extramedullary hematopoiesis in the adult. There are case reports on the occurrence of myeloblastic infiltrations in the peripheral lymph nodes in patients with chronic granulocytic leukemia (Urasiński et al., 1972). It is not known whether a portion of these myeloblasts may mature into neutrophils.

BIOLOGIC SITES OF NEUTROPHIL DISINTEGRATION

The mechanisms of neutrophil disintegration in the tissues of man *in vivo* have been the subject of only a few reports. It is known that some portions of the neutrophil pool enter the urine. In patients with pyelonephritis, the passage of neutrophils into the renal canaliculi is increased. These cells also occur in small numbers in the saliva. In subjects with inflammatory lesions of the oral cavity, the neutrophils in the saliva are more numerous. The elimination of neutrophils via the lungs, liver, and spleen has long been known. Quantitative data on these routes of neutrophil elimination are not known. A number of neutrophils leave the body via the digestive tract. The mechanisms of neutrophil passage through the capillaries are also little known; these mechanisms are not related to lysosomal granule lysis or the digestion of the capillary walls, since neutrophils exhibit no degranulation in experiments on the passage of these cells through the capillaries. There are almost no reports on this subject in man.

MECHANISMS CONTROLLING THE PRODUCTION OF NEUTROPHILS

Information on the control of neutrophilopoiesis in man is scanty. Most studies in this field have been on experimental models and observations *in vitro*. Among the more important regulators of neutrophilopoiesis chalones, colony-stimulating activity, the neutrophilia-promoting factor, and hormonal factors should be mentioned.

Chalones

Chalones are low-molecular-weight peptides synthesized intracellularly which inhibit the entrance of neutrophil precursors into the DNA synthesis phase (Rytömaa, 1975; Rytömaa et al., 1976). Their action mainly affects the G_1 phase or the borderline between the G_1 and S phases. Chalones do not exhibit species specifity, though their action is cell-specific; they act on all cells of the neutrophilic series that are capable of mitotic divisions. The biologic counterparts of chalones are antichalones. Antichalones are characterized by a higher molecular weight than that of chalones. The complex interaction between chalones and antichalones is probably of fundamental importance in the control and regulation of cellular cycles and the production of neutrophils.

A characteristic feature of chalones is the fact that these substances are produced by the same cells of which they inhibit the proliferation. As far as chalones of neutrophils are concerned, the following general properties should be noted: 1) they inhibit prolifaration of cells through a negative feedback loop; 2) their selectivity is restricted solely to immature cells of the neutrophilic series; 3) their effect is reversible and not toxic to cells (Paukovits et al., 1975; Rytömaa et al., 1976). Studies on the structure and composition of chalones have not hitherto resulted in the isolation of purified chalones. The molecular weight of chalones is about 4000 (Paukovits et al., 1975). The majority of recent investigations on chalones were performed on animals (Rytömaa, 1973). The presence of chalones was found not only in normal cells but also in leukemic cells isolated from the blood of patients with acute myeloblastic or chronic granulocytic leukemia (Maiolo et al., 1975). It seems worth mentioning that no differences in the content of chalones have been found between normal and leukemic cells. This fact has given rise to the concept that leukemic cells are probably insensitive to the inhibitory and controlling action of chalones. This concept needs detailed studies.

The Colony-Stimulating Factor

The colony-stimulating factor (CSF) is present in various cells and tissues as well as in the serum and urine. Human neutrophils also probably are cells excreting CSF. CSF isolated from neutrophils stimulates marrow cultures more strongly than that from urine. CSF activity in myeloblasts from patients with acute myeloblastic leukemia is very low (Robinson et al., 1970). CSF is also present in neutrophils from patients with chronic granulocytic or myelomonocytic leukemia (Golde et al., 1974). CSF isolated from urine is a glycoprotein with a molecular weight of 40,000.

The significance of this factor in man has not been fully elucidated. According to some opinions CSF influences neutrophilopoiesis. The reason why some leukemic cells produce CSF and others do not is not known; neither is it known whether the presence or absence of CSF in leukemic cells influences the clinical course of the disease. The relationship between CSF activity *in vitro* and the extent of neutrophilia *in vivo* has not been clarified (Galbraith et al., 1974). It has been suggested that the degree of neutrophilia affects not only neutrophil release from the bone marrow but also myelocyte proliferation.

The Neutrophilia-Promoting Factor

The neutrophilia-promoting factor (the granulocytosis-promoting factor, GPF) has been isolated from mammary tumors in mice. This factor probably differs from the leukocytosis-inducing factor (LIF), which has been demonstrated in rat urine.

Hormonal Regulation of Neutrophil Production

Hormonal regulation of neutrophil production is documented by the following facts:

1. The neutrophil count increases during the second half of the menstrual cycle (Polishuk et al., 1973). This increase is accompanied by activation of the alkaline phosphatase in these cells.

2. Physiologic concentrations of testosterone stimulate neutrophilopoiesis *in vitro* (Rosenblum et al., 1974). In patients treated with this hormone, the number of neutrophils and the alkaline phosphatase activity in these cells increase (Lisiewicz et al., 1975). Similar increases are noted in patients with chronic granulocytic leukemia (Janicki et al., 1977).

3. Epinephrine may induce a biphasic increase in the neutrophil count in the blood (Samuels, 1951).

4. The circadian variations of the mitotic index in the bone marrow and the daily cycles of the neutrophil count are probably due to hormonal stimulation (Sabin et al., 1925; Mauer et al., 1965).

MOBILIZATION OF NEUTROPHILS

Mobilization in the Blood

In patients with various bacterial infections, the neutrophil count in the circulating blood increases. This increase varies in its dynamics, depending on the type of infection and the individual reactivity of the host. The mechanisms of the rapid changes in the neutrophil count have not been fully elucidated. It has already been mentioned that there is a bone marrow reserve of these cells which may undergo mobilization in a very short time before the stimulation of proliferative mechanisms. In normal conditions, after the injection of labeled thymidine, maximum radioactivity, corresponding to the entrance of mature neutrophils into the blood, is noted between the fourth and eighth day (Perry et al., 1968). This phenomenon shows that between the first and the fourth day after the application of the marker the more mature cells of the neutrophilic series, capable of DNA synthesis, have incorporated the marker, completed DNA synthesis, undergone mitosis, finished maturation, and entered the circulating blood.

In patients with acute infections, labeled neutrophils appear in the blood strikingly sooner than in healthy subjects. In patients with severe bacterial infections, these cells are detectable in the peripheral blood after 48 hours, and in those with less severe infections after 72 hours (Fliedner et al., 1964). More rapid mobilization of neutrophils is also observed in patients with leukemoid reactions and after the injection of endotoxin in dogs and of etiocholanolone in man. In patients with chronic infections the mobilization time of neutrophils is similar to that in healthy subjects.

There are several agents stimulating the bone marrow neutrophil reserve. An increase in the neutrophil count in the blood is noted after the administration of prednisolone (Strausz et al., 1967). The mobilization of neutrophils is weaker in patients with leukopenia, pernicious anemia, or infectious mononucleosis (Strausz et al., 1968). The mechanism of the prednisolone-induced mobilization of neutrophils is obscure.

The awareness of factors increasing neutrophil mobilization has found practical application in patients treated for malignant growth by antimitotic drugs or radiotherapy. The administration of bacterial endotoxins to these patients results in a transient mobilization of neutrophils in the blood. A similar increase in the neutrophil count is observed in some patients with acute leukemias in whom bacterial abscesses have developed.

The regulating factors of both the kinetics and mobilization of neutrophils are the level of leukocytosis and the extent of elimination of leukocytes from the blood. As previously mentioned, neutropenia induces an action stimulating neutrophil production. A factor increasing the neutrophil count occurs in the plasma of patients with neutropenia (Marsh et al., 1971). This factor has not yet been fully characterized. It has been shown that repeated leukopheresis in rats, like injections of typhoid or paratyphoid vaccine, induces the appearance of the leukocytosis-promoting factor in the serum (Gordon, 1964). This factor differs from the so-called granulocytopoietin described in mice (Bierman et al., 1972). The significance of these factors or even their existence in man has not been fully established.

Local Mobilization (Migration)

Local mobilization of neutrophils (LMN) occurs owing to the migratory capacity of these cells. The capacity to migrate is one of the most important elements determining neutrophil functions. The term "migration of neutrophils" refers to the active movement of these cells, especially in the presence of an inflammatory focus, into which they enter from the surrounding tissue spaces and capillaries. The mobilization of neutrophils in the blood and their chemotactic properties are inherent attributes of effective directional migration and phagocytosis of microbial agents or other objects. There have been reports on cases with defective LMN associated with deficiency in the plasma of the physiologic antagonists of the inhibitor of neutrophil mobility (Soriano et al., 1973).

Phagocytosis in a site of inflammation depends on several events, which will be briefly summarized: 1) local irritation due to the effect of microbial agents in the tissues; 2) the appearance of metabolites or products of microbial agents which enter the blood; 3) the mobilization of the extramedullary and bone marrow neutrophil reserves and the increase in the neutrophil count in the blood; 4) the penetration of neutrophils into the sites of inflammatory lesion; and 5) their interaction with microbial agents or components of the affected tissues resulting in phagocytosis.

There are only a few studies on neutrophil viscosity, which is an important feature of these cells (Brubaker, 1974). Neutrophil viscosity is lowered in patients with chronic granulocytic leukemia or acute myeloblastic leukemia; it also decreases under the influence of prednisone or alcohol. This biologic feature of neutrophils requires further investigation.

FACTORS ACTIVATING NEUTROPHIL MIGRATION

Only some of the so far known factors activating neutrophil migration are of importance in human pathology (Table 14). In natural conditions a significant stimulatory effect is induced by pyrogens of various origin, products of tissue disintegration, and substances isolated from the serum proteins, albumins, gamma globulins, and the complement components. Epinephrine, histamine, and prostaglandins induce a similar effect. The efficiency of action of all these substances depends on their local concentrations. Small amounts may have a stimulatory effect on neutrophil migration, but very high concentration frequently result in inhibition of migration. Vasoactive factors such as bradykinin, serotonin, and several antihistaminic agents may also alter the migratory capacity of neutrophils.

The neutrophil migratory capacities may be studied by several methods. One of those frequently used is that of Rebuck, the so-called skin window technique (Rebuck et al., 1955). This technique consists in the superficial scarification of the skin and the use of covering glasses which adhere to the irritated area. The accumulation of migrating cells on the glasses and its periodic changes enable the dynamic evaluation of cellular events in inflammatory exudate during various intervals of time. This method, however, permits

TABLE 14. Agents influencing neutrophil migration.

Agents enhancing neutrophil migration	References	Agents inhibiting neutrophil migration	References
Etiocholanolone	Vogel et al., 1967	Ethanol	Brayton et al., 1964
Bacterial pyrogens	Senn, 1972	Phenylbutazone	Senn et al., 1975
Plant pyrogens (echinacin)	Senn, 1972	Indomethacin	Senn et al., 1975
Dexamethasone	Senn et al., 1975	Prednisone	Senn et al., 1975
Leukoegresin (degradation product of IgG)	Yoshinaga et al., 1972	Histamine	Senn, 1972
Extracts of leukocytes, tissues, crude subfractions	Beaver et al., 1963 Borel et al., 1969 Gowland, 1964 Hurley, 1964	Epinephrine	Senn, 1972
Leukotactic factor of lymphocytes	Ward et al., 1969		
Fractions of serum containing IgG	Senn et al., 1975		
Autologous serum	Senn et al., 1975		
Magnesium ions	Senn, 1972		
Calcium ions	Senn, 1972		

rather the evaluation of local reaction against a foreign body (glass) than an insight into the migratory abilities of neutrophils. The use of plastic chambers that cover the irritated site of the skin enables a more accurate quantitative evaluation of neutrophil migration to be made (Senn, 1972; Senn et al., 1967, 1969, 1975). This method may also be used to determine the neutrophil clearance from the blood in various conditions.

It has been shown that monocytes in the presence of hydrocortisone produce a factor stimulating neutrophil migration in a cell culture (Stevenson, 1974). Lymphocytes do not exhibit a similar effect in the same conditions. The monocytic factor has no yet been fully described. The complex interaction between monocytes and lymphocytes, on the one hand, and neutrophils, on the other, needs further explanation, especially in the light of the fact that lymphocytes may produce factor-inhibiting chemotaxis (Jirillo et al., 1976).

FACTORS INHIBITING NEUTROPHIL MIGRATION

Natural inhibitors of neutrophil migration which are capable of provoking severe defects in this activity are not known; neither is it known whether defects in migration differing from those of chemotaxis occur. Neutrophil migratory activity is diminished in patients intoxicated with ethanol (Brayton et al., 1964). This effect is probably related to the influence of ethanol on the bone marrow neutrophil reserve (McFarland et al., 1963; Lindenbau et al., 1969) which diminishes under the influence of this agent. LMN is also inhibited by indomethacin and phenylbutazone (Senn et al., 1975).

Information on the effects of the corticosteroids on neutrophil migration is controversial. Several authors have observed a stimulatory effect of these hormones, but others have not confirmed these observations. A difference in this respect between the actions of prednisone and dexamethasone has been noted; prednisone inhibits LMN, dexamethasone activates LMN (Senn et al., 1975). Epinephrine and histamine introduced into the plastic chambers according to Senn's method inhibit LMN (Senn, 1972). The prostaglandin effect on neutrophil migration needs further investigation (Zurier, 1974). Similarly, the effect of IgG degradation products, appearing after digestion with papain, is not quite clear (Yoshinaga et al., 1972).

An inhibitory effect on neutrophil migration may be provoked by various products of protein degradation appearing in the blood owing to the action of proteolytic enzymes released from the pancreas in patients with acute pancreatitis or from the leukocytic mass in patients with endotoxic shock. Disturbances in neutrophil migration in patients with neutropenia are a separate problem. The relationships between the mechanisms of neutropenia and those of abnormal neutrophil migration are not clear. As already mentioned, the importance of the lymphocytic factor inhibiting neutrophil migration is not clear (Jirillo et al., 1976).

ABNORMALITIES IN NEUTROPHIL MIGRATION

Disturbances in neutrophil migration as separate clinical entities have been described mainly in patients with defective chemotaxis accompanying the Chediak-Higashi syndrome and in other congenital defects of chemotaxis. Disturbed neutrophil migration has also been observed in patients with hemocytopathies and diseases of the liver.

Myeloproliferative Diseases

In patients with chronic granulocytic leukemia, neutrophil migration exhibits some abnormalities (Banerjee et al., 1972; Senn, 1972; Jungi et al., 1974). Various disturbances in neutrophil migration have been reported in patients with aplastic anemia, pancytopenia (Senn et al., 1975), plasma cell myeloma, and acute myeloblastic leukemia (Holland et al., 1971; Senn et al., 1975). During remissions in patients with acute leukemias defects in neutrophil migration disappear, and both LMN and neutrophil clearance normalize (Perillie et al., 1964; Senn et al., 1971). In patients treated with prednisone, defective LMN is more evident than in others.

Lymphoproliferative Diseases

A decrease in LMN has been noted in patients with chronic lymphocytic leukemia (Senn et al., 1975). In patients with Hodgkin's disease the results of studies have been less conclusive; probably these patients exhibit defective neutrophil clearance rather than defective neutrophil migration. In other entities in the lymphoproliferative group of diseases, neutrophil migration has not hitherto been studied.

Diseases of the Liver

In alcoholics with cirrhosis of the liver, the neutrophil migrative capacity has been found to diminish (Senn, et al., 1975). Patients with viral hepatitis or malignant metastases in the liver exhibit no alterations in this regard.

Other Diseases

Disturbed neutrophil migration has been observed in patients with disseminated lupus erythematosus, diseases of the central nervous system, diabetes (Kontras et al., 1968; Jansa, 1973), paroxysmal nocturnal hemoglobinuria, and viral or bacterial infections (Senn, 1972).

Alterations in neutrophil mobility during hemodialysis in patients with renal insufficiency may depend on the material used for the production of dialyzable membranes. Diminished random mobility of neutrophils occurs both *in vitro* and *in vivo* in the presence of cellulose membranes; polysulfone membranes do not give this effect (Henderson et al., 1975).

LEUKERGY

Leukergy is a phenomenon consisting in the adhesion of leukocytes to one another and the formation of leukocyte aggregates which are usually composed of cells of one type. Neutrophils form more of these aggregates than lymphocytes, monocytes, or basophils (Fleck et al., 1957). Leukocyte aggregates are formed in citrated blood after incubation at 37°C during 1 to 3 hours. Leukergy is an expression of the biologic activation of leukocytes. The mechanism of leukergy has not so far been discovered. The phenomenon probably depends on the surface changes and adhesion mechanisms preceding phagocytosis. The normal course of leukergy is conditioned by the presence of magnesium and calcium ions in the cellular environment (Allison et al., 1964). Leukergy may be provoked by the injection of typhoid vaccine, the leukocytosis-promoting factor (Menkin's factor), and tuberculin. It has been suggested that leukergy depends *inter alia* on the control of the central nervous system and represents part of the alarm reaction associated with an increase in ACTH and corticoid contents in the blood (Michałowicz, 1967). In healthy subjects leukergy is not observed except in pregnant women. Increased leukergy is noted in patients with fever, infections, or inflammatory diseases, and is usually accompanied by elevated leukocytosis. Leukergy is also noted in patients with typhoid fever characterized by leukopenia.

The phenomenon of leukergy has been noted in patients with rheumatic fever, pertussis, syphilis, lung or skin tuberculosis, and after BCG vaccination in tuberculous subjects (Aleksandrowicz et al., 1976). In a healthy subject tuberculin does not provoke leukergy. In the premature infant the degree of leukergy is parallel to the stage of biologic maturation. Normalization of the leukergy index proceeds more rapidly in female infants, characterized by higher resistance to infections and a higher survival index, as compared with males (Bryniak et al., 1974).

CHAPTER 4

PHAGOCYTIC PROPERTIES OF NEUTROPHILS

Phagocytosis is one of the basic elements of nonspecific resistance of the body to microbial invasion. In the circulating blood of man, phagocytic properties are exhibited by neutrophils, monocytes, and eosinophils (Leder, 1967; Aleksandrowicz et al., 1976; Szczeklik et al., 1976). The initial phase of phagocytosis is the directional migration of neutrophils toward the object to be engulfed. Direct contact between the neutrophil and the phagocytized object, surface changes in the cell membrane, engulfment of the object, formation of a phagocytic vacuole, intracellular killing of microbial agents, and decomposition of their biochemical components represent the subsequent stages of the process of phagocytosis.

The term phagocytosis refers to the phenomenon of engulfment of a given object, most frequently a microbial agent, by a neutrophil. The term pinocytosis refers to engulfment of soluble material. There has been a proposal to use the term endocytosis for both phagocytosis and pinocytosis (Jacques, 1969), but so far this term has not been generally accepted. Similarly, other terminologic equivalents of phagocytosis proposed by various authors have not entered into common use. Among these terms atrocytosis, chromopexis, colloidopexis, cytopempsis, endomembranosis, micellophagosis, micropinocytosis, phagotrophy, rhopheocytosis, ultraphagocytosis, and ultramicrophagocytosis may be mentioned (Jacques, 1969).

The phagocytic properties of neutrophils have been the subject of numerous articles and reviews (Rabinovitch, 1968; Jacques, 1969; Douglas, 1970; Lehrer, 1971; Spitznagel, 1975; Souillet et al., 1975; Sbarra et al., 1976; Aleksandrowicz et al., 1976). The close dating of 1968–1976 for these publications is due to the unusual progress of research in this field. The main advances in the knowledge of phagocytosis are related to the intracellular mechanisms of killing and biochemical decomposition of microbial agents by neutrophils. The neutrophil antimicrobial systems were presented in detail in the chapter on the biochemistry of these cells.

Neutrophils exhibit phagocytic ability against various biologic objects. These cells phagocytize most bacteria, fungi, and microbial agents of the genus *Mycoplasma* (Parkinson et al., 1975; Baehner, 1975). Viruses, protozoa, and encapsulated bacteria are phagocytized, in contrast, by the macrophages of the reticuloendothelial system. Neutrophils are also capable of phagocytizing cellular remnants, fibrin, fibrinogen, and fibrinogen degradation products (Běleš et al., 1972). Latex, iron particles, and several other substances may also be phagocytized by neutrophils. There is little information on the mechanisms by which the neutrophils can differentiate objects that can be phagocytized from those that cannot. The term autophagocytosis refers to engulfment of the body's own materials and products. Neutrophil autolysis is also included in autophagocytosis. Phagocytosis of foreign objects such as microbial agents is defined as heterophagocytosis.

During phagocytosis neutrophils release pyrogen into their environment. The febrile reactions induced by this pyrogen may be of significance in the mobilization of the neutrophilic cell series as a whole. Pyrogen may induce increased production of neutrophils in the bone marrow and an increased efflux of these cells from reservoirs into the circulating blood. A detailed description of pyrogen action on the neutrophil system was given in the chapter on the biochemistry of the neutrophil. The phagocytic process involves three separate stages: 1) chemotaxis, i.e., directional movement of neutrophils toward the object to undergo phagocytosis; 2) engulfment and the formation of a phagocytic vacuole; and 3) intracellular degradation and the destruction of the microorganisms. These three stages of phagocytosis represent elements that are separately controlled and depend on different biochemical mechanisms. The clinical manifestation of defective phagocytosis may be related to each of these stages. Complex defetcs of phagocytosis characterized by the abnormality of more than one of these stages have also been reported.

There is not much information on the general conditioning of the neutrophil phagocytic properties. Little is known of the effects of the general state of the body and its temperature on phagocytosis. In experiments *in vitro* it has been noted that the phagocytic activity of neutrophils does not change at temperatures from 33°C to 41°C (Mandell, 1975). It is not known whether the circadian variations in phagocytic activity are associated with the temperature cycles. Physical training increases the phagocytic activity of neutrophils (Górski et al., 1969; Eberhardt, 1971). There is only scanty information on the different degrees of resistance of various microorganisms to phagocytosis. It is known that several subtypes of gonococci are phagocytized to different extents by neutrophils (Dilworth et al., 1975).

96

CHEMOTAXIS

The chemotactic properties are among the basic biologic properties of neutrophils and form an element of their phagocytic function. Despite numerous studies, the main mechanisms of chemotaxis remain obscure. The mechanism by which neutrophils differentiate chemotactically between active and nonactive objects still remains obscure. The directional movement of neutrophils toward objects that are to be phagocytized should by conditioned by the presence of the neutrophil surface of receptors capable of differentiating very small concentrations of substances activating chemotaxis and excreted by these objects. In this way the neutrophil would direct its movement toward the areas of highest concentration of these substances. There is, however, an almost total lack of information on the characteristics of these theoretic surface receptors. There are numerous clinical examples of defective chemotaxis associated with lowered resistance to bacterial infections. Numerous substances activating or inhibiting chemotaxis have been described.

The term chemotaxis refers to the directional movement of neutrophils toward definite biologic objects, most frequently bacteria, and so has a different meaning from the expression general mobility of neutrophils, which refers to indirectional movement. The directional movement of neutrophils is evaluated by various methods, most frequently by means of the Boyden chamber; the indirectional movement may be studied by the capillary tube or filter technique. Attention has been called to the fact that there are defects in neutrophil mobility detectable only by the use of one of these methods, whereas others do not show the defect. Methods of neutrophil chemotaxis evaluation by means of cells labeled with ^{51}Cr (Goetzl et al., 1972) and agarose gel (John et al., 1976) have been reported.

Mechanisms of Chemotaxis

The fundamental problems of the molecular mechanism of chemotaxis and the structural changes in the neutrophil membrane during directional movements have not yet been solved. Very little is known of the alterations occurring in the membrane during the reception of the chemotactic stimulus or in the course of directional movement. It has been stated that neutrophil maturation is closely related to adaptation to active movements and chemotaxis. The fact that the cellular membrane of the mature neutrophil is less rigid than that of the myeloblast confirms this concept (Lichtman, 1970). These observations suggest that changes in the cell membrane taking place during the maturation of neutrophils enable these cells to pass from the bone marrow sinuses into the circulating blood. Investigations on the effects of ATP, ADP, cAMP, and GMP on the cell membrane have given new opportunities to elucidate the mechanism of chemotaxis (Miller, 1975).

Factors Activating Chemotaxis

Many factors activating chemotaxis also affect neutrophil migration. The main factors are listed in Table 14. It seems worth emphasizing that in many cases there is a lack of correlation between the activity *in vitro* and *in vivo* of a given agent influencing neutrophil chemotaxis. In experimental conditions corticoids decrease the chemotactic activity of neutrophils (Ward, 1966), though patients treated with large doses of these hormones do not exhibit alterations in this activity. Some of the results reported on the effect of some agents, e.g., colchicine, on chemotaxis are controversial (Baum, 1975). In man, the following groups of agents activating neutrophil chemotaxis are of importance:

1. The chemotactic system of kallikrein and of the plasminogen activator. Kallikrein and plaminogen activator induce a chemotactic effect on neutrophils. The generation of these agents is closely related to the activation of the Hageman factor (Cochrane et al., 1972; Kaplan et al., 1972, 1973; Goetzl et al., 1974). Activation of this factor occurs in inflammatory areas and on the basal membrane of injured vessels as well as on unveiled collagen fibrils.

2. Chemotactically active components of complement. Activation of complement by immune complexes, by polysaccharides, or by walls of bacterial cells results in the formation of chemotactically active fragments of the complement components C_{3a} and C_{5a} and of the chemotactic complex $C_{5,6,7}$ (Ward et al., 1969; Lachman et al., 1970; Ruddy et al., 1972).

3. The eosinophil chemotactic factor of anaphylaxis (ECF-A). This factor is formed during the IgE-dependent immunologic activation of mast cells (Kay et al., 1971; Goetzl et al., 1974; Czarnetzki et al., 1975). ECF-A is an acid peptide with a molecular weight of about 500 produced by the blood basophils, mast cells, and tissues rich in mast cells. It has a chemotactic effect on eosinophils. A separate chemotactic factor has been reported in neutrophils which is active against both eosinophils and neutrophils (Zigmond et al., 1973). This factor is generated from neutrophils during the phagocytosis of aggregated gamma globulin. The clinical significance of the eosinophilotactic factors produced by neutrophils requires further study.

4. Immunoglobulin G. IgG induces a chemotactic effect after digestion with papain (Yoshinaga et al., 1972). This action depends on the structural specificity of IgG. IgG_2 and IgG_4 isolated from sera of patients with plasma cell myeloma induce a stronger chemotactic effect than normal IgG. The substance

released from IgG by papain and responsible for the chemotactic effect has a molecular weight of about 14,000, and in this respect resembles leukoegresin, the chemotactic agent isolated from inflammatory areas. It is not known whether the selective release of beta-glucuronidase from neutrophils, induced by IgG$_1$, IgG$_2$, IgG$_3$, IgG$_4$, IgA$_1$, and IgA$_2$, is of significance in chemotactic phenomena (Henson et al., 1972).

Not much is known of the chemotactic properties of various tissues and organs in which inflammatory changes are observed. It has been shown that extract of supragingival dental plaque exhibits a stronger chemotactic effect (Helldén et al., 1973). It has also been demonstrated that chromatographically purified fractions of this substance increase vascular permeability and neutrophil migration from the granulation tissue vasculature.

Chemotactic Specificity of Leukocytes

The reaction of neutrophils to various chemotactic factors varies. These cells exhibit an evident specificity, though they may also react to factors that are chemotactically active in relation to other cells as well. It is known that chemotactic factors, derivatives of C$_{5a}$ and C$_{3a}$, attract not only neutrophils but also eosinophils and monocytes (Goetzl, 1975). The biologic role of the eosinophil chemotactic factor isolated from neutrophils has not been precisely defined (Czarnetzki et al., 1975).

Inhibitors of Chemotaxis

The chemotactic actions of neutrophils are controlled by means of cybernetic feedback loops. The subtle interaction of various feedback mechanisms is associated with factors inhibiting chemotaxis. It has been shown that in some cases only diluted plasma has chemotactic properties and undiluted plasma has no chemotactic effect (Keller et al., 1974). This observation may be of significance in interpreting the results given in many papers. The clinical significance of particular inhibitors of chemotaxis has not been closely defined (Ward, 1972). Some of these inhibitors play a role in the local mobilization of neutrophils. Several drugs, including antibiotics, inhibiting chemotaxis may diminish the immunologic reactivity of the body (Majeski et al., 1975). The major inhibitors of chemotaxis so far known are as follows:

1. Thr-lys-pro-arg tetrapeptide. This peptide, named tuftsin, is released from human gamma globulin degraded by the proteolytic enzyme present in neutrophils (Nishioka et al., 1972; Najjar et al., 1972). This peptide inhibits chemotactic activity neutrophils after stimulation by kallikrein (Goetzl, 1975). The peptide may also stimulate the phagocytic properties of neutrophils.

2. The neutrophil immobilizing factor (NIF). This factor is formed during incubation of neutrophils with endotoxin or with particles which may be phagocytized (Goetzl et al., 1972; Goetzl, 1975). The molecular weight of the factor is about 4000 to 5000. The factor inhibits both migration and chemotaxis in neutrophils and eosinophils. The phagocytic properties and viability of these cells are not altered by the factor.

3. Plasma gamma globulin. It has been demonstrated that $alpha_2$-macroglobulin may induce a strong inhibitory effect on chemotaxis (Goetzl, 1975).

4. Cytochalasin B. This factor inhibits neutrophil chemotaxis after stimulation with chemotactically active bacterial agents (Becker et al., 1972). Simultaneously, cytochalasin B inhibits neutrophil bactericidal activity against *Streptococcus pyogenes* during the early phase of interaction between the neutrophil and the bacteria, and also inhibits the translocation of myeloperoxidase-positive granules into the phagosomes within these cells (Okuda, 1975).

5. Streptolysin O. This agent is a strong inhibitor of neutrophil chemotaxis (Anderson et al., 1972). It also retards the rate of migration in neutrophils.

6. The leukocyte inhibitory factor (LIF). This factor is released by antigenically stimulated lymphocytes, and its molecular weight is about 68,000. LIF selectively inhibits the mean migration of neutrophils but has no effect on monocytes (Rocklin, 1975). The factor differs from that inhibiting macrophages (MIF), produced also by lymphocytes.

7. Viral agents. Influenza virus strains A and B inhibit neutrophil chemotaxis *in vitro* (Schlesinger et al., 1976). It has been suggested that this phenomenon is associated with the penetration of the viruses into the cells. Deactivation of chemotactic factors may be of definite biologic importance. The inhibition of chemotactic activity in kallikrein by C_1INH or by $alpha_2$-macroglobulin may be mentioned here (Goetzl, 1975).

8. Tobacco smoking. Whole tobacco smoke, gas phase of smoke, and water-soluble fraction are potent inhibitors of neutrophil chemotaxis (Bridges et al., 1977). It is suggested that the major inhibitory effects of tobacco smoke probably result from the direct action of oxidants and/or thiol-reactive substances on neutrophils.

OPSONIZATION

Opsonization of bacteria by complement or by specific antibodies is well known to be important in the subsequent degradation of bacteria by neutrophils. Interaction between the complement components and the specific antibodies may also result in the opsonization of bacteria. There are agents involved in the opsonization of streptococcal capsules which do not take part in the phagocytosis of other bacteria (Stollerman et al., 1963). A satisfactory description of these agents has not yet been given.

Opsonized bacteria are fixed on the surface of neutrophils, which contain receptors for both IgG and C_3. Only after this immunoadherence are there conditions for the invagination of the external membrane of the neutrophil and engulfment of bacteria. ATP is utilized and some components of the membrane, e.g., lipids, are translocated during the formation of the phagocytic vacuole. Other biochemical phenomena of phagocytosis, such as the activation of antimicrobial systems, lysosomal enzymes, peroxidase, and hydrogen peroxide, take place after these surface events.

Phagocytic activity in neutrophils is stimulated by IgG isolated from human serum (Christie et al., 1976). It has been shown that the Fc fragment is of importance not only for the course of phagocytosis but also for intracellular bacteriolysis. Fragment $F(ab')_2$ exhibits no stronger action in this respect. The stimulatory effect of IgM is weaker. In some instances the interaction between IgG, on the one hand, and neutrophils and their phagocytic properties, on the other, is more complex. Evidence has been shown that the serum from patients with a high titer of antibodies against *Candida albicans* antigens induces inhibitory action on the fungicidal properties of neutrophils (Laforce et al., 1975). The serum does not exert any inhibitory action on the bactericidal properties of neutrophils.

Increased phagocytosis is noted in the presence of subclasses of IgG—IgG_1, IgG_2, IgG_3, and IgG_4 (Leffell et al., 1975). This is associated with degranulation of granules containing myeloperoxidase and lactoferrin. The high degree of extracellular release of lactoferrin in these conditions suggests that the biologic role of this agent is played outside the neutrophils. The presence of surface receptors for antibodies of the IgG type in neutrophils is significant in erythrophagocytosis and thrombocytophagocytosis (Handin et al., 1974; Zipursky et al., 1974). It has been supposed that phagocytosis of erythrocytes and platelets covered with specific antibodies may be of importance in the clearance of these cells in patients with erythrocytopenia or thrombocytopenia. Some bacteria may be phagocytized without the presence of serum and without preliminary opsonization. Most bacteria, however, are not phagocytized before opsonization.

The term opsonization refers to the action of the serum factors that modify the surface of the bacterial cells in a manner enhancing or enabling phagocytosis. It has just been said that the main factors taking part in opsonization and present in the serum are antibodies and complement components. Opsonizing antibodies belong to various classes of immunoglobulin, but especially to IgG. Deficiency of the complement components, mainly C_3 and C_4, results in defective opsonization and subsequently defective phagocytosis. Attention has been called to the fact that during an interaction between gamma globulin particles and an opsonized object, molecular and physicochemical changes may occur in the particles (Davies et al., 1975). The nature of these changes has not, however, been defined. A more detailed presentation of the problems related to immunoglobulin and complement deficiencies as a basis of defective phagocytosis is given in the next chapter.

THE STAGE OF ENGULFMENT AND FORMATION
OF THE PHAGOCYTIC VACUOLE

The chemotactic movement of neutrophils results in the maximal approach to the object to be phagocytized and its subsequent engulfment. The intracellular formation of a phagocytic vacuole represents the next stage. Before the start of engulfment there is a short period of direct contact between the object and the outer membane of the neutrophil. During this period no neutrophil movements are noted. After this, a complex process of surface changes takes place—the formation of a neutrophil membrane wall around the object, and its engulfment into the intracellular spaces. During the first period the neutrophil membrane wall forms a hollowed-out space where the phagocytized object is located. The invagination of this craterlike structures is associated with the formation of a phagocytic vacuole. The inner walls of the vacuole subsequently consist of that part of the neutrophil external membrane which primarily formed the crater where the phagocytized object was situated. In this manner, the outer membrane of the neutrophil is translocated into the inner spaces of the cell, and the membrane surface that previously faced the cell cytoplasm now forms the external membrane of the phagocytic vacuole. The complex interaction between the membrane of the phagocytic vacuole, the lysosomal granules, the lysosomal enzymes and the other antimicrobial systems of the neutrophil represents the primary step in the further stages of phagocytosis, consisting of the inactivation and degradation of the phagocytized object (Fig. 12).

The process just described represents the approach to phagocytosis. There are numerous methods of evaluating the phagocytic capacity of neutrophils. Some of these methods enable the simultaneous determination of the extent of intracellular killing. Since a detailed presentation of these methods is beyond the scope of this monograph, only general data in this regard will be presented.

Methods of Investigating Phagocytosis

Methods of investigating the phagocytic capacity of neutrophils are mainly based on the determination of the numbers of phagocytizing cells and of phagocytized bacteria after incubation *in vitro*. Some authors propose the use of high concentrations of antibiotics or of phenylbutazone, which inhibit the various modes of the intracellular killing of bacteria (Solberg, 1972). New modifications of these methods have recently been proposed.

1. The method of simultaneous determination of the extent of phagocytosis and of intracellular killing of *Staph. aureus* by means of agar pour plates (Castro et al., 1972). The lysis of neutrophils in blood samples incubated with bacteria prior to plating in agar in this method enables the release and subsequent growth of bacteria which were phagocytized but not killed. The difference between the total number of bacteria growing in colonies from a lysed sample and the total number of bacteria from a control sample enables the intracellular bactericidal activity indices to be calculated. There are several variants of this method (Koch, 1974).

2. The method based on the fact that bacteria remaining alive within neutrophils are capable, after incubation, of incorporating ^{3}H-thymidine, whereas killed or nonreplicating bacteria do not exhibit this capacity (Cline, 1973).

3. The method based on the determination of radioactivity after incubating neutrophils with bacteria labeled with ^{54}Ca (Suzuki et al., 1971).

4. The method based on the isolation of phagocytic vacuoles from neutrophils (Stossel et al., 1971). These vacuoles may be subjected to structural and enzymatic studies at given intervals after phagocytosis.

5. Immunofluorescent methods. These enable phagocytized fibrinogen, fibrin, or products of fibrin degradation to be demonstrated within neutrophils (Bělěs et al., 1972). Attempts have been made to apply these methods in the early detection of venous and arterial thromboses.

6. The method of simultaneous determination of bactericidal activity and of glucose utilization in neutrophils (Territo et al., 1974). This method enables a rapid determination of the glucose oxidation stimulated by phagocytosis.

7. Recently, trials have been made of a statistical method for the evaluation of phagocytosis (Hoffman et al., 1973). The method takes into consideration the variables inherent within different test microorganisms such as *E. coli* and *Staph. aureus*, the different preparations of the assay medium, and the distribution of normal results as a logarithmic function, and permits the comparison of bactericidal tests between laboratories and at different points in time within the same laboratory. Similar trials have been made using models of theoretical formulas and the mathematical approach to experimental results (Capo et al., 1974).

8. There has also been a marked development of methods permitting the quantitative estimation of H_2O_2 production by phagocytizing neutrophils. Recently, an automated method has been presented in which H_2O_2-induced oxidation of nonfluorizing leukodiacetyl-2,7-dichlorfluoroscein to a fluorizing compound in the presence of peroxidase is used (Homan-Müller et al., 1975).

The Surface Events

The initial phenomena of phagocytosis consist in the adherence and clumping of neutrophils. The phenomena are associated with changes in the cell surface. The nature of these changes is not yet known. It has been shown that neutrophil agglomeration depends on the presence of bivalent cations, including magnesium and calcium (Allison et al., 1964). It has also been demonstrated in these studies that sublethal doses of dinitrophenol inhibit neutrophil agglomeration, which indicates the participation of glycolytic mechanisms in this phenomenon. The biologic role of neutrophil agglomeration during phagocytosis is not clear. It has been suggested that proteolytic enzymes appearing in the blood after trauma or bacterial invasion alter the functional state of the neutrophil surface, activate these cells, and increase their adhesion and agglomeration, resulting in the facilitation of phagocytosis (Allison et al., 1964).

One of the enzymes of the neutrophil membrane is leukokinase (Najjar et al., 1970). The enzyme splits off a small tetrapeptide from the Fc fragment, which represents part of the gamma globulin Fab fragment with properties activating phagocytosis in neutrophils. The interaction of this tetrapeptide, named tuftsin (L-threonyl-L-lysyl-L-prolyl-L-arginine), with the neutrophil membrane during the period of its phagocytic activation is a little-known aspect of the surface alterations accompanying phagocytosis.

It has been demonstrated that trypsin induces surface changes in neutrophils resulting in the blockage of the phagocytic and adhesive properties of these cells (Allison et al., 1965), but the nature of these surface changes under the influence of this enzyme has not been elucidated.

These observations refer to data indicating that phospholipase C, incubated with neutrophils, induces an increase in the hexose monophosphate shunt activity, in the incorporation of acetate-1-^{14}C into lipids, and in the NADP/NADPH index (Kaplan et al., 1972). There is still lack of information on surface changes in neutrophils at the molecular level. There have been assumptions that the biochemical properties of the membrane of neutrophils enable these cells to differentiate between materials that can undergo phagocytosis and those that cannot. The chemical alterations on the neutrophil surface during the initial phases of phagocytosis are not well known. It is known only that these alterations are accompanied by characteristic changes in cell metabolism, mainly

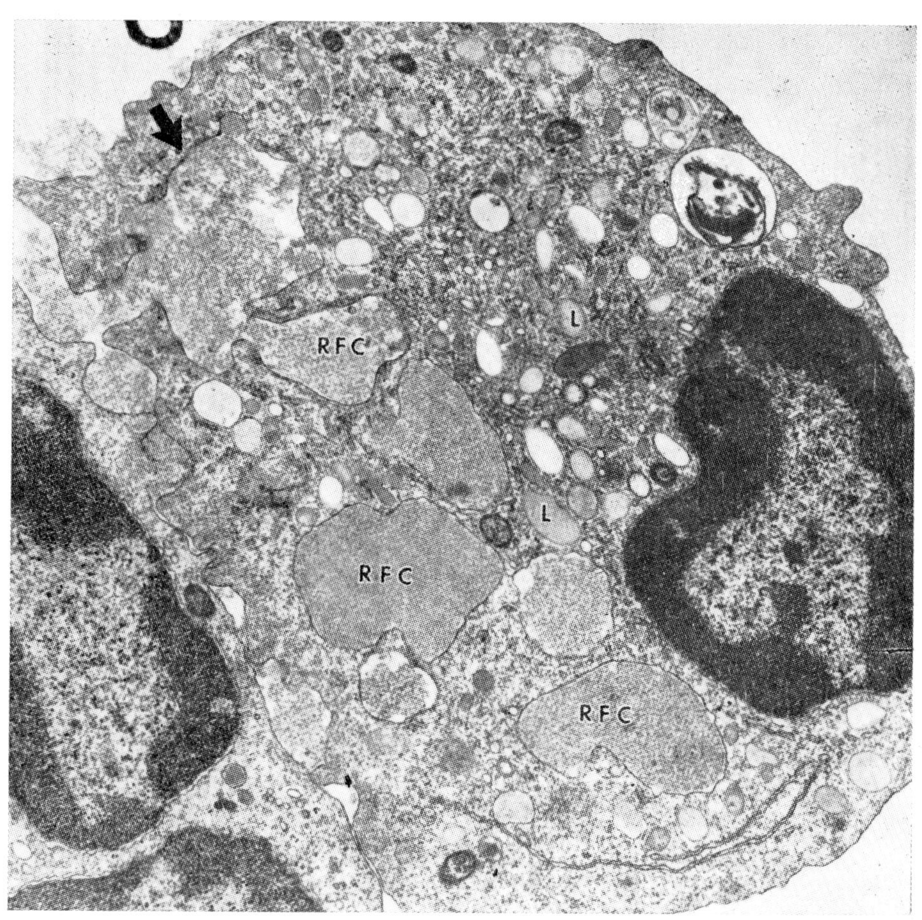

Fig. 12. A human peripheral blood neutrophil exposed *in vitro* to rheumatoid factor complex (RFC). Several phagocytic vacuoles containing RFC are visible in the cytoplasm as well as intact primary lysosomes (L). RFC can also be seen adhering to the cell membrane. The arrow indicates a phagocytic vacuole in the process of formation. × 16,000. (Courtesy of Dr. Sylvia Hoffstein, New York University Medical Center)

consisting in an increased oxygen uptake and enhanced carbohydrate and lipid metabolism (Graham et al., 1967). Similar changes have been noted in neutrophils after contact with some surface-active substances such as digitonin and the cholic acids (Karnovsky, 1968).

An important role in the surface phenomena occurring during phagocytosis is played by sialic acid. After digestion of the neutrophil outer membrane by a *Vibrio cholerae* extract containing sialidase, the phagocytic acitivity of the cells decreases (Fischer et al., 1956). This phenomenon is accompanied by a significant lowering of the intracellular glucose content due to the inhibition of the conversion of 6-phosphoglucose into 6-phosphofructose. It is not certain, however, whether there is a direct link between this phenomenon and the biochemical alterations (Karnovsky, 1968).

Formation of the Phagocytic Vacuole

During phagocytosis microbial agents are first engulfed by the neutrophil through invagination of the cell membrane. The second stage of phagocytosis consists in the accumulation of lysosomal granules around the phagocytic vacuole, the degranulation of these granules, and the introduction of the lysosomal enzymes into the inner spaces of the phagocytic vacuole.

Scanning electron microscopy enables a more detailed insight into the morphologic events during the first phases of phagocytosis (Bessis, 1973). It is known that the phagocytized object is actively introduced into the inner spaces of the neutrophil cytoplasm. The forces responsible for this active transport are not definitely known. The main result of the phagocytic events is the isolation of the phagocytized microbial agent from the surrounding liquid cytoplasm by means of the phagocytic vacuole membrane. In a very short time, active grouping of the lysosomal granules takes place around the phagocytized microbial agent within the vacuole. The degranulation of these granules is one of the most important events during phagocytosis (Hirsch et al., 1960). Direct contact between the outer membrane of the phagocytic vacuole and the lysosomal granules results in the lysis of the latter and the transport of their enzymatic contents into the inner areas of the vacuole. This renders it possible for the lysosomal enzymes to act directly on the phygocytized object. The morphologic details of the fusion of the lysosomal granules with the phagocytic vacuole membrane are known   rather well (Lockwood et al., 1963; Horn et al., 1964; Zucker-Franklin et al., 1964), but we have not yet a satisfactory knowledge of the biochemistry of this fusion. There have been suggestions that the pH values decrease at the sites of fusion.

Not much is known about the time-related sequence of the lysis of particular subgroups of lysosomal granules during fusion with the phagocytic vacuole. In experiments on rabbits it has been shown that during the first minutes after phagocytosis of *E. coli* or *Staph. aureus* the earliest enzymes to be released are those in the specific granules; the enzymes in the azurophilic granules are released 2 to 3 minutes later (Bainton, 1973). Analogous observations on man have not yet been made. Such observations will be of interest because the intracellular localization of some enzymes differs in human and rabbit neutrophils.

The Morphology of Destructuralization of Microbial Agents

The sequence of destructuralization of engulfed microbial agents within neutrophils has been the subject of only a few reports. It is not known which of the neutrophil enzymes first attack particular components of the microbial cells. The complex interaction between the neutrophil enzymes, on the one hand, and the components of the microbial structure, on the other, is the result of a prolonged evolutionary process. Little is known on the phylogenesis of this interaction. The species of agent phagocytized is, of course, of basic importance in this regard.

Structural analysis of the events accompanying phagocytosis indicates the almost immediate appearance of surface changes in the microbial agents after the lysosomal enzymes have fused with the phagocytic vacuole (Lockwood et al., 1963; Horn et al., 1964; Zucker-Franklin et al., 1964). Several morphologic features of microbes are changed in these conditions; the disintegration of particular substructures of these agents is due not only to the action of lysosomal enzymes but also to the effect of other neutrophil antimicrobial systems, such as myeloperoxidase, lysozyme, hydrogen peroxide, or cationic antimicrobial proteins. There is still a scarcity of reports on structural analogues of the disintegrating action of these systems.

Neutrophil Antimicrobial Systems

After the phagocytic vacuole has been formed and the engulfed microbial agent killed, the process of biochemical degradation of the microbial components starts. The neutrophil has at its command a complex antimicrobial system operating through independently acting subsystems capable of oxidation, iodination, hydrolysis, and the enzymatic breakdown of phagocytized material. The system was presented in detail in the chapter on the biochemistry of the neutrophil; here only a brief summary of knowledge in this field will be given (DeChatelet, 1975; Sbarra et al., 1976; Aleksandrowicz et al., 1976).

The oxidative reactions directed against the phagocytized microbial agents induce paralysis of the majority of the respiratory enzymes in the microbial cells and stop the processes of respiration, oxygen uptake, and glucose utilization at various levels. These reactions depend on the presence and production of free hydrogen peroxide and singlet oxygen in neutrophils.

Neutrophils are capable of hydrogen peroxide synthesis. There are two main antimicrobial systems within the neutrophil. The first is oxygen-dependent and the second oxygen-independent. The oxygen-dependent system involves myeloperoxidase, H_2O_2, halides, singlet oxygen, and superoxide anions. The oxygen-independent system involves the lysosomal enzymes, antibacterial cationic proteins, and lactoferrin. The lysosomal enzymes provoke the biochemical decomposition of microbial components such as lipids, lipoproteins, cell membrane proteins, cytoplasmatic proteins, nucleic acids, carbohydrates, and many other substances. In this way the total destructuralization of the microbial agent is possible. Cooperation between various enzymes enables the microbial components to be degraded at varying levels, e.g., the breakdown of microbial RNA through ribonuclease results in the appearance of mononucleotides and oligonucleotides, which are consecutively degraded through phosphatases and diphosphoesterases; the final degradation of RNA derivatives is due to the action of nucleosidase, deaminase, and oxidase.

The phagocytosis process is accompanied by an increase in the activity of several enzymes, including the acid and alkaline phosphatase, beta-glucuronidase, 5-nucleotidase, cholinic dehydrogenase, the alkaline and acid lipases, and esterases.

NEUTROPHIL METABOLISM DURING PHAGOCYTOSIS

The initial phases of phagocytosis in neutrophils are characterized by several biochemical alterations leading to an increased supply of energy, greater utilization of oxygen and glucose, and the production of carbon dioxide. These changes are associated with the increased energy requirements of the cell starting serious biologic efforts to phagocytize and kill an invasive microbial agent. The biochemical changes also include DNA and RNA synthesis.

Numerous observations refer to cytochemical alterations within the neutrophil during phagocytosis. Though the general importance of these observations is less than that of biochemical investigations, the clinical use of cytochemical methods of evaluating neutrophil reactivity during phagocytosis makes it desirable to present data from cytochemical studies also.

Energy Supply

The phagocytosis process and inactivation of engulfed objects, most frequently microbes, are associated with an increase in energy metabolism and with alterations in the activity of several enzymes regulating this metabolism. The source of intracellular energy in the neutrophil is the breakdown of 6-phospho-glucose (6-PG), which originates from glycogen or is supplied from the cell environment. In normal conditions only a small percentage of 6-PG is metabolized in the pentose cycle and the major part of this compound, i.e., about 90%, is metabolized in the Embden-Meyerhof glycolysis cycle (Sznajd et al., 1969). Most of the cells in the body in aerobic conditions perform glycolysis through oxidative phosphorylation and do not produce lactic acid. In contrast, mature neutrophils in the presence of oxygen, in addition to oxidative phosphorylation, produce lactic acid. This phenomenon, named oxidative glycolysis, is a characteristic feature of cells in the neutrophilic series, probably associated with their adaptation for the production of energy in anaerobic conditions.

During phagocytosis an increase in glucose metabolism is observed. This increase is due to the respiratory processes, the production of lactic acid, and the enhancement of metabolic processes in the pentose cycle. The absence of oxygen or the inhibition of respiratory processes by inhibitors only slightly diminishes the phagocytic activity. In contrast, the inhibition of the glycolytic processes results in the loss of the neutrophil capacity of active phagocytosis. Hence the basic feature of the phagocytizing neutrophil is the fact that the source of intracellular energy may derive from the anaerobic breakdown of 6-PG in both aerobic and anaerobic conditions (Karnovsky, 1968). The increase in oxygen utilization and in hydrogen peroxide production during phagocytosis depends on the nature of the particles engulfed. During phagocytosis of bacteria, this increase is greater than during phagocytosis of latex particles (Mandell, 1971).

During phagocytosis an increase is observed in the cell respiratory activity, oxidation of glucose-1-^{14}C and glucose-6-^{14}C, and lactate production (Selvaraj et al., 1967). In patients undergoing radiotherapy the extent of these changes is smaller. This phenomenon is, however, noted only *in vivo*; irradiation of neutrophils *in vitro* does not cause a decrease in these processes.

Another characteristic feature of phagocythosis is the activation of the pentose cycle. Resting neutrophils metabolize only about 2% of glucose in this cycle. Phagocytizing cells, however, metabolize about 40% of glucose in the pentose cycle. This is accompanied by a significant increase in oxygen uptake. The increase in oxygen utilization and the extent of pentose cycle activation are proportional to the number of particles phagocytized and to the number of neutrophils taking part in phagocytosis (Sbarra et al., 1959; Karnovsky, 1968).

The activation of the pentose cycle is the most striking event during phagocytosis in neutrophils. This phenomenon is of special interest since neither the mechanism of this activation nor the biologic basis for the enhancement of this pathway of glucose metabolism has yet been fully elucidated.

Among the enzymes within the neutrophil cytoplasm involved in catalyzing processes in the pentose cycle, the lowest activities are exhibited by 6-

phosphogluconic dehydrogenase and transketolase. From the theoretical standpoint, these two enzymes may be limiting factors influencing the intensity of metabolism in the whole cycle. If during the disintegration of lysosomes and degranulation accompanying phagocytosis additional amounts of these two enzymes are released into the cell cytoplasm, the cause of the significantly increased intensity of the pentose cycle would be elucidated to a greater degree, but it has been shown that the activity of these two enzymes is similar in resting and in phagocytizing cells (Stjernholm, 1968). Hence these data argue against the concept that the increased activity of the pentose cycle during phagocytosis is due to an increase in the activity of these two enzymes (Table 15).

The pentose cycle is a source of cellular NADPH. The conversion of NADPH into NADP, resulting in the appearance of large amounts of NADP, influences the rate of metabolism within the whole cycle. In neutrophils there

TABLE 15. Values of pentose enzymes in neutrophils.* (According to Stjernholm, 1968)

Enzyme	Resting	Phagocytizing
Glucose-6-phosphate dehydrogenase	14.8	15.7
6-phosphogluconic dehydrogenase	5.5	5.9
Ribose-5-phosphate isomerase	34.6	45.5
Xylulose-5-phosphate-3-epimerase	35.4	50.7
Transketolase	4.3	4.3
Transaldolase	11.8	13.7

* Results expressed in mols per hour per 10^8 cells.

is a separate enzymatic system synthetizing hydrogen peroxide with the participation of O_2 and NADP (Iyer et al., 1961). During phagocytosis the amounts of H_2O_2 produced are from twice to four times as much (McRipley et al., 1967). Probably the factor responsible for this increase in the rate of the pentose cycle is NADPH oxidase; the release of this enzyme into the cytoplasm during degranulation may increase the amount of available NADP (McRipley et al., 1967).

Oxygen Uptake

The amounts of oxygen taken up and used by phagocytizing neutrophils in the pentose cycle have been calculated in detail (Karnovsky, 1968). It has been shown that about 80% of the oxygen taken up is contained in the hydrogen peroxide produced. This indicates that the increase in oxygen uptake is not exactly parallel either to the increase in intensity of oxidative phosphorylation or to the respiratory processes in the neutrophil. The uptake of oxygen in highly purified suspensions of neutrophils differs from that in suspensions of these cells with an admixture of other leukocytes (Weening et al., 1974).

It was previously assumed that the cause of the increase in metabolic processes in the pentose cycle was the increased requirement of NADPH during the synthesis of lipids accompanying the formation of the phagocytic vacuole. Radioisotopic studies, however, have demonstrated that the uptake of NADPH does not increase for the synthesis of fatty acids.

A characteristic product of the pentose cycle in neutrophils is hydrogen peroxide. During its synthesis it is possible that NADPH is used in the process of reoxidation with the participation of the oxygen molecule (Karnovsky, 1968). The enzyme initiating this synthesis is NADPH oxidase. During degranulation the activity of this enzyme increases. This results in an immediate increase in the NADPH requirement and in hydrogen peroxide production, after which the activation of all processes involved in the pentose cycle occurs. The hydrogen peroxide produced forms, with myeloperoxidase and Cl^- ions, a strong antibacterial system degrading bacterial toxins (McRipley et al., 1967; Zatti et al., 1968), amino acids, peptides, and nucleotides (Karnovsky, 1968; Zgliczyński et al., 1968, 1975). The hypothesis that activation of the metabolic processes in the pentose cycle is associated with increased production of hydrogen peroxide has been confirmed by the observation that neutrophils of patients with chronic granulocytic leukemia are capable of engulfing foreign particles and of normal oxygen uptake, but that during phagocytosis they do not show either an increased oxygen uptake or activation of the pentose cycle. It has been shown that these leukemic cells are depleted of NADPH activity.

Lipids

In addition to the alterations already mentioned, the phagocytic process in neutrophils is accompanied by enhanced lipid synthesis. An increased incorporation of nonorganic phosphates into phosphatides (Karnovsky et al., 1961; Karnovsky, 1968), an increased turnover of phosphatidic acid, phosphatidylinositol, and phosphatidylserine, and an intensified incorporation of lysoleucine into lecithin (Elsbach et al., 1969) have also been noted in phagocytizing neutrophils. It is supposed that the increase is associated with the synthesis of the phagosome capsule walls. There is a lack of information on the possible association between lipid metabolism and the changes in the composition and properties of the neutrophil cell membrane.

110

RNA Synthesis

The increase in the synthesis of enzymatically active proteins during phagocytosis is accompanied by enhanced RNA metabolism, expressed in the elevated RNA breakdown rate, the diminution of the cell nucleotide pool, and the
increased synthesis of new RNA. All these events lead to an increased uptake of
RNA precursors (Cline, 1966, 1975).

SUBSTANCES ACTIVATING PHAGOCYTOSIS

Despite numerous experimental studies, only a few agents that activate
phagocytosis and are of clinical importance are known. Investigations on
drugs capable of increasing phagocytic activity in neutrophils seem to be of
special interest.

Magnesium Ions

The elevation of the neutrophil count after the application of magnesium
salts (Delbiase) has been observed in patients with chronic lymphocytic leukemia (Aleksandrowicz et al., 1970). Neutrophil acid phosphatase activity also
increases in these patients. It seems that clinical use of magnesium salts for
patients with a lowered neutrophil count is still insufficient.

Clofazimine (B 663)

Clofazimine (B 663) is a phenazine derivative used in the treatment of
leprosy. Administered perorally this drug increases the phagocytic activity of
neutrophils (Brandt, 1972). This effect reaches its maximum between the 4th
and 11th days of treatment. A similar effect is induced by clofazimine in
patients with chronic granulocytic leukemia.

Antithyroid Drugs

Some agents used in cases of hyperthyroidism, such as propylthiouracil
and methimazole, induce an effect enhancing the pentose cycle in neutrophils (Tsan et al., 1975). This effect is observed solely during phagocytosis;
resting cells do not respond to the action of these drugs. Antithyroid agents
do not affect phagocytosis.

SUBSTANCES INHIBITING PHAGOCYTOSIS

Little is known on the physiologic regulators of neutrophil phagocytic properties. The role of the particular immunoglobulin classes in this regard is not clear. There have been controversial reports on the effect of IgG on the phagocytosis of *Streptococcus viridans* by neutrophils; some authors have observed the inhibition of phagocytosis by IgG_1, IgG_2, and IgG_3 (MacLennan et al., 1973). Others, however, have not noted this effect as far as IgG_2 is concerned (Messner et al., 1970).

There is a large group of substances exhibiting an inhibitory action on phagocytosis in experimental conditions. Some of these substances influence the initial steps of phagocytosis, i.e., chemotaxis; other have an inhibitory effect on the engulfment and subsequent intracellular killing of microbial agents. The practical significance of these substances has recently increased owing to the fact that some widely used drugs, e.g., antibiotics, may exhibit such effects. There are few physiologic substances inhibiting phagocytosis present in the blood. Among them $alpha_1$-acid glycoprotein (orosomucoid) should be mentioned (Oss et al., 1974).

Hydrocortisone

This hormone does not affect the engulfment of foreign objects by neutrophils, but has an inhibitory effect on the intracellular killing of bacteria (Mandell et al., 1970). This effect is not associated with disturbances in neutrophil degranulation. It is accompanied by a decrease in NADPH oxidase activity, oxygen uptake, H_2O_2 production, and NBT reduction. It has been remarked that these alterations resemble those noted in patients with chronic granulomatous disease. The effect of hydrocortisone on neutrophils depends on its concentration. High concentrations of hydrocortisone may inhibit both phagocytosis and the intracellular killing of *Klebsiella pneumoniae* and enterococci *in vitro* (Olds et al., 1974). Methylprednisone used for a short time in large doses does not disturb the intracellular killing of these bacteria.

Cytostatics

Numerous cytostatics used in the treatment of leukemias and cancer inhibit the phagocytosis of *Candida albicans* by neutrophils (Goldfinger et al., 1965; Whittaker et al., 1975). Among these agents colchicine, vincristine, vinblastine, cytosine arabinoside, busulfan, and daunorubicin should be mentioned. The practical significance of this observation has not been finally established; in particular it is not known whether the therapeutic use of some of these drugs alters neutrophil phagocytic activity.

Cytochalasin B

This agent is a metabolic product of *Helminthosporium dematioideum* inhibiting the engulfment of bacteria by neutrophils (Davis et al., 1971). The agent does not exhibits any influence on the opsonization of bacteria.

Antipyretic Agents

Aspirin and phenylbutazone induce an inhibitory effect on the phagocytic activity of neutrophils (Whittaker et al., 1975). The mechanism of action of these drugs in this respect is not known.

Sodium Cyanate

Sodium cyanate is a substance inhibiting the intracellular killing of *E. coli* and *Staph. epidermidis* by neutrophils (Ratzan et al., 1975). This effect is associated with a decrease in the production of carbon dioxide from glucose and in the iodination of bacteria. It is supposed that sodium cyanate interferes with the oxidative metabolism of glucose via the pentose cycle and decreased production of hydrogen peroxide. The general vitality of neutrophils, the engulfment of the bacteria mentioned, and the killing of *Streptococcus faecalis* are not affected by this agent.

EFFECT OF IRRADIATION ON PHAGOCYTOSIS

It is well known in practice that radiotherapy causes a fall in the neutrophil count and subsequently a lowered antibacterial immunity. High doses of irradiation also inhibit chemotactic and phagocytic activity in neutrophils (Holley et al., 1974). Despite the wide use of radiotherapy, only a few reports on the effect of irradiation on neutrophil function in man have been published. The effect of irradiation on neutrophil phagocytic activity might be of importance in subjects exposed occupationally to irradiation.

The following main effects of irradiation on neutrophilic system should be considered:

1. The diminution of the total neutrophil pool is of special importance in patients heavily irradiated on account of cancer or other malignancies.

2. High doses of irradiation may induce total destruction of the neutrophilic system in the blood and bone marrow. This effect depends, of course, on the dose of irradiation applied. The phagocytic functions of neutrophils have never been systematically studied in subjects heavily irradiated by atomic bomb explosions or accidental exposure to gamma rays.

3. Disturbed phagocytic functions in the neutrophils are noted in patients after radiotherapy (McRipley et al., 1967). The decrease in phagocytic activity refers in the first instance to the phagocytosis of *E. coli*, *Pseudomonas aeruginosa*, and *Staph. aureus*, and includes the abnormal killing of these bacteria.

The mechanism of abnormal phagocytosis in irradiated subjects is not known in detail. Experiments on mice indicate that this abnormality may be related to alterations in the neutrophil lysosomal apparatus and a decrease in the activity of some lysosomal enzymes (Aleksandrowicz et al., 1976). In patients irradiated for splenomegaly and leukemias, an increase in the activity of neutrophil cholinic dehydrogenase has been noted (Merker et al., 1965). In irradiated mice a transient decrease in both acid phosphatase-positive and phosphatase-negative neutrophils has been observed (Aleksandrowicz et al., 1976). Two months after irradiation a reactive increase in the neutrophil count has been seen in these animals.

CHAPTER 5

IMMUNOGENIC PROPERTIES OF NEUTROPHILS

Like other body cells, neutrophils exhibit a definite antigenic structure. Most studies have hitherto dealt with the characteristics of the surface antigens of these cells. Neutrophil antigens differ from those of lymphocytes. A knowledge of the antigenic structure of neutrophils has become of more practical importance since the introduction of blood cell separators into the therapy of various hematologic diseases (Lisiewicz, 1978). The transfusion of neutrophils requires proper typing of donors and recipients. During the transfusion of neutrophils or of blood containing these cells the immunization of the recipient and the appearance of antineutrophilic antibodies may take place (Szmigiel, 1967). Another problem is the production of autoantibodies against neutrophils. Some cases of neutropenia may be of an autoimmunologic character. The mechanisms of autoaggresion in patients with neutropenias are still insufficiently known. Neutropenia may be a result of complex fetomaternal interaction. There is a possibility of reciprocal immunizing effects between the fetus and the mother. The reactions of the immune system to leukemic cells of the neutrophilic series in patients with chronic granulocytic or acute myeloblastic leukemia have been the subject of only a few reports. The detection of antineutrophilic antibodies by various methods has formed a basis for the clinical diagnosis of neutropenias and for typing neutrophil donors.

ANTIGENIC STRUCTURE OF NEUTROPHILS

Neutrophils possess surface antigens which are potentially capable of immunizing the recipient (Jeannet, 1976). The appearance of circulating antibodies against antigenic components may cause the rapid disintegration of the donor neutrophils transfused into a recipient. This may result in clinically inefficient neutrophil transfusions and the release of pyrogens from these cells, which may induce febrile reactions. The surface antigens of neutrophils may be classified in three separate groups: ABO antigens, HLA antigens, and cell-specific antigens.

ABO Antigens

Neutrophils are carriers, like erythrocytes, platelets, and other leukocytes, of ABO system antigens (Jeannet, 1976). The basis of donor typing is the establishment of ABO compatibility. Suspensions of neutrophils may also contain an admixture of erythrocytes, and so the need for ABO compatibility is obvious. It is also desirable to determine the presence of anti-A and anti-B hemolysins in the donor serum. A negative red blood cell crossmatch is a basic examination before neutrophil transfusion. It seems worth emphasizing that there is a lack of more detailed studies on the ABO and other antigenic determinants in neutrophils as far as their composition and molecular structure are concerned.

HLA Antigens

Like other cells of the human body, with the exception of erythrocytes, neutrophils possess an HLA antigenic system which is the main histocompatibility system in man. The HLA system is exceptionally complex and contains over 50 different antigens controlled by four different loci (A, B, C, and D) localized in chromosome 6 (Table 16). This is the basis for the occurrence of

TABLE 16. Antigens of the HLA system depending on four various loci (A, B, C, D) of chromosome 6 in man. (According to Jeannet, 1976)

Locus A		Locus B		Locus C	Locus D
A1	AW23	B5	BW15	CW1	DW1
A2	AW24	B7	BW16	CW2	DW2
A3	AW25	B8	BW17	CW3	DW3
A9	AW26	B12	BW21	CW4	DW4
A10	AW30	B13	BW22	CW5	DW5
A11	AW31	B14	BW35	C	DW6
A28	AW32	B18	BW37		
A29	AW35	B27	BW38		
	AW34		BW39		
	AW36		BW40		
	AW43		BW41		
			BW42		

very numerous phenotypes, about 30,000, in a human population. In this situation the typing of fully compatible donors and recipients of neutrophils is impossible in practice (Jeannet, 1976). The most convenient method is to type donors from among the brothers and sisters of a given patient. The mode of the HLA genetic system transmission indicates that in such conditions, the

116

chances of typing a proper donor are 1 in 4. The selection of donors from among the immediate members of a family also diminishes the possibility of allergization to antigens other than those beloging to the HLA system. The degree of serologic compatibility is also of importance. Usually the selection of identical donors is not possible; hence the typing of donors depends on the degree of HLA compatibility. The greater this degree, the better the clinical results of neutrophil transfusion, i.e., an increased neutrophil count and the absence of febrile complications. It has been observed that the best results of neutrophil transfusion are obtained when neuthophils from siblings are used. There is an inverse relationship between the degree of serologic discordance between donor and recipient as far as the components of the HLA system are concerned, as well as the elevation in the neutrophil count one hour after the transfusion of donor cells (Mishler et al., 1975). It was stated in these studies that in selected unrelated, parent and sibling donors possessing mean serologic discordances of 33%, 22% and 16% there were posttransfusion neutrophil increments of 10%, 46% and 117%, respectively.

Specific Neutrophil Antigens

The main antigens in neutrophils belong to the histocompatibility complex, and there are also numerous surface antigens belonging to the HLA system. These cells have yet another group of specific antigens independent of those belonging to the HLA system (Lalezari et al., 1974). The clinical significance of these cell-specific antigens remains obscure, and their list is shorter than that of the HLA antigens (Table 17). The nomenclature of the specific

TABLE 17. Specific surface antigens of neutrophils. (According to Lalezari et al., 1974)

Locus	Gene	Localization	Clinical importance
5	5a, 5b	varying	?
NA	NA_1, NA_2	neutrophils	neonatal neutropenias
NB	NB_1	neutrophils	autoimmune neutropenias
V_{az}	NC_1	neutrophils	posttransfusion shock
9	9a	neutrophils eosinophils	?

neutrophil antigens is simple. N denotes the specificity of the neutrophil, the next letter (e.g., A, hence NA) refers to the genetic locus in the chronologic order of its discovery, and the arabic numeral (e.g., NA_1) identifies the alleles. Two such loci have so far been discovered, NA and NB. The NA system is composed of NA_1 and NA_2; the NB system contains only NB_1 (Lalezari et al.,

1974). The V_{az} (NC$_1$) system has also been described. The relationship between this last system and other neutrophil specific antigen systems is not known. The NA$_1$ and NA$_2$ antigens occur less frequently than NB$_1$ and NC$_1$. Group-specific human neutrophil antigens were detected on a cell line of CGL origin which beared a Ph$_1$ marker (Drew et al., 1977).

The clinical significance of these neutrophil specific antigens has not been the subject of any extensive studies. A patient was observed in whom a febrile reaction occurred after a neutrophil transfusion containing antigen NA$_1$ (Lalezari et al., 1974). This reaction was associated with pulmonary infiltrations and the presence of anti-NA$_1$ antibodies in the patient's blood.

There have been some reports indicating that neutrophil specific antigens, e.g., NA$_1$ and NB$_1$, may be of importance in fetal-maternal immunization and the appearance of neutropenia in a certain percentage of newborns. In some patients with neutropenia of the autoimmune type, anti-NA$_2$ antibodies could be detected. The role of the neutrophil specific antigens in posttransfusion reactions and in neutropenias due to repeated neutrophil transfusions has not been definitively elucidated. It is, however, worth noting that some cases of neutropenia are not associated with immunization against the antigens of the HLA system and so might be involved in immunization against neutrophil specific antigens (Jeannet, 1976).

ANTINEUTROPHILIC ANTIBODIES

The frequency of neutropenia due to the presence of circulating antibodies in the human population is not known, nor is the clinical entity corresponding to this state. In addition, the antineutrophilic antibodies have not been definitively classified. The laboratory techniques hitherto used do not enable the structural characteristics and other properties of these antibodies to be studied.

In the diagnosis of antineutrophilic antibodies several methods have been used, e.g., leukoagglutination, the complement fixation test, leukoprecipitation, the phagocytosis inhibition test, the antibody consumption test, and leukotoxic tests. The frequent occurrence of neutropenias in patient who have received many transfusions suggests an immunologic mechanism for this complication. In subject exibiting antineutrophilic antibodies the transfusion of neutrophils from healthy donors or donor-patients with chronic granulocytic leukemia may result in febrile reactions, nausea, vomiting, or even hypotension (Schwarzenberg et al., 1975). The symptoms resemble those noted after serologically incompatible blood transfusions. On the other hand, neutropenia does not occur in some patients with antineutrophilic antibodies. Analysis of previous reports does not enable isoantibodies to be distinguished from autoantibodies in patients with immunoneutropenia. The functional state of the neutrophils in patients with antineutrophilic antibodies has been the subject of only a few reports. Decreased NBT reduction (Moroni et al., 1976) and abnormal phagocytosis (Coiffier et al., 1976) have been seen in these patients.

Studies on specific antineutrophilic antibodies are associated with the production of the respective antisera and the obtaining of fully purified neutrophil suspensions. The specificity of these antibodies is related not only to mature cells in the granulocytic series—i.e., neutrophils, eosinophils, and basophils—but also to the immature forms of these cells. Antisera containing antibodies against myeloblasts might be ineffective against mature neutrophils, and vice versa (Mahmoud et al., 1974). This favors the concept that the antigenic structure of cells may be associated with mitotic cycles and cell development.

Antineutrophilic antibodies are frequently reported in patients with collagenoses, lupus erythematosus, rheumatoid arthritis, Felty's syndrome, and leukemias.

A very important observation on the biologic effects of antineutrophilic antibodies is that the neutrophil survival time in patients exhibiting the presence of leukoagglutinins in the blood, studied by means of DF-^{32}P marker, is evidently shortened. This fact may affect the efficiency of neutrophil transfusions (Goldstein et al., 1971). In many patients in whom leukoagglutinins are present, the simultaneous occurrence of splenomegaly, which may be responsible for neutropenia, is noted. The increase in the neutrophil count in these patients after splenectomy is also difficult to explain, since it may be a result either of a smaller degree of neutrophil destruction or of a diminished antibody production due to the elimination of the spleen, which produces large amounts of immunoglobulins.

The mechanism of action of antineutrophilic antibodies has not been explained in detail. Corticotherapy may induce a lowering in the level of these antibodies (Lalezari et al., 1975). This suggests that antineutrophilic antibodies may increase the clearance of neutrophils by mononuclear phagocytes (Boxer et al., 1975). The effect of antineutrophilic antibodies on the functions and metabolism of neutrophils has seldom been studied. Small doses of IgG containing these antibodies increase phagocytosis, while large doses have the opposite effect (Boxer et al., 1974). These antibodies may also increase glucose oxidation by neutrophils. These results are closely connected with observations on the effect of IgG and its components on opsonization. It has been found that a strong opsonizing effect is induced only by the Fc fragment, whereas the Fab and F(ab')$_2$ fragments show no such activity (Oss et al., 1973). It is not known which component of IgG present in antineutrophilic serum changes the function and metabolism of neutrophils. Receptors for Fc and C_3 on the surface of the neutrophil membrane have recently been demonstrated (Wong et al., 1975).

SELECTION OF NEUTROPHIL DONORS

The criteria for typing neutrophil donors are now well established, though further progress in this field is still needed. Among the most important criteria the following should be noted: 1) compatibility of the ABO system; 2) a negative lymphocytotoxicity test; 3) negative leukoagglutination; 4) a negative neutrophilotoxic test using cells labeled with ^{51}Cr. The clinical significance of the detection on antineutrophilic antibodies by means of neutrophils labeled with ^{51}Cr is a subject of current studies (Jeannet, 1976). It should be emphasized that full HLA compatibility is needed only in strongly immunized patients. Now there is a tendency to type donors in whom most of the HLA components are compatible (Mishler et al., 1975).

The importance of compatibility in the NA, NB, and NC systems is still under investigation. Currently leukoagglutination tests and microcytotoxicity testing are largely used in various centers specializing in neutrophil transfusions. The negativity of these tests is critical in the selection of donors. The simultaneous performance of leukoagglutination tests and tests of HLA compatibility is based on the fact that leukoagglutinating antibodies and antibodies against particular components of the HLA system occur in the blood independently (Hester et al., 1975).

There are, of course, general criteria of the donor typing related to the clinical state, results of basic laboratory findings, and tests for syphilis, viral hepatitis (HB_sAg, HB_cAg), cytomegaly, and toxoplasmosis.

TECHNIQUES OF NEUTROPHIL COLLECTION

The two main methods of neutrophil collection for transfusions for patients with neutropenia now available are continuous flow centrifugation (CFC) and filtration leukopheresis (FL). These techniques are presently the subject of intensive clinical studies (Goldman et al., 1975; Stryckmans et al., 1975). The wide use of these methods is an example of progress in the therapy of immunologic deficiencies in the neutrophil system.

120

<h1 style="text-align:center">Continuous Flow Centrifugation</h1>

The technique of CFC consists in continuous centrifugation of the donor blood in a closed separator system enabling leukocytes, mainly neutrophils, to be obtained while returning other components to circulating blood. Among the separators now in use, the Aminco cell separator, the NCI-IBM blood cell separator, and the IBM 2991 blood cell processor should be mentioned. Other separators, such as the Haemonetics model 10 blood cell separator or the Haemonetics model 30 blood processor, are also used, mainly in Europe. The costs of operating these last separators, however, are higher than for the other mentioned, owing to the need for exchangeable parts of the apparatus. The relatively low efficiency of various separators has given rise to the use of numerous substances that, when applied to donors, increase the neutrophil count in the blood before collection. Among these substances prednisone, dexamethasone, hydrocortisone, and other corticosteroids should be mentioned; agents enhancing the erythrocyte sedimentation rate such as hydroxyethyl starch are also useful for this purpose (Mishler et al., 1975; Huestis et al., 1975). It has been found that the administration of hydrocortisone with simultaneous physical excercise results in a greater elevation of the neutrophil count than the application of each of these stimuli separately (Söderlund et al., 1975). In the clinical evaluation of the CFC technique, such advantages as the technical simplicity of operation, the short time taken by the procedure, the fact that it is unnecessary to heparinize or premedicate donors, as well as the feasibility of collecting platelets and leukocytes separately, might be advanced. The mechanical trauma to the neutrophils transfused is only slight. The effects of CFC on donors are not of any great importance, though such alterations as a decrease in the total protein content, albumin level, and IgG, IgA, and IgM levels, an increase in the fibrinogen level, and a slight decrease in the hemoglobin, leukocyte, and platelet levels may occur to a certain degree. Local tenderness at the site of injection is the main side effect noted in donors. Chills, headache, and nausea are observed only on rare occasions. Repeated numerous leukophereses do not show any important effects. The laboratory findings mentioned do not differ in donors who undergo leukophereses more or less frequently. The anemia occurring in a certain percentage of donors is a result of the constant loss of reticulocytes accompanying leukophereses.

Filtration Leukopheresis

This technique consists in the collection of neutrophils on scrubbed nylon-fiber filters and reversible leukoadhesion. The leukopherators used are characterized by the constant pressure propulsion in contrast to the constant volume propulsion of the rotor pumps of the CFC system (Djerassi et al., 1975). The mechanism of the reversible adhesion of neutrophils and monocytes as well as of a small number of sticky lymphocytes has not been fully elucidated. The FL technique enables large quantities of neutrophils to be collected without any marked admixture of other cells. The number of neturophils collected by means of the FL technique is greater than that obtained by the CFC technique (Higby et al., 1975), though there are data indicating that neutrophils collected by the FL technique undergo several inconvenient alterations, among which ultrastructural abnormalities and disturbances in chemotaxis and phagocytosis, including intracellular killing of bacteria, should be mentioned (Wright et al., 1975; Ts'ao et al., 1976; Zaharia et al., 1976; McCullough et al., 1976).

In patients undergoing transfusion of FL-collected neutrophils, febrile reactions and chills are observed. These complications are due to the release of pyrogens from cells in the course of cell separation or to the antigen-antibody reaction. Attention has been called to the fact that the first fraction of FL-collected neutrophils does not exhibit any alterations in the phagocytic properties or morphologic abnormalities (Fliedner et al., 1974). The FL technique does not affect the neutrophil capacity to release the beta-glucuronidase and beta-galactosidase activities from the lysosomes (Medenica et al., 1976). Several types of leukopherators are in use, with constant technical improvement (Goldman et al., 1975). Among the advantages of the FL technique, the clinical efficiency of the transfused neutrophils and the low costs of the basis equipment are emphasized. The need of large amounts of anticoagulants, the extracorporeal circulation of a large volume of blood, an its prolonged immobility are undesirable aspects of the FL technique. The effect of FL on donors is only slight. The hemoglobin and platelet contents transiently decrease after the collection of cells, and the neutrophil count increases after 24 hours. Only a small percentage of donors exhibit such symptoms as debility, nausea, or local pain at the site of injection. Transient neutropenia is noted only during the first 30 min of FL. As compared with CFC, FL enables the collection of five to eight times as many neutrophils from donors.

EFFECT OF NEUTROPHIL TRANSFUSION ON RECIPIENTS

Good clinical results are noted only in those patients who have received more than three neutrophil transfusions. The mean survival time of the transfused neutrophils is from 8 to 12 hours. In inflammatory exudates in patients with neutropenia the transfused neutrophils do not appear before 2 hours (Goldman et al., 1975). Neutrophils from donors show an animated phagocytic activity in the organism of the recipient. Neutrophil transfusions have been used in patients with acute myeloblastic leukemia, or acute lymphoblastic leukemia in which neutropenia occurred during the course of the disease. In patients transfused with neutrophils the control of infections is easier, the frequency of remissions is greater, and the survival time is longer (Hill et al., 1975). Neutrophils are transfused into patients with various neutropenias, agranulocytosis, or aplastic anemia. Especially beneficial results have been noted in patients with severe neutropenia exhibiting less than 500 neutrophils per cu mm. Frequent posttransfusion reactions are a serious clinical problem in patients in whom neutrophils collected by the FL technique have been transfused. These reactions occur in about 50% of patients treated by the FL system as compared with 7% in those treated by the CFC system.

TRANSFUSION OF NEUTROPHILS FROM THE BLOOD OF PATIENTS WITH CHRONIC GRANULOCYTIC LEUKEMIA

Several trials of collection and tansfusion of neutrophils from the peripheral blood of patients with chronic granulocytic leukemia have been made by means of the FL and CFC techniques. These leukemic cells exhibit adequate phagocytic activity despite several abnormalities of their enzymatic activities as compared with normal cells. It is emphasized that leukemic donors of neutrophils should be patients exhibiting no infections and having no alloantibodies of the antierythrocytic or antineutrophilic type; patients with cytomegaly, toxoplasmosis, or viral hepatitis should be immediately eliminated (Bussel et al., 1975). The criteria for the clinical use of neutrophils from patients with chronic granulocytic leukemia have not been unequivocally established. It should be noted that leukemic donors represent a richer source of neutrophils than healthy subjects (Lowenthal et al., 1975), but posttransfusion reactions appear more frequently after transfusions of leukemic neutrophils as compared with cells from healthy donors. It has not been established whether leukemic neutrophils should be irradiated prior to transfusion. Irradiation causes injury to neutrophils and diminishes their phagocytic activity. On the other hand, irradiation of leukemic neutrophils lessens the risk of occurrence of the GVH reaction. It has been suggested that patients with neutropenias and infections that do not react to antibiotic therapy should receive transfusions of neutrophils every day or every second day for one or two weeks. Transfusion of leukemic neutrophils may result in the occurrence of functioning bone marrow homograft in the recipient. The presence of neutrophil precursors undergoing mitoses can be demonstrated in the recipient with the use of chromosomal markers—chromosome Ph_1 and sex chromatin (Coltman et al., 1975). On rare occasions, after transfusion of neutrophils from patients with chronic granulocytic leukemia, a remission has been observed in patients with acute leukemias. The explanation of this phenomenon is not known as yet. Transfusion of neutrophils exibiting a greater degree of histocompatibility results in more frequent remission than transfusion of histoincompatible neutrophils (Cooper et al., 1975).

LEUKOPHERESIS IN THE TREATMENT OF ACUTE AND CHRONIC LEUKEMIAS

Attempts have recently been made to treat leukemias by leukopheresis. It should be emphasized that in patients with acute myeloblastic leukemia, leukopheresis may result in greater susceptibility to chemotherapy. In patients with chronic granulocytic leukemia, leukopheresis brings about a decrease in the total leukocyte count, especially evident in patients resistant to treatment with cytostatics. Not all patients with this leukemia, however, react to leukopheresis (Goldman et al., 1975). In some cases the leukemic leukocytosis is elevated after leukopheresis, so that the clinical use of this mode of treatment should be the subject of more intensive studies.

NEONATAL ISOIMMUNIZATION NEUTROPENIA

This entity is regarded as a result of fetomaternal neutrophil incompatibility and the transplacental passage of leukoagglutinins from mother to fetus (Braun et al., 1960; Jensen, 1960; Halvorsen, 1965; Lalezari et al., 1960, 1966, 1971, 1974). The mechanism of the transplacental passage of fetal neutrophils into the mother's blood is not known. The specific antibodies involved belong to the IgG class. Immunization against the specific neutrophil antigens NA, NB, and NC is less frequent than that against HLA antigens. Cases have been reported in which anti-NA_2 antibodies occurred solely in the child and were not detectable in the mother (Lalezari et al., 1975). The frequency of neonatal immunization neutropenia in the total population is not known (Lalezari et al., 1974). The disease is noted more often in children born from women with more numerous pregnancies. It has been shown that antineutrophilic antibodies

124

from both these mothers and their affected children are capable of agglutinating neutrophils from the respective fathers.

The duration of neutropenia in newborns depends on the length of the time that maternal antibodies are present in their blood.This averages about 7 weeks, exhibiting individual fluctuations ranging from 2 to 17 weeks (Lalezari et al., 1974).

The clinical effects of neutropenia of this type vary. The majority of children affected show increased susceptibility to infections, though some do not undergo more frequent microbial invasions. The occurrence of leukoagglutinin in mothers may not affect children to any great extent (Halvorsen, 1965; Payne, 1964). In individual cases it is difficult to establish whether neutropenia is a result of the action of antineutrophilic antibodies or of concurrent infection. It has been shown that neutropenia of newborns may result not only from the transplacental passage of leukoagglutinins but also from not properly identified leukotoxic factors (Stefanini et al., 1958; Seip, 1960).

AUTOALLERGIC NEUTROPHIL REACTIONS

The suggestion has been put forward that neutrophils may take part in the autoallergic reactions of the body against kidney tissue antigens in patients with acute or chronic pyelonephritis (Spector et al., 1975). The participation of these cells in allergic reactions has not been fully elucidated. The possible use of the neutrophil damage test in the diagnosis of allergy to pathogenic factors in some bacterial and fungal infections has been advanced (Stepanova, 1975). Allergic alterations in neutrophils may be used to evaluate occupational allergic reactions to antibiotics, especially penicillin (Filyushina, 1974).

Reactivity to tuberculin is also reflected by alterations in the neutrophilic system. Using the neutrophil damage test, it has been shown that the serum of patients with lung tuberculosis potentializes the neutrophil reaction to tuberculin (Zhuklis, 1975). Abnormal results of this test have also been reported in patients with tuberculous meningoencephalities (Nazarenko, 1975).

IMMUNOADHERENCE OF NEUTROPHILS

The phenomenon of the erythrocyte and platelet adherence to neutrophils was reported only recently. This adherence is morphologically expressed by the formation of rosettes of erythrocytes and platelets around neutrophils.

The spontaneous formation of these rosettes of erythrocytes has been observed in patients with autoimmunologic hemolytic anemia with the presence of anti-erythrocytic antibodies of the IgG and IgM types (Marmont et al., 1976). The formation of the rosettes is not accompanied by phagocytosis of erythrocytes by neutrophils. It has been suggested that the phenomenon of immunoadherence is associated with the presence of the complement component C_{3b} on the surface of the erythrocytes; probably it reflects the activation of C_3 convertase by antierythrocytic antibodies.

Immunoadherence of platelets to neutrophils has been observed in patients with lupus erythematosus, but it may also be noted in subjects exhibiting no detectable pathologic alterations (Zeigler, 1974). The phenomenon of platelet adherence to neutrophils might be a reason for discrepancies in estimating the platelet count with an electronic counter and in direct calculation from blood smears. The adherence of platelets to neutrophils causes the electronically calculated number of platelets to be lower than that calculated from blood smears (pseudothrombocytopenia). It has been shown that adherence depends on a plasma factor which is a component of IgG.

The mechanism of the immunoadherence phenomenon has not been elucidated. It is not known whether this phenomenon is related to the stimulation of neutrophils by aggregates of immunoglobulins or to the presence on the neutrophil surface of receptors for IgG and other immunoglobulins (Henson et al., 1975; Lawrence et al., 1975). In certain conditions immunoglobulin production by neutrophils may be activated via released elastase and cathepsin G (Bretz et al., 1976). It is not known whether this effect is related to the immunoadherence mechanisms.

The results of these studies are related to observations on the conversion of the complement component C_3 to C_{3b} and C_5 to a C_{5b}-like fragment by neutrophil elastase and on the conversion of C_3 by the collagenase of these cells. The interaction of the complement system with the neutrophil enzymes has not been the subject of major studies, and the clinical aspect of this interaction is obscure. Probably corticoids may influence the interaction (Sneiderman et al., 1975). Moreover, attention has been drawn to the fact that the complement globulin binding on the surface of neurophils may play a role in the pathogenesis of Schultze's agranulocytosis (Hartl et al., 1972). The biologic role of various receptors on the surface of neutrophils is not yet clearly known (Beckmann, 1974).

It has been assumed that the recognition and specific binding of a given particle to the outer neutrophil membrane is the initial phase of phagocytosis. The biochemical description of the neutrophil receptors participating in phagocytosis is inadequate. While endeavoring to find these receptors, it has been shown that the sites of surface binding of ricin and concanavalin A on neutrophils are not identical with the sites of the receptors participating in phagocy-

tosis (Baggiolini et al., 1976). Concanavalin A, however, inhibits the phagocytosis of neutrophils (Berlin, 1972).

The relationships between the factors stimulating the lymphoid and neutrophil systems are not clear. It cannot be excluded that both systems have
common functional stimulators. In favor of this concept there are data showing
that thymus extracts cause neutrophil stimulation accompanied by an increase
in lysosomal acid phosphatase (Lisiewicz et al., 1976).

CHAPTER 6

NEUTROPHILS IN BLOOD COAGULATION

The role of neutrophils in the phenomena of blood coagulation and fibrinolysis has been the subject of intensive studies during past ten years. It has been demonstrated that these cells play an important role in the formation and lysis of thrombi. Neutrophils possess procoagulant and antiheparin activities, are the biologic site of plasminogen synthesis and possibly of factor VIII, and are capable of releasing several proteolytic enzymes which may in certain conditions affect the hemostatic system. Despite these data, there is little direct information on the part played by neutrophils in the phenomena of hemostasis in physiologic conditions in man. Much more is known about the role of these cells in hemostatic disturbances in patients with leukemic proliferation of the neutrophilic system (Lisiewicz, 1978).

HEMOSTATICALLY ACTIVE SUBSTANCES IN NEUTROPHILS

Procoagulant Activity

The leukocytic mass isolated from the blood of healthy subjects exhibits procoagulant activity in various laboratory tests. It has been shown that crude extracts of these leukocytes may substitute platelets in the thromboplastin generation test, increase thrombin generation in the plasma, and shorten the plasma recalcination time (Lisiewicz, 1965; Kuznik, 1966; Erdogan, 1968; Alnikov, 1973). The main defect of these observations was that the cell suspensions used in experiments were mixtures of various cells such as neutrophils, lymphocytes, eosinophils, and others. In later studies it was shown that the majority of these cells exhibit similar procoagulant properties *in vitro*.

The effect of cells in the neutrophilic series isolated from the blood of patients with chronic granulocytic leukemia on hemostatic tests *in vitro* has been the subject of numerous but, to a certain degree, controversial studies. On the one hand, it has been noted that extracts of these cells increase the prothrombin consumption in the serum and show procoagulant activity in other hemostatic tests (Eiseman et al., 1954; Tropeano et al., 1957; Manai et al., 1961), but, on the other, these extracts have been observed to prolong the recalcination and plasma prothrombin times (Martin et al., 1951). These discrepant results may be due to the use of cellular material of varying composition. It is well known that during the various stages in the clinical evolution of chronic granulocytic leukemia a leukocyte pellet from patients with this disease may contain an important percentage of eosinophils or basophils containing large quantities of heparin and histamine. A relationship has been found between the percentage of basophils in a population of leukocytes from patients with chronic granulocytic leukemia and the effect induced by an extract of leukocytic mass on the plasma prothrombin and plasma recalcination times (Kuznik et al., 1969). It is not known whether this effect depends only on the presence of heparin in the basophils, since in these experiments extracts of chronic granulocytic leukemia leukocytes did not prolong the plasma thrombin time and their effect was not neutralized by the addition of toluidine blue.

The presence of procoagulant activity in samples of neutrophils from patients with chronic granulocytic leukemia free from admixture of other cells has been found in numerous studies. It has been remarked that the activity is weaker in these neutrophils than in the myeloblasts of acute myeloblastic leukemia or in lymphocytes from patients with chronic lymphocytic leukemia (Fortynova et al., 1964). We have shown that neutrophils from patients with chronic granulocytic leukemia, like normal leukocytic mass, increase thrombin formation in the plasma *in vitro* and may be used as a substitute for platelets in the thromboplastin generation test (Lisiewicz, 1968, 1969). The procoagulant activity of leukemic neutrophils is similar to that of leukocytic mass from healthy subjects, but is weaker than that of platelets. The intracellular localization of the procoagulant activity in leukemic neutrophils has not so far been the subject of any very detailed studies. In neutrophils from suppurative pleural exudate the activity is localized mainly in the lysosomal granule fraction and in the fraction containing mitochondria, ribosomes, endoplasmic reticulum, and the Golgi apparatus (Szpilman et al., 1969).

The lack of homogeneity in the composition of leukocytes from patients with chronic granulocytic leukemia makes it difficult to interpret the results obtained. Some blood coagulation factors may also be absorbed on the surface of these cells (Fortynova et al., 1764). We have, however, demonstrated a striking similarity between the procoagulant activity of highly purified leukemic neutrophils and that of brain thromboplastin (Lisiewicz et al., 1973). Among the main features of the procoagulant subtance of leukemic neutrophils in our study, the following should be mentioned:

— the major part of the procoagulant activity was in the protein fraction with a molecular weight of more than 200 (Fig. 13);

— the activity was not resistant to heat; after 6 to 8 minutes of heating at 60°C and 100°C, extracts of cells obtained by means of a Sephadex G-200 chromatographic column showed a significant decrease in activity;

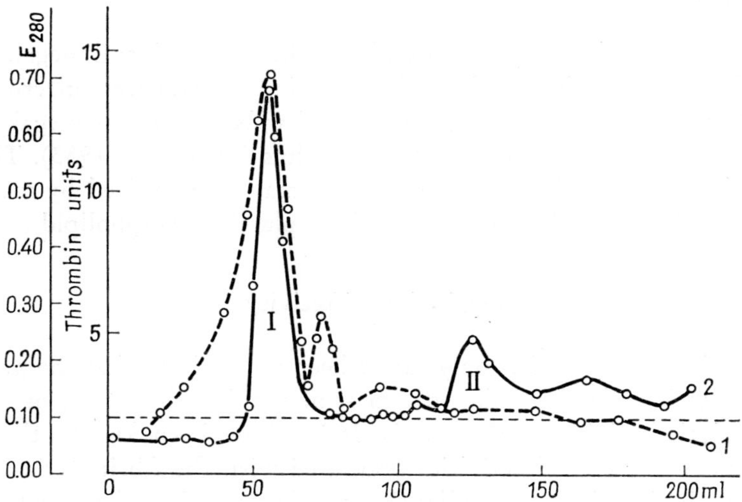

Fig. 13. Filtration of a neutrophil supernatant from a patient with chronic granulocytic leukemia through a Sephadex G-200 column. The thromboplastic activity (*1*) of these cells is concentrated in fraction *I* of the eluated proteins (*2*). (According to Lisiewicz et al., 1973)

— changing the hydrogen ion concentration from pH 7.3 to pH 3.0 resulted in a decrease in procoagulant activity parallel to the decrease in the total protein content in the sample;

— the most active procoagulant material was obtained after extraction with a mixture of methanol and chloroform; extraction with ethyl alcohol and *n*-butanol was less effective.

There is a complete lack of information on the differences between the degree of procoagulant activity of mature neutrophils and that of their precursors in healthy subjects. There is much information, in contrast, on the procoagulant activity of leukemic myeloblasts. Extracts of these cells induce an increase in prothrombin consumption in the serum (Eiseman et al., 1954). Procoagulant activity in myeloblasts has also been demonstrated by means of the plasma recalcination test and the thromboelastographic method *in vitro* (Alpidovskii, 1967; Zukovskaya et al., 1973). The activity is exhibited by both mechanically injured and uninjured cells (Fortynova et al., 1964). The activity of homogenized cells is higher than that of intact cells, which indicates its intracellular localization. This activity may also be demonstrated by many other hemostatic methods such as the thrombin generation and thromboplastin generation tests (Lisiewicz, 1968). The degree of procoagulant activity in leukemic myeloblasts is similar to that in platelets and lymphocytes. Preliminary studies carried out in our laboratory have indicated that the characteristics of this activity are similar to those of brain thromboplastin. This activity is also present in the promyelocytes of patients with promyelocytic leukemia (Quigley, 1967).

The interaction between neutrophils, on the one hand, and megakaryocytes and platelets, on the other, as far as hemostatic processes are concerned, is not clear. Attention has been called to the fact that bone marrow megakaryocytes frequently show the phagocytosis of neutrophils (Blicharski, 1953). The hypothesis has been advanced that the neutrophil may be reutilized by megakaryocytes during the formation of procoagulant platelet phospholipids.

Fibrinolytic Activity

In previous studies it has only rarely been pointed out that the presence of proteolytic activity in the leukocytic mass may affect the results of studies on the fibrinolytic activity of these cells. It has long been known that human leukocytes contain several activities associated with the fibrinolytic system. It has been emphasized in these studies that the fibrinolytic and proteolytic activity of leukocytes isolated from the blood of healthy subjects differs from that of plasminogen (Gans, 1964; Sinakos et al., 1965). In the mass of normal leukocytes the presence of both the activator of plasminogen-to-plasmin conversion and an activity inhibitory to plasmin have been shown (Goldstein et al., 1971; Wünschmann et al., 1970). It has been found that the activity of the plasminogen activator in normal leukocytes is localized in the lysosomes (Goldstein et al., 1971). The activity increases under the influence of bacterial endotoxins and is inhibited by Trasylol and EACA. There have been suggestions that in leukocytes there also occurs another activator of plasminogen, resistant to EACA and localized in extralysosomal areas (Bleyl, 1967).

There are some similarities in the characteristics of the plasma and the neutrophil plasminogen which have given rise to the concept that neutrophils may represent a source of plasma plasminogen. Some authors, however, have not confirmed the presence of plasminogen in peripheral blood neutrophils (Ohlsson, 1971). Despite these controversies, the actual role of neutrophils in fibrin digestion and their antifibrinolytic system are still a subject of intensive studies (Prokopowicz, 1968; Prokopowicz et al., 1968; Wołosowicz et al., 1970; Wołosowicz, 1978). The term leukofibrinolysis has been proposed to define the process of fibrin engulfment and degradation by neutrophils (Lewis et al., 1972).

The fibrinolytic activity of neutrophils and their precursors in leukemic patients has frequently been studied. The use of this activity to mark cells in

132

the neutrophilic series has been proposed (Kirchmayer et al., 1970). Leukemic cells deriving from the neutrophilic series, like myeloblasts or micromyeloblasts, in contrast to cells in the lymphocytic series, exhibit this activity.

In leukemic as in normal neutrophils there occur numerous proteolytic enzymes, such as aminotripeptidase, glycylglycine dipeptidase, glycylleucine dipeptidase, imidodipeptidase, iminodipeptidase (Haschen et al., 1966). In these studies, leukemic neutrophils exhibited higher neutral proteinase and catheptic carboxypeptidase activities than normal leukocytic mass. The aminotripeptidase and iminodipeptidase activities were only slightly increased in leukemic cells. In contrast, all the other enzymes mentioned exhibited lower activity in leukemic than in normal cells. It has been pointed out that neutrophils from patients with chronic granulocytic leukemia have a high gamma-glutamyl-transpeptidase activity (Kotlarek-Haus, 1970). The real significance of all these differences between normal and leukemic neutrophils is obscure. It is not known to what extent these differences are responsible for the abnormal functioning of leukemic neutrophils. In addition, the complex interrelationship between disturbances of various metabolic pathways in leukemic cells and the decreased or increased rate of synthesis of these enzymes is not clearly understood. A more detailed insight on these problems is given in studies on the comparative characteristics of various enzymes. It has been shown, e.g., that the acid phosphatase isolated from leukemic neutrophils does not differ, as far as the isoenzymatic characteristics and various biochemical properties are concerned, from that in normal cells (Pajdak et al., 1972). On the other hand, several differences have been found between ribonuclease from normal and from leukemic neutrophils (Sznajd et al., 1969; Sznajd, 1972).

For a long time it was supposed that the increase in the fibrinolytic activity of the blood in patients with acute myeloblastic leukemia was due to the fibrinolytic properties of leukemic leukocytes (Creveld et al., 1960; Cattan et al., 1966). In our own studies we have demonstrated that there is a relationship between the degree of leukemic leukocytosis and the fibrinolytic activity of the blood (Lisiewicz et al., 1975). A similar correlation has also been observed by other authors (Krasik et al., 1972). The correlation between the uric acid level and the degree of fibrinolytic activity in patients with leukemias has also been stressed (Girolami, 1967). It is worth mentioning, however, that the results of some investigations have not confirmed the existence of any correlation between leukocytosis, leukocyte fibrinolytic activity, and the fibrinolytic activity of the blood (Holemans et al., 1967; Tatarsky et al., 1967).

It seems that the conditions for the release of fibrinolytic activity from neutrophils should be the subject of more detailed studies in the future. It is difficult to interpret the available literature on the fibrinolytic activity of neutrophils, since it is not easy to distinguish the fibrinolytic from the proteolytic activity in various experiments. It has been shown that fibrin clot dissolution by human leukocytes depends on protease action and not on plasminogen activity (Astrup et al., 1967).

The presence of lytic activity of the activator type directed against fibrin has been demonstrated both in myeloblasts from patients with acute myeloblastic leukemia and in myeloblasts from patients with myeloblastic exacerbation of chronic granulocytic leukemia (Tatarsky et al., 1967). Activity of this type is also present in mature leukemic neutrophils.

The fibrinolytic activity of leukemic myeloblasts is localized in the lysosomal fraction (Cattan et al., 1968). Significant individual variability in this activity has been noted in patients with acute leukemia. Myeloblast activity is not inhibited by inhibitors of proteolytic enzymes, such as EACA or methyl-aminocyclohexanocarboxylic acid (Cattan et al., 1968). It has therefore been suggested that the fibrinolytic activity of myeloblasts differs from that of plasmin.

The total proteolytic activity of myeloblasts is lower than that of leukocytes from the blood of healthy subjects (Gonciarz et al., 1970). Low myeloblast proteolytic activity has also been demonstrated in experiments on the antithrombin effect of an extract of these cells (Lisiewicz, 1968). Leukemic myeloblasts have a significantly lower effect than neutrophils from patients with chronic granulocytic leukemia and healthy subjects.

In comparison with normal leukocytic mass, the myeloblasts of acute myeloblastic leukemia exhibit lower activities of neutral proteinase, aminotripeptidase, glycylglycine dipeptidase, and iminodipeptidase (Haschen et al., 1966). In contrast, the activities of catheptic carboxypeptidase, leucinaminopeptidase, glycylleucine dipeptidase, and imidodipeptidase are higher in myeloblasts than in leukocytic mass from healthy subjects.

Fibrinolytic activity is also present in promyelocytes isolated from the blood of patients with acute promyelocytic leukemia (Cattan et al., 1966). The fibrinolytic and proteolytic activities of these cells exhibit significant individual variations (Gralnick et al., 1973). Leukemic promyelocytes are probably capable of phagocytizing fibrin fibrils (Matsuoka et al., 1969). This observation, like the suggestions on the release of trypsin (Hillestad, 1957) or of plasminogen activator (Gupta et al., 1969) from promyelocytes, needs further confirmation. Data on the occurrence of fibrinolytic and proteolytic activities in leukemic myeloblasts and promyelocytes cannot be extrapolated, of course, to the analogous neutrophil precursors present in the bone marrow of healthy subjects.

Antiheparin Activity

The presence of antiheparin activity in leukemic leukocytes has long been known (Fekete et al., 1958; Lisiewicz, 1965). Extracts of neutrophils from patients with chronic granulocytic leukemia exhibit higher antiheparin activity than those of myeloblasts in acute leukemia or lymphocytes in chronic lymphocytic leukemia (Fig. 14) (Lisiewicz, 1968). The nature of the antiheparin activity of leukemic neutrophils has been elucidated in our studies carried out on chromatographic columns, Sephadex CM A-50, Sephadex G-75, Sephadex G-100, and DEAE A-50 (Lisiewicz et al., 1966; Sznajd et al., 1969). We have shown in these studies that the antiheparin activity of leukemic neutrophils depends on the presence within these cells of numerous cationic proteins with a molecular weight from 6000 to 100,000 (Fig. 15). Antiheparin activity

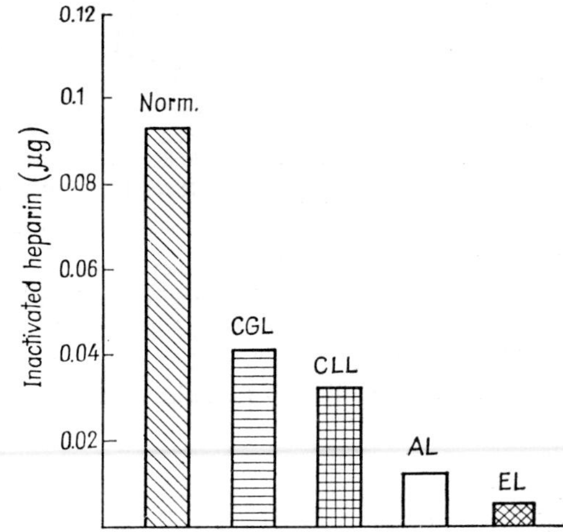

FIG. 14. Comparison of antiheparin activity of neutrophils from patients with chronic granulocytic leukemia (CGL), lymphocytes from patients with chronic lymphocytic leukemia (CLL), myeloblasts from patients with acute myeloblastic leukemia (AL), eosinophils from a patient with eosinophilic leukemia (EL), and normal leukocytic mass (Norm.). (According to Lisiewicz, 1968)

is also exhibited by some cationic enzymatically active proteins such as myeloperoxidase and ribonuclease (Fig. 16). The antiheparin activity of myeloperoxidase depends on the presence of protein in the sample studied and not on enzymatic activity. The antiheparin activity of ribonuclease is weaker than that of myeloperoxidase. The nonspecific character of the antiheparin activity of myeloperoxidase is also suggested by the fact that inactivation of the enzyme activity by potassium cyanate does not result in any change in its antiheparin activity. In 1962, we demonstrated the antiheparin activity of ribonuclease isolated from the pancreas (Gaertner et al., 1962).

The results of our studies on the antiheparin activity of cationic proteins in neutrophils have been confirmed by American authors, who showed the

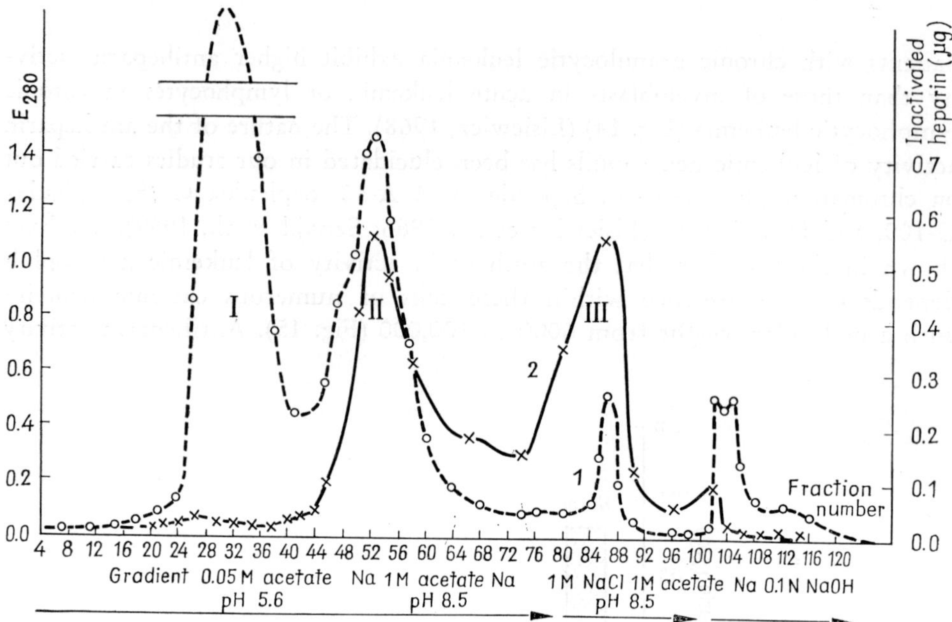

FIG. 15. Chromatographic fractionation of chronic granulocytic leukemia neutrophil proteins on a Sephadex CM A-50 column. Fractionation into three main fractions has been obtained (*I, II, III*) (*1*). Fraction *III* was followed by a small fraction of denatured proteins, which appear in the eluate only after the addition of NaOH. Antiheparin activity (*2*) was present in fractions *II* and *III*). (According to Lisiewicz et al., 1966)

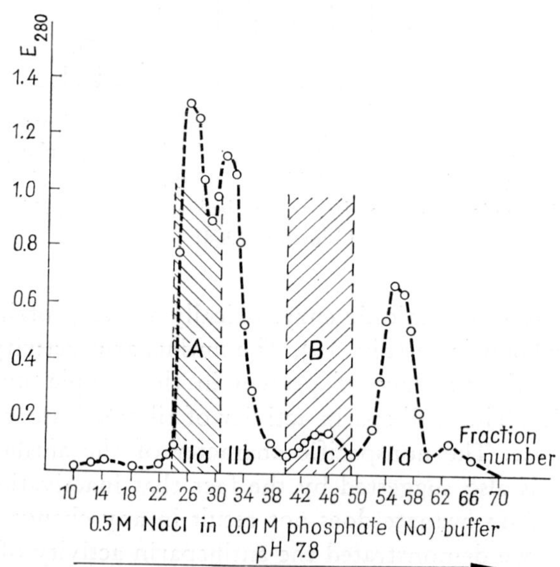

FIG. 16. Fraction *IIa* and fraction *IIc* obtained by molecular filtration on a Sephadex G-100 column of fraction *II*, which was obtained by filtration on a Sephadex CM A-50 column (see Fig. 15), contained ribonuclease (*A*) and myeloperoxidase (*B*). (According to Sznajd et al., 1969)

136

presence of this activity in rabbit neutrophils (Saba et al., 1968). It was also shown that the antiheparin activity of pleural exudate neutrophils is localized in the fraction containing ribosomes, endoplasmic reticulum, and mitochondria (Popławski et al., 1969). The localization of the activity in leukemic cells is not known. The results of our studies as well as those of other authors indicate that the antiheparin activity of various substances exhibiting enzymatic activity is directly associated with its cationic properties. Myeloperoxidase, which is an enzyme more cationic than ribonuclease, exhibits higher antiheparin activity. Indirectly, the results of our studies may be of importance for the confirmation of previous studies on the antiheparin platelet factor (platelet factor 4). Despite the fact that purified samples of this factor were obtained, the possible admixture of nonspecific cationic proteins or enzymes such as ribonuclease has not been excluded.

The biologic significance of the antiheparin activity in neutrophils is not clear. It may be assumed that various cationic antiheparin proteins released by these cells, especially in patients with chronic granulocytic leukemia, perhaps inactivate traces of heparin in the circulating blood and affect the homeostatic balance of the blood coagulation system.

Antithrombin Activity

This activity is present in neutrophils of patients with chronic granulocytic leukemia and in leukocytic mass from healthy subjects (Lisiewicz, 1968). This activity is apparently a result of the effect of the nonspecific proteolytic activity of these cells or may depend on the presence of various known proteolytic enzymes. Antithrombin activity in neutrophils differs from the antithrombin activity of heparin since it has progressive action and is not inactivated by protamine sulfate. Ether inactivates this activity. Antithrombin activity is high in normal leukocytic mass and in neutrophils from patients with chronic granulocytic leukemia, but is much smaller in the myeloblasts of acute myeloblastic leukemia and the lymphocytes of chronic lymphocytic leukemia (Fig. 17). The biologic significance of these activities has not hitherto been fully clarified.

Fibrinogen, Fibrin, Factor VIII

In patients with thrombotic complications as well as in experimental conditions, a certain percentage of neutrophils in the circulating blood exhibit the presence of fibrinogen, fibrin, and fibrin degradation products (Barnhart,

1965). It has been suggested that this phenomenon reflects neutrophil involvement in thrombolysis, consisting in neutrophil penetration into the thrombus, the engulfment of part of the thrombotic matrix, and the return of the cells in the circulating blood. It is not known, however, whether the presence in neutrophils of fibrin degradation products may not indicate that these cells

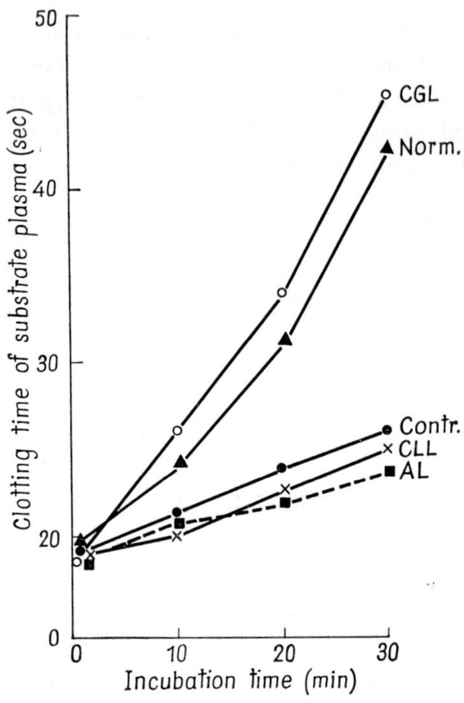

Fig. 17. Incubation of thrombin solution with extracts of chronic granulocytic leukemia neutroblasts of acute myeloblastic leukemia (AL) do not exhibit such an effect. (According to prolongation of the clotting time of substrate plasma. Compared with the control with buffer (Contr.), extracts of chronic lymphocytic leukemia lymphocytes (CLL) and extracts of myeloblasts of acute myeloblastic leukemia (AL) do not exhibit such an effect. (According to Lisiewicz, 1968)

play a part in the physiologic phenomena of the metabolism of blood coagulation factors (Gibiński et al., 1970, 1971). The problem of the biologic site of factor VIII synthesis has not been solved. The presence of this factor has been demonstrated in neutrophils (Szmitkowski, 1973). It is known, however, that factor VIII also appears in cultures of lymphocytes, fibroblasts, and liver cells (Zacharski et al., 1969).

138

NEUTROPHILS AND THE MECHANISMS OF THROMBOLYSIS

Neutrophils are an integral part of thrombi and emboli. They participate in the formation of thrombi and exhibit phagocytic and migratory properties influencing thrombolysis.

Thrombus Formation

The development of thrombi is characterized by several morphologic alterations within the thrombus body, associated with biologic activity in the neutrophils and lymphocytes, as well as in the basophils and monocytes. During the first phase the intravascular thrombus undergoes changes leading to its consolidation and structural fixation to the vessel wall (phase of thrombus organization). During the second phase the thrombus undergoes gradual lysis (phase of thrombolysis) which results in the final recanalization of the vessel.

An intravascular thrombus is a global biologic object consisting of a fibrin net and aggregates of leukocytes and platelets. The platelet aggregates form part of the thrombus structure only during the initial stages of thrombus formation. The presence of a thrombus within the lumen of a vessel, where a constant flow of blood occurs, affects the thrombus structure which as a result consists of a frontal part, composed of platelets, neutrophils, lymphocytes, and other white blood cells (white thrombus). This frontal part is fixed to the vascular wall by the cells of the vascular endothelium, which proliferate and migrate to the thrombus margins; this results in the characteristic histologic appearance. The end of the thrombus is a freely moving taillike structure containing mainly erythrocytes and long fibrin fibrils. The macroscopic appearance of thrombi depends on local anatomic conditions.

Thrombolysis

In an experimentally induced thrombus a rapid increase in the number of neutrophils within the thrombus is noted (Henry, 1965). These neutrophils migrate from the circulating blood. During the first few days, neutrophils are first seen in the thrombus, while eosinophils and basophils are less numerous. After some days, fibroblasts appear and consolidate the structure of the thrombus, forming junctions with the vessel wall. The morphologic evolution of a thrombus is due to alterations in the cytologic composition, i.e., thrombus organization. These alterations are associated with the biologic activity of various leukocytes.

During migration through the thrombus, the neutrophils phagocytize fibrin fragments and prepare the subsequent recanalization of the vessel

(Barnhart, 1965). The mechanism of the chemotactic migration of neutrophils into the inner space of the thrombus has not been fully clarified. The immuno-fluorescent techniques has enabled the demonstration of fibrin, fibrinogen, and fibrinogen degradation products within these neutrophils. This is an argument for the concept that after phagocytosis of the thrombus components, the neutrophils leave the thrombus and migrate back to the circulating blood. Despite these data there are still several unsolved problems concerning the part played by neutrophils in thrombolysis. Neutrophils are capable of intracellular and extracellular digestion of fibrin fibrils (Riddle et al., 1964, 1965), but these experimental observations require confirmation in man. The thrombolytic mechanism of the neutrophil action may be due to the mechanical loosening of the thrombus structure during migration, to phagocytosis and fibrin fibril digestion, or to the release of lysosomal proteolytic enzymes capable of digesting the fibrin network, which occurs at the time of neutrophil destruction and death. Monocytes, lymphocytes, and basophils also take part in the morphologic evolution of thrombi. This problem is dealt with in detail in another monograph by the present author (Lisiewicz, 1976). Here it seems proper to emphasize that there have been very few studies on neutrophil participation in thrombus formation in man. It is striking that thrombi obtained from humans and caused by arterial or venous surgery have not previously been a subject of interest.

THROMBOHEMORRHAGIC PHENOMENA AND NEUTROPHILS

The term thrombohemorrhagic phenomena refers to states characterized by the simultaneous presence of microthrombi and hemorrhagic lesions in small vessels. The hemorrhagic thrombus is a common element occurring in patients with various clinical entities. These entities include acute or chronic leukemias, tumors, several hemorrhagic diatheses, complications after surgical and obstetric operations, and some diseases of the kidneys or digestive tract.

Sanarelli-Shwartzman Phenomenon

The Sanarelli-Shwartzman phenomenon is an example of thrombohemorrhagic phenomena. The phenomenon represents a kind of thrombohemorrhagic lesion elicited by two consecutive (preparatory and provocative) injections of determined bacterial endotoxins. The local variant of the Sanarelli-Shwartzman phenomenon is elicited by a preparatory injection directly to a given tissue, most frequently the skin, and the generalized variant is elicited by an intravenous preparatory injection. In both cases the provocative injection is intravenous. The term thrombohemorrhagic phenomena is broader than the term Sanarelli-Shwartzman phenomenon, since the former refers not only to various clinical conditions but also to experimental conditions in which pathologic alterations are induced not solely by microbial agents but also by agents of other origin. Both local and generalized thrombohemorrhagic lesions are of clinical imporance. Among the generalized variations of thrombohemorrhagic phenomena in man, disseminated intravascular coagulation is a subject of special interest.

A characteristic feature of the Sanarelli-Shwartzman phenomenon is the 24-hour interval between the preparatory and the provocative injection necessary to elicit the thrombohemorrhagic lesion, though this time may vary on account of the experimental conditions. It is supposed that during this interval alterations take place which affect the reactivity of a given organ or are related to the condition of the hemostatic system. In experimental conditions thrombohemorrhagic phenomena may be elicited not only by bacterial products but also by other agents. The first agent is preparatory (e.g., polysaccharide or a metal) and influences the reactivity of tissues or affects the general predisposition. The second agent is provocative (e.g., catecholamines, ACTH) and causes local or generalized thrombohemorrhagic alterations (Selye, 1966). The majority of the studies on thrombohemorrhagic phenomena in animals have no counterpart in man.

The part played by neutrophils in these phenomena has been the subject of relatively numerous studies. A suggestion has been put forward that the procoagulant factor taking part in the mechanism of the Sanarelli-Shwartzman phenomenon originates in the neutrophils (Horn et al., 1968). It has also been demonstrated that neutropenia prevents the occurrence of the phenomenon (Forman et al., 1969). These data are in accordance with the results of our studies on the procoagulant activity in neutrophils, which is capable of provoking thrombohemorrhagic lesions in some experimental conditions (Lisiewicz. 1968; Malkiewicz et al., 1971; Lisiewicz et al., 1973). We have shown that a local Sanarelli-Shwartzman phenomenon may be induced in the skin of rats by the local injection of a suspension of cells of the neutrophilic series obtained from the blood of patients with chronic granulocytic leukemia and the intravenous injection of *E. coli* endotoxin (Lisiewicz et al., 1973). The effect of leukemic myeloblasts in this respect is stronger than that of leukemic lymphocytes or neutrophils. The duration of the skin reaction is also longer after the injection of myeloblasts (Table 18). Histologic examination of the thrombohemorrhagic lesions elicited in rat skin has shown that when myeloblasts are injected there is a larger local hemorrhage than that caused by neutrophils. The purpose of this difference is obscure. It is probable that the stronger effect of myeloblasts is due to their high procoagulant activity (Lisiewicz, 1968).

TABLE 18. Characterization of the local Sanarelli-Shwartzman phenomenon provoked in the skin of rats by preparatory injection of neutrophils from the blood of patients with chronic granulocytic leukemia, myeloblasts from the blood of patients with acute myeloblastic leukemia, and lymphocytes from the blood of patients with chronic lymphocytic leukemia). (According to Lisiewicz et al., 1973)

Leukemic cell type	Number of animals	Number of positive reactions	Time of appearance of local reaction in hr (arithmetic mean)	Time of duration of local reaction in hr (arithmetic mean)
Neutrophils of chronic granulocytic leukemia	10	2	60	41.0
Myeloblasts of acute myeloblastic leukemia	10	6	44.6	83.6
Lymphocytes of chronic lymphocytic leukemia	10	7	57.7	42.1

Disseminated Intravascular Coagulation

Disseminated intravascular coagulation (DIC) is clinically manifested by a generalized hemorrhagic diathesis which takes a severe course, especially in patients with acute leukemias and in those with obstetric complications. Observations on DIC in patients with acute myeloblastic leukemia and chronic granulocytic leukemia have enabled a better understanding of the part played by leukemic leukocytes derived from the neutrophilic series in the mechanism of this hemorrhagic syndrome. It is of interest that in some patients hemostatic laboratory findings typical of DIC do not lead to the clinical appearance of hemorrhage (Huth et al., 1968). DIC is a relatively frequent complication of acute myeloblastic leukemia (Sultan et al., 1972).

Among the theoretic possibilities of neutrophil participation in the mechanisms of DIC the following should be mentioned:

1. The release of procoagulant substances from leukemic cells into the circulating blood, resulting in the initiation of DIC, has been a suggested mechanism from data on the high procoagulant activity of leukemic myeloblasts and neutrophils, which are also capable of eliciting thrombohemorrhagic lesions in experimental conditions (Lisiewicz et al., 1973). Furthermore, in patients with acute myeloblastic or acute promyelocytic leukemia who exhibit a low neutrophil count, the eliciting of the Sanarelli-Shwartzman phenomenon is difficult (Komp et al., 1970). In patients with acute myeloblastic leukemia, DIC is noted more frequently than in those with other forms of leukemia (Logoida, 1970). This may be related to the high procoagulant activity of neutrophils.

2. Bacterial pyrogens released into the blood of patients with septic shock may induce the disruption of leukemic cells and a subsequent efflux of proco-

agulant activity into the blood. In patients with bacterial sepsis, DIC is frequently observed (Ekert, 1969). Another mechanism has been suggested by experiments in which the anticoagulant action of bacterial mucopolysaccharides has been shown (Freeman, 1952).

3. Attention has been drawn to the fact that in contrast to neutrophils, leukemic myeloblasts and lymphoblasts are not capable of phagocytosis or the elimination of fibrin, fibrinogen, and fibrinogen degradation products from the blood. Hence an accumulation of these factors in the blood may be expected, resulting in the initiation of regulatory hyperfibrinolysis or of blood coagulation consumption mechanisms (Lisiewicz et al., 1975).

The mechanisms of DIC are probably much more complex. The roles of endothelial lesions, reticuloendothelial system blockade by products of the disruption of leukemic cells, the interaction between pyrogens of bacterial or leukocytic origin, on the one hand, and chemotherapeutical agents, on the other, are still under discussion.

The frequent occurrence of DIC in patients with acute promyelocytic leukemia deserves separate discussion. It has been noted that in patients with this leukemia, hypofibrinogenemia is very frequent (Bernard et al., 1963; Ryder, 1966). The relatively frequent occurrence of local or disseminated thrombotic changes in these patients has given support to the supposition that the main mechanism of these complications is due to DIC (Albarracin et al., 1971; Polliack, 1971; Rachmilewitz et al., 1972). A possible relationship between the high activity of thromboplastic substances in the promyelocytes and the thrombohemorrhagic lesions occurring in these patients has also been suggested (Quigley, 1967). The high frequency of microthrombi in the capillaries and the frequent occurrence of DIC favor the concept that leukemic promyelocytes may play an important role in initiating alterations in the hemostatic system in these patients (Cattan et al., 1966; Sultan et al., 1969; Piquet et al., 1969).

On the contrary, several authors have emphasized that microthrombi occur only in relatively few patients with this leukemia (Didisheim et al., 1964, 1969; Laws et al., 1968). Similarly, a low fibrinogen level is not observed in all patients (Cattan et al., 1966; Huth et al., 1968). Heparin therapy for DIC is efficient only in some patients with promyelocytic leukemia, suggesting that not in all cases are the hemostatic disturbances related solely to DIC. Again, strong thromboplastic activity is observed not only in promyelocytes but in several other leukemic cells (Lisiewicz, 1968; Malkiewicz et al., 1971).

The functional state of neutrophils in patients with DIC has been the subject of only a few reports. It has been noted that during shock accompanying DIC the neutrophilc exhibit abnormalities in phagocytosis (Roth et al., 1975). The significance of this phenomenon requires further study.

CHAPTER 7

QUANTITATIVE CHANGES IN NEUTROPHILS

Despite the incessant production and turnover of neutrophils in the body, the number of these cells in the circulating blood in healthy subjects remains within a definite physiologic range. Relatively little is known of the mechanisms of maintaining a constant neutrophil count in the blood; they were discussed in the chapter on the production and kinetics of neutrophils. It should merely be mentioned here that an increasing amount of data indicates that the regulation of the neutrophil count in the blood depends on subtle cybernetic mechanisms involving both positive and negative feedback loops.

The neutrophil count in the blood undergoes changes related to the stage of ontogenic development, the hormonal cycles, and biologic cycles such as the lunar, the solar, and the circadian. Several factors associated with the state of the central nervous system, the temperature of the environment, and nutrition influence neutrophil count. In patients with infectious diseases this count exhibits characteristic variations related to the phase of the disease. The neutrophil count is strongly affected by drugs. Some, e.g., the cytostatics, induce depression of the neutrophil production system; others, e.g., the corticoids, stimulate the system and increase the number of circulating neutrophils.

From the practical point of view a knowledge of the alterations in the neutrophil count during maturation in various periods of life—i.e., in the premature and the term infant, the child, and the adult—is of obvious importance. Changes related to aging are also of significance.

The estimation of the absolute neutrophil count in the blood is more important than evaluation of the total and differential leukocyte counts. A false interpretation of the total leukocyte count frequently leads to errors in diagnosis. It is well known that elevated leukocytosis accompanying abdominal symptoms resembling appendicitis may be related not to a local inflammation but to a leukemic process. On the other hand, a simple increase in the neutrophil or lymphocyte percentage in the differential leukocyte count may give rise to a premature diagnosis of chronic granulocytic or chronic lymphocytic leukemia, respectively. Elevation of the neutrophil or lymphocyte percentage in the differential leukocyte count may, of course, be due to simple inflammatory irritation of the upper respiratory tract or tonsils, and is closely connected with the stage of the inflammatory process. It may also be stressed that the differential leukocyte count, total leukocyte and absolute neutrophil counts reflect only a small, and at any given moment incidentally observed, frame of a long biologic film which, as far as the white blood cell system is concerned, corresponds to a given stage of the pathologic process.

EFFECTS OF AGE, SEX, AND BIOLOGIC CYCLES

The maturation and aging of the body comprise a long chain of processes which also involve the neutrophil system. Alteration in this system observed in human fetuses during various periods of intrauterine maturation were discussed in the first chapter. The period of development between birth and biologic maturity is characterized by complex changes in the neutrophil system which are of importance for pediatricians. The long period of the adult age is not associated with more evident changes involving neutrophils, and major alterations in this respect are not observed before advanced age. Information on the neutrophil system in the last periods of human life is scanty.

The period of pubescence is characterized by numerous alterations in the neutrophil system associated with hormonal maturation. The differences between sexes, so far as neutrophils are concerned, are of major importance only during pregnancy and in relation to the ovulatory cycle. In women treated with estrogens, the neutrophil count in the blood increases (Cruickshank et al., 1972).

Biologic cycles have been the subject of numerous studies in man, though few have been related to the neutrophil system. The mechanisms of these cycles are not yet clearly known, and the biologic chronometers regulating neutrophils are rather a subject of speculation than of fact. Little is known of the circadian, lunar, and solar cycles and the influences of general natural phenomena such as meteorologic changes, seasonal variability, or environmental and geographic factors on the neutrophil system.

Single reports on circadian variations in the phagocytic activity of neutrophils have recently been published. The complex interaction of various factors such as the supply of food components, or trace metals and their effect on neutrophils, has not been exhaustively studied. In healthy subjects, a ten-day fast results in a decrease in both the neutrophil alkaline phosphatase activity and the bactericidal activity of these cells against *Staphylococcus aureus* (Palmblad, 1976). These changes do not depend on iron deficiency.

Alterations in the Neutrophil System after Birth

A characteristic feature of the quantitative changes in neutrophils is the great variability of individual results. The neutrophil count after birth ranges from 4000 to 20,000 per cu mm. The factors influencing this variability are not known in detail. It has been observed that prolonged delivery is usually accompanied by the occurrence of a higher absolute neutrophil count in newborns. During the first day after birth an increased number of mature neutrophils and stabs is frequently noted. The first hours after birth are characterized by a transient increase in leukocytosis and in the neutrophil absolute count.

During the first week of life a gradual decrease in the neutrophil count is observed. This tendency increases during the second week. These alterations are characterized in Table 19 (according to Altman et al., 1961). The percentage

TABLE 19. Alterations of the number of mature neutrophils and stabs during first two weeks of life. (According to Altman et al., 1961)

Time after birth	Directly after birth	7 days after birth	14 days after birth
Leukocytosis			
$\overline{X}$	18,100	12,200	11,400
range	9.0–30.0	5.0–21.0	5.0–20.0
Absolute neutrophil count (total)			
$\overline{X}$	11,000	5500	4500
range	6.0−26.0	1.5−10.0	1.0−9.5
%	61	45	40
Absolute stab count			
$\overline{X}$	1600	830	630
%	9	6	5.5
Absolute mature neutrophil count			
$\overline{X}$	9400	4700	3900
%	52	39	34

of neutrophils in the differential leukocyte count during the subsequent period, i.e., between the fourth week and the second year of life, is about 30%. This percentage increases between the 3rd and 4th years, and gradually reaches a value of more than 50% between the 8th and 10th years of life. Between the 12th and 20th years neurophils represent 52%–56% of the differential leukocyte count.

These alterations are accompanied by changes in the percentage of the neutrophilic cell series in the bone marrow during various periods after birth. During the first month of life the percentage of neutrophils in the marrow varies greatly, from 10% to 45%. After the first three months this percentage reaches values from 2.0% to 24% (Gairdner et al., 1952). The percentages of myeloblasts, promyelocytes, myelocytes, and metamyelocytes undergo various but less characteristic changes during this period of life.

Normal Neutrophil Values in the Adult

There are no great differences between the total leukocyte values in male and female healthy blood donors (Majda et al., 1965). In both sexes neutrophils form about 61% of the cells in the differential leukocyte count; the percentage of stabs in both women and men is about 2% (Table 20). In healthy

TABLE 20. Total leukocyte count and percentage of cells in the neutrophilic series in the peripheral blood of 1002 healthy blood donors. (According to Majda et al., 1965)

	Total leukocyte count (thousands per cu mm)	Stabs (%)	Mature neutrophil (%)
Men 670 subjects	6.15	2.11	61.45
Women 332 subjects	6.20	2.16	61.17

subjects the circulating blood contains no metamyelocytes, myelocytes, or myeloblasts. Subsequent phlebotomies in blood donors result in a slight decrease in total leukocytes (Majda et al., 1965). Even five or six phlebotomies do not alter the neutrophil percentage, and the stab percentage is only slightly lowered.

Biologic Rhythms in Neutrophils

Cyclic changes in the neutrophil count in the peripheral blood as well as in the biologic activity and phagocytic capacity depend on mechanisms controlling biologic rhythms. Some of these changes are related to variations in the hormone levels in the blood, mainly those of the corticoids.

Circadian rhythm. The neutrophil count increases gradually in healthy subjects during the day and reaches maximal values in the evening (Sharp, 1960;

Hume et al., 1975). It is a characteristic feature that about 90 min after awakening the neutrophil count exhibits almost no change and does not increase for some hours. This observation indicates that the regulation of the neutrophil count differs from that of the lymphocytes and eosinophils, which undergo a transient decrease in the early morning. The stab count shows more intensive diurnal variations; at 4 o'clock in the afternoon, the number of these cells is about twice as high as in other circadian periods. In subjects with a reverse circadian rhythm of sleeping and waking, correspondingly reverse cycles of the white blood cell count are noted. A reverse rhythm in the neutrophil count is observed not earlier than 3 to 6 days, starting from the onset of the experiment, in contrast to other white blood cells, which are characterized by a reverse rhythm in less than 3 days.

Regulation of circadian variability in the neutrophil count in the blood partially depends on insolation. Keeping subjects in darkness during the morning hours resulted in a transient decrease in the neutrophil count for some hours (Sharp, 1960). It is not known whether the differences in the mean values of the neutrophil count among populations living in various geographic regions are related to the degree of insolation and the length of day. The prospects for the use of information on circadian rhythm in neutrophil precursor mitotic activity for the purposes of "chronotherapy" and the consequent obtaining of better effects of cytostatic therapy through more accurate interference with cell cycles are a subject of current discussion (Hume et al., 1975).

There have also been some reports on diurnal variations in the enzymatic composition and the leukocyte RNA content (Kohler et al., 1972; Ashkenazi et al., 1973), but these are of minor importance for the knowledge of neutrophils, which were not separated in these studies from other leukocytes. The variability of individual results has suggested the effect of lunar or solar cycles.

Sexual cycles. During observations lasting from 3 to 4 weeks no very marked variations were noted in the neutrophil count (Maughan et al., 1973). In women, the variations noted were related to the menstrual cycle, and in the period after ovulation there were increases in the neutrophil alkaline phosphatase activity (Radwańska et al., 1971; Polishuk et al., 1973). This phenomenon is probably related to changes in the blood estrogen level, since the activity of this enzyme is higher in women than in men. Elevated activity of the enzyme has also been observed in pregnant women. More details concerning this last problem are given in Chapter 11.

It should be mentioned that cyclic variations in the neutrophil and other white blood cell counts, lasting from 50 to 60 days, have been observed in patients with malignant proliferation of this cell system, i.e., with chronic granulocytic leukemia (Chikkappa et al., 1976), but nothing is known as yet about the mechanisms controlling this phenomenon.

NEUTROPHILIA

The term neutrophilia denotes states characterized by elevation of the absolute neutrophil count in the peripheral blood. A synonym of this term is neutrophilic leukocytosis. In assessing the degree of neutrophilia the percentage of neutrophils in the differential and absolute leukocyte counts should both be taken into consideration. It is known that in patients with chronic lymphocytic leukemia, neutrophils frequently represent only 5% to 10% of the differential leukocyte count, whereas the actual absolute count of these cells may significantly exceed the normal values, especially in patients who have leukocytosis within the range of 100,000 to 200,000 per cu mm.

The mechanisms of the rapid reactions of the neutrophil system and the mobilization of neutrophils from reservoirs are discussed in the chapter on the production and kinetics of these cells. Here only the basic mechanisms regulating the increase in the neutrophil count will be briefly presented.

Mobilization from the Bone Marrow and Other Sources

The bone marrow is the main source of neutrophils in the body. Rapid mobilization of the marrow neutrophil pool conditions the increased number of these cells in the circulating blood and tissues. The marginal neutrophil pool is another reservoir of these cells. The duration of the mobilization reaction depends on the kind of stimulus, the time of exposure to the stimulus, and the individual reactivity of the body.

Increase in Production

Increase in neutrophil production is another mechanism which raises their number in the circulating blood. It is reflected in an increase in the neutrophilic cell series, mainly precursors, in the bone marrow. The evaluation of bone marrow smears may be difficult in patients with increased neutrophil production and a strong reaction of the neutrophilic system resembling that in patients with chronic granulocytic leukemia. Additional laboratory examinations are necessary in these cases. Usually the increase in the mitotic index and the number of myeloblasts in the bone marrow is proportional to the activity of the stimulatory agents.

Prolonged Survival Time

The disturbed mechanisms of neutrophil elimination from the blood are only rarely considered to be a cause of neutrophilia. This phenomenon may be of importance in patients with chronic granulocytic leukemia characterized by a significant accumulation of leukemic neutrophils in the blood. The prolonged survival time of neutrophils as a mechanism of neutrophilia has not so far been the subject of extensive investigations.

Agents Inducing Neutrophilia

These agents were discussed in detail in the chapter on neutrophil kinetics. Among the most important are endotoxins, etiocholanolone, and various toxic substances. Neutrophilia may also be caused by several hormones, such as the corticosteroids, noradrenaline, or epinephrine (Clemmensen et al., 1976). Neutrophilia-stimulating factors present in the plasma of some patients with neutropenia will not be described in detail (Marsh et al., 1971).

Clinical Classification of Neutrophilia

From the clinical standpoint there is no generally accepted classification of neutrophilia. The mechanisms of neutrophilia have not been studied in many morbid entities, and the only information available in many cases is that neutrophilia is present in the blood (Table 21).

TABLE 21. Conditions associated with neutrophilia in the peripheral blood.

Infections	**Malignancies**
acute and chronic diseases of bacterial origin	cancers of various organs
infections with protozoa, fungi, or parasites	chronic granulocytic leukemia
in the digestive tract	leukemoid reactions
Inflammations	primary polycythemia
postsurgical or puerperal states	myelofibrosis
local ischemia, necroses	bone marrow metaplasia
infarcts (myocardial, brain, pulmonary, renal)	**Physiologic states**
thromboses, hypersensitivity reactions	after marked physical effort
Intioxcations	after epinephrine injection
metabolic disorders, mainly	paroxysmal tachycardia
uremia, diabetes, eclampsia	newborns after birth
intoxications with chemicals,	**Miscellanea**
drugs, lead, digitalis,	chronic idiopathic neutrophilia
snake or insect venoms	states accompanied by increase in the
Acute hemorrhages	blood corticosteroids
in the digestive tracts, due to trauma	
hemolytic crisis	

Infections and Inflammations

The majority of bacterial infections and local inflammations, mainly acute, are accompanied by an elevation of the neutrophil count in the blood (Aleksandrowicz et al., 1976). The list of these diseases and states is long. The occurrence of neutrophilia in patients with infectious diseases is discussed in detail in Chapter 12. Among inflammatory states characterized by neutrophilia the following should be mentioned: glomerulonephritis, colitis, pancreatitis, thyroiditis, and inflammatory states of the vessels.

Pregnancy

Neutrophilia is a characteristic pattern in pregnant women (Kuvin et al., 1962). Neutrophil mobilization during pregnancy is a result of complex hormonal and immunologic reactions. It is associated with the intracellular enzymatic mobilization of neutrophils and increased acid and alkaline phosphatase activities in the cells. The transient additional increase in the neutrophil count observed in women during the puerperal period is probably of inflammatory origin (Lisiewicz et al., 1974).

Tumors

Neutrophilia is frequently noted in patients with cancers of the stomach, lungs, pancreas, or uterus. It is also noted in patients with tumors of the brain, melanoma, or cancer of the larynx (Lisiewicz et al., 1976).

Hematologic Diseases

An increased neutrophil count in the peripheral blood is observed above all in patients with chronic granulocytic leukemia. It is also observed in patients with primary polycythemia, osteomyelosclerosis, leukemoid reactions, or thrombocythemia.

Metabolic Diseases

Neutrophilia may also be observed in patients with eclampsia, uremia, necrosis of the liver, thyrotoxic crisis, or diabetes (Bogusz et al., 1968; Cline, 1975).

Leukemoid Reactions

Leukemoid reactions of the neutrophil system may be due to various basic diseases and factors. They are discussed in Chapter 9.

Neutrophilia may be caused by several physical stimuli, among which trauma, exercise, and heat may be mentioned (Athens, 1966). An electric shock may cause a significant increase in neutrophilic leukocytosis (Rey et al., 1968). A similar effect may be provoked by acute cerebral hypoxemia (Cress et al., 1943). Neutrophilia is also observed in patients with anxiety, pain, nausea, or vomiting, and various emotional states (Milhorat et al., 1942). Ether anesthesia may also be a cause of neutrophilia. The degree of neutrophilic leukocytosis associated with exercise, e.g., a marathon race, probably depends on the intensity of the exercise and to a lesser extent on its duration. There are single reports on the occurrence of neutrophilia in patients with urticaria (Tindall et al., 1969), lipidosis of the spleen (Burdick, 1965), and phocomelia (Dignan et al., 1967).

NEUTROPENIA

The term neutropenia denotes a diminution in the absolute neutrophil count in the peripheral blood. The term granulocytopenia in practice is a synonym of neutropenia. According to the traditional definition, granulocytopenia includes a decreased count not only of neutrophils but also of other granulocytes, e.g., eosinophils and basophils. The term agranulocytosis is used of states of neutropenia characterized by a severe clinical course and a significant decrease in the neutrophil count. In practice it is generally accepted that if the absolute neutrophil count falls below 500 per cu mm, the risk of bacterial infections may rise significantly. A neutrophil count between 1000 and 500 per cu mm also represents a risk pattern, but of a lesser degree. There is a relationship not only between the neutrophil but also the monocyte count and resistance to bacterial invasions. The functional state of neutrophils in patients with neutropenias has not been the subject of many studies. Most children with congenital neutropenias exhibit abnormal neutrophil phagocytic functioning and diminished activities of the phosphatases and dehydrogenases in these cells (Ageikin et al., 1973).

A general assessment of neutrophil production in patients with neutropenia is difficult. Investigation on the neutrophil precursor count in the bone marrow in the phase of DNA synthesis (S) and on the neutrophil colony-forming capacity have given no conclusive results (Greenberg et al., 1973).

General Mechanisms of Neutropenia

Among the main mechanisms of neutropenia the following should be mentioned:

1. The increased passage of neutrophils from the circulating blood to the tissues as a result of reaction against infection or inflammation.

2. The shortened survival time of neutrophils in the peripheral blood, which may be due to the presence of agents toxic to neutrophils, of antineutrophilic antibodies, or of hyperactivity of the spleen and reticuloendothelial system.

3. The shift of circulating neutrophils to the marginal pool of these cells.

One of the main causes of neutropenia is the diminished release of mature neutrophils from the bone marrow into the peripheral blood. The source of these alterations may lie in a decrease in the total neutrophilopoiesis, ineffective but increased neutrophilopoiesis, or the disturbed passage of neutrophils from the bone marrow pool to the circulating blood poll.

The functional classification of neutropenia includes five main types: 1) diminished production of neutrophils; 2) increased but ineffective production of neutrophils; 3) shortened survival time of neutrophils; 4) various combinations of types 1 and 2 neutropenia, on the one hand, and of type 3, on the other; and 5) pseudoneutropenia.

Diminished Production of Neutrophils in the Bone Marrow

Diminished production of neutrophils in the bone marrow causes the absolute count of these cells produced by the bone marrow and released into the peripheral blood to be too small to maintain the neutrophil count within normal limits and to balance their constant elimination from the circulation. The result of this mechanism is to lessen the total turnover of neutrophils in the body despite their normal survival time. The local mobilization of neutrophils in areas of inflammatory lesions is also diminished in these conditions. Decreased neutrophil production is usually accompanied by marked morphologic changes within the marrow cavities. These changes may consist in malignant proliferation, mainly of the leukemic type, fibrosis, or other abnormalities. Defective maturation of cells in the neutrophilic series is most often related selectively to this series and does not involve monocytes or eosinophils. Models of disturbances of this type *in vitro* have been presented (L'Esperance et al., 1973).

One of the most frequently noted causes of diminution in bone marrow neutrophil production is damage to the precursors provoked by physical factors or irradiation. It is also well known that the majority of cytostatic drugs exert a neutropenic effect. The most frequent mechanism of action of these drugs is the disturbance of DNA synthesis, shown in the decreased uptake of labeled thymidine both *in vivo* and *in vitro*. The three main subtypes of neutropenia caused by diminished neutrophil production in the bone marrow are:

1. Drug-induced cytolytic marrow damage.

2. Drug-induced blockage of the metabolic pathways important in neutrophil proliferation; the blockage is caused mainly by drugs interfering with the metabolism of purines and pyrimidines.

3. Drug-induced defective neutrophil production of unknown mechanism.

The intensity of drug-induced neutropenia, as far as cytostatic drugs are concerned, depends on the dose and on the time during which the drug is administered. Inhibitory action on the nucleic acid synthesis in the neutrophil precursors may be provoked by chloramphenicol (Yunis et al., 1960). It is not known, however, whether the neutropenia appearing after the administration of this drug is due to the mechanisms mentioned. Despite the fact that chloramphenicol is frequently cited as a drug causing neutropenia, in practice the occurrence of this complication is less frequent after this drug (Casey, 1968) than after the drugs used in the therapy of hyperthyroidism (Bogusz et al., 1968) or after therapy with sulfonamides (Huguley, 1966).

Ineffective Increased Neutrophil Production

Neutropenia of this type is due to defective maturation of the neutrophil precursors, toxic effects on these cells within the marrow cavity, and the decreased release of mature neutrophils from the marrow. Effective neutrophil production results in a sufficient release of mature cells from the marrow into the blood. In contrast, ineffective neutrophil production is characterized by an increase in the proliferation rate of the precursor cells in response to the decreased survival rate of the precursors within the marrow cavity, while the release of cells from the marrow into the blood is diminished. In the mechanism of this type of neutropenia the main role is played by decreased neutrophil counts within the circulating, marginal, and marrow pools. Frequently the survival time of neutrophils in these conditions may be shortened (Mauer et al., 1964). The myelogram of patients with this type of neutropenia is characterized by an increase in the number of mitotic figures, increased total cellularity, morphologic features of abnormal maturation of the neutrophil precursors reflected in the vacuolization of the cytoplasm, the occurrence of dense nuclear chromatin, macrocytosis, and degenerative alterations. The model of total ineffective neutropenia is shown in the neutropenia caused by drugs blocking the utilization of folic acid during DNA synthesis (methotrexate) or by drugs disturbing the absorption of substances utilized during DNA synthesis (diphenylhydantoin).

Shortened Survival Time of Neutrophils

Increased destruction of neutrophils in the blood and the shortening of their survival time result in an increased total production of these cells in the bone marrow and an increased release of mature neutrophils into the circulating blood.

The upsetting of the balance between the extent of extramedullary neutrophil destruction and intramedullary neutrophil production causes neutropenia. Among the factors influencing the occurrence of neutropenia, the presence of antineutrophilic antibodies, neurotoxins, increased sequestration of neutrophils in the spleen, and intensive phagocytosis of neutrophils in the reticuloendothelial system should be mentioned. The antineutrophilic antibodies are described in the chapter on the immunogenic properties. In patients with this type of neutropenia the neutrophil survival time is evidently shortened (Greenberg et al., 1967). Another aspect of neutropenia is shown in the diminishing of the total body neutrophil reserve and of the number of neutrophils migrating into inflammatory areas. In a certain percentage of patients with neutropenia of this type, the presence of antineutrophilic antibodies or leukotoxin is demonstrable (Tullis, 1958; Walford, 1960). One of the effects of the shortened survival time and increased lysis of neutrophils is a rise in the lysozyme level in the patient's serum (Vietzke et al., 1968). Neutropenia of this nature may result in total depletion of the bone marrow reserve of neutrophil precursors. An example of neutropenia due to shortened cell survival time is aminopyrine-induced neutropenia, which is associated with the formation of the aminopyrine-haptene-antibody complex (Moeschlin et al., 1952).

The role of autoimmunologic mechanisms in the pathogenesis of neutropenia has recently been emphasized. Several observations have confirmed the importance of these mechanisms:

1. Specific antinuclear antibodies to neutrophils are present in those patients with rheumatoid arthritis in whom neutropenia occurs (Wiik et al., 1974).

2. Autoallergic damage to neutrophils in the presence of soluble antigen for heart muscle tissue is much greater in patients with chronic tonsillitis or metatonsillar rheumocarditis than in patients showing no alterations in the state of the heart (Levin et al., 1971).

3. In patients with nonspecific pyelonephritis or renal tuberculosis, the phenomenon of autoallergization to kidney tissue may occur. The autoallergization is detectable by means of the neutrophil damage test, using kidney antigen (Spector et al., 1975).

156

Pseudoneutropenia

The occurrence of neutropenia of this type is associated with a shunt between the circulating neutrophil pool and other pools of these cells. Alterations of this type may be the result of increased hemolysis, various hemodynamic factors, or hypersensitivity. Pseudoneutropenia is characterized by the absence of functional and morphologic abnormalities in the neutrophils.

Clinical Characteristics of Neutropenias

Among the neutropenic conditions caused by decreased neutrophil production familial neutropenia, infantile genetic neutropenia, neutropenia with dysglobulinemia, and pancreatic insufficiency neutropenia should be listed. This group of neutropenias also includes neutropenia with constitutional defects, neutropenia with bone marrow hypoplasia, and various drug-induced neutropenias. A separate form of neutropenia is that associated with stem cell defect. Conditions frequently associated with neutropenia are presented in Table 22.

TABLE 22. Conditions associated with neutropenia in the peripheral blood.

Infectious diseases
  typhoid fever, paratyphoid
  fever, brucellosis, tularemia,
  inflluenza, measles, varicella,
  dengue, yellow fever, malaria,
  kala-azar, rickettsialpox
	Diseases of the blood
	  aplastic anemia,
	  pernicious anemia,
	  chronic iron-
	  deficiency anemia
	  splenomegaly

Conditions associated with exposure
to physical agents, chemicals, drugs
  ionizing radiation,
  benzene, nitrogen mustard,
  urethane, cytosiatics,
  antimetabolites, several
  antitumor drugs, antithyroid
  drugs, anticonvulsants,
  antihistaminics, tranquilizers,
  antimicrobial agents
	Congenital and hereditary diseases
	  cyclic neutropenia,
	  chronic hypoplastic
	  anemia, hereditary
	  infantile agranulocytosis,
	  primary splenic neutropenia
	
	Other diseases
	  Banti syndrome, Felty's
	  syndrome, Gaucher's
	  disease, lupus erythematosus,
	  cachexia, alcoholism,
	  posttraumatic shock,
	  anaphylactic shock

Neutropenia with Stem Cell Defect

The occurrence of this neutropenia favors the concept that there is a common stem cell for all white blood cells. In the literature, neutropenia of this type is termed neutropenia with alymphocytosis, reticular dysgenesis, or the de Vaal-Seynhaeve syndrome (de Vaal et al., 1959). Some authors are of the opinion that congenital alymphocytosis occurring together with thymic aplasia should be included in this group of cytopenic defects (Gitlin et al., 1964). The de Vaal-Seynhaeve syndrome has been described in only a few cases, and its hematologic description is very unsatisfactory. The syndrome is accompanied by neutropenia and lymphocytopenia, and its prognosis is fatal owing to decreased immunity.

Chronic Neutropenia with Constitutional Defects

Cases of familial pancytopenia occur with congenital dyskeratosis (Bryan et al., 1965). This syndrome is a sex-linked, hereditary, recessive trait observed solely in men. The bone marrow in the patients is hypoplastic, and the main hematologic feature is a lowered neutrophil count in the blood. The prognosis of the syndrome is fairly hopeful, and patients mature and age normally. The relationship of this syndrome to familial pancytopenia of the Fanconi type has not been well established, and in many cases the occurrence of simultaneous monocytosis and sometimes splenomegaly makes its appropriate classification difficult.

Cyclic Neutropenia

This disease is frequently inherited as an autosomal dominant trait (Morley et al., 1967). Usually symptoms of the disease occur during childhood, but several cases have been reported in which the onset took place later (Duane, 1958; Hahneman et al., 1958; Evans et al., 1968). The disease is characterized by a lowered neutrophil count and increased susceptibility to infections. A striking feature of this form of neutropenia is its occurrence in cycles at intervals of about 3 weeks. This periodicity has not yet been explained. In some subjects the periodicity ranges between 15 to 35 days. When neutropenia appears, it lasts from 3 to 4 days. It is accompanied by frequent fever, skin infections, and ulcerations of the oral cavity. The first reported case of this disease was characterized by recurrent furunculosis (Leale, 1910). The degree of neutropenia varies greatly. In some instances neutrophils may totally disappear from the blood. Infectious complications do not usually appear in patients before the neutrophil count decreases to a value of about 500 per cu mm. In numerous patients compensatory monocytosis has been noted; in these cases infections are less frequent.

The nature of cyclic neutropenia is not clear as regards either the periodicity or the mechanism involved in lowering the neutrophil count. During remissions no abnormalities in neutrophil kinetics are noted (Meuret et al., 1974). Relapses are characterized by a significant shortening of the neutrophil survival time and an increase in the cell marginal pool. Only on rare occasions has the presence of leukoagglutinins in the serum of patients been shown. The therapeutic efficiency of testosterone indicates the possible participation of hormonal disregulation in the mechanism of this neutropenia (Barkve, 1967). In some cases changes in the colony-stimulating activity (CSA) in the urine have been correlated with the neutrophil count (Mangalik et al., 1973). Almost half the patients exhibit an increased neutrophil count after splenectomy (Page et al., 1957; Morley et al., 1967). This last observation indicates the possible role of the spleen in the mechanism of cyclic neutropenia.

Familial Benign Neutropenia

This disease is characterized by moderate neutropenia and is inherited as an autosomal dominant trait. The cases hitherto reported have taken a benign clinical course (Djaldetti et al., 1961; Cutting et al., 1964). The diagnosis of the disease is freguently made in an advanced period of the patient's life; sometimes concurrent monocytosis and eosinophilia are observed. Some cases may take a less benign clinical course with more frequent infections (Hitzig, 1959; Levine, 1959; Bjure et al., 1962). In these patients a deficiency of mature neutrophils and compensatory monocytosis are often noted. In a few cases hypergammaglobulinemia or obscure implications has been reported.

Infantile Genetic Agranulocytosis

This disease is inherited as an autosomal recessive trait. The onset occurs in early childhood, and infections and fever are frequent (Kostman, 1956). The lowered neutrophil count is usually compensated by increased monocytosis (Rodin et al., 1973). In individual cases the normal neutrophil survival time has been noted (Wriedt et al., 1966). A characteristic feature of the disease is the absence of reactvity of the neutrophil precursors in the bone marrow to neutropenia and their incapability of operating through a functional feedback loop, as shown by the absence of cells of the neutrophilic series in the S phase in the bone marrow (Olofsson et al., 1976). The relationship of the disease to preleukemic states is of special interest. In some cases chromosomal aberrations corresponding to the Philadelphia chromosome (Ph_1) have been seen (Matsaniotis et al., 1966). It is known that this chromosome is a characteristic feature of chronic granulocytic leukemia. A case of transformation of this agranulocytosis into acute leukemia has been observed (Gilman et al., 1969). All these data refer to the discussion on the relationship between neutropenia and agranulocytosis, on the one hand, and preleukemic states, on the other.

Neutropenia with Dysgammaglobulinemia

Relatively numerous familial cases of this neutropenia have been observed (Lonsdale et al., 1967). Both increased and decreased gamma globulin levels have been seen in the patients. In a few cases the occurrence of macroglobulin has also been reported (Hong et al., 1962; Ackerman, 1964).

Pancreatic Insufficiency Neutropenia

More than 20 cases of this syndrome have been reported (Burke et al., 1967; Pringle et al., 1968). The neutrophil count in these patients ranges from 200 to 400 per cu mm. The absence of compensatory monocytosis and the relatively stable neutrophil count in individual patients are characteristic signs of the disease. Pancreatic insufficiency is reflected by the lowered level of pancreatic exocrine enzymes in the serum and fatty stools.

Drug-Induced and Postirradiation Neutropenias

Drug-induced neutropenias are of serious practical significance. A large number of different drugs may cause neutropenia and subsequent infections, some of which may be fatal. Drug-induced neutropenia is of special importance in patients with leukemias and tumors treated with cytostatics and irradiation. There have been numerous reports on the neutropenic effect of various drugs (Table 23). The recent use of various radiomimetic drugs, such as alkylating agents, antagonists of purines and pyrimidines, various antibiotics, phenothiazines, antithyroid drugs, etc., has increased the chance of drug-induced neutropenia occurring in the human population.

Ionizing radiation. The neutropenic effect of ionizing radiation has been known for a long time. In patients treated for various reasons by radiotherapy, neutropenia has serious clinical implications. Adequate dosage of irradiation and periodic control of leukocytosis prevent the development of more severe forms of neutropenia. A single high dose of irradiation provokes damage to the bone marrow and subsequent neutropenia within a few days, depending on the size of the dose. Only a few studies have referred to the effect of irradiation on neutrophils in humans.

Antimetabolic drugs. In practice antimetabolic drugs are used almost exclusively in patients with leukemias and tumors. Most of these drugs are known to exert a neutropenic action. Despite numerous studies on the mechanism of action of these drugs and on DNA synthesis in various cells, not many investigations have been made using cells of the neutrophilic series.

160

TABLE 23. Classification of drug-induced neutropenias. (According to Williams et al., 1977; Wintrobe et al., 1975)

Drug-induced antimetabolic neutropenia
6-mercaptopurine, 5-fluorouracil, 6-thioguanine, azathioprine, azaserine, duazomycin, methotrexate, hydroxyurea, arabinoside cytosine, 5-iododeoxyuridine

Drug-induced cytolytic-type neutropenia
nitrogen mustard, cyclophosphamide, chlorambucil, busulfan, alkeran, thio-TEPA, triethylene melamine, vinblastine, vincristine, colchicine, ionizing radiation

Drug-induced idiosyncratic-type neutropenia
indomethacin, allopurinol, thiazides, phenylbutazone, procainamide, sulfonamides, antithyroid compounds, quinine, quinidine, plasmochin, amodiaquin, chloramphenicol, benzene, gold salts

Drug-induced ineffective production of neutrophils
methotrexate, arabinoside cytosine, diphenylhydantoin, pyrimethamine, postirradiation, chloramphenicol, postagranulocytosis

Drug-induced neutropenia associated with the presence of antineutrophil antibodies
aminopyrine, amidopyrine, dipyrine, phenylbutazone, mercuhydrin, sulfapyridine

Drug-induced phenothiazine-type neutropenia
phenothiazines (mepazine, promazine, chlorpromazine), dibenzazepine compounds (imipramine, desimipramine, desmethylipramine), antithyroid compounds (carbimazole, methimazole, all thiouracil derivatives), sulfonamides (sulfathiazole, sulfapyridine, sulfadiazine, dapsone, sulfonureas, acetazolamide, chlorothiazide derivatives), antibiotics (ampicillin, cephaloridin, griseofulvin, gentamicin, lincomycin, methicillin, streptomycin, metronidazole, ristocetin), anticonvulsants (phenobarbital, thalidomide, tridione, ethosuximide), other drugs and agents (penicillamine, thioglycollic acid, DDT, tibione, dinitrophenol, phenindione, ethacrynic acid)

Antibiotics. Among antibiotics exhibiting a neutropenic effect chloramphenicol should be mentioned in the first instance (Fraumeni, 1967). The mechanism of action of this antibiotic on neutrophils is still obscure. Neutropenia has also been reported in patients treated with gentamicin, lincomycin, ampicillin, ristocetin, and streptomycin. The majority of case reports on antibiotic-induced neutropenia fail to deal with the action of these drugs on neutrophil function and metabolism (Newton et al., 1958; Brun et al., 1967; Graf et al., 1968).

Antithyroid drugs. There is ample literature on the effects of these drugs on the occurrence of neutropenia and agranulocytosis (Bogusz et al., 1968). It has been pointed out that in untreated patients with hyperthyroidism the leukocyte values are lower than in healthy subjects. Spontaneous leukopenia occurs in about 10% of these patients. Leukopenia is noted in about 19% of subjects treated with methimazole and iodine. Treatment with thiouracil and propylthiouracil results in the occurrence of leukopenia in from 1.1% to 4.4% of cases, according to statistics presented by various authors (Bogusz et al., 1968). Neutropenia is a little less frequent and occurs in from 0.36% to 2.9% of patients treated. The rarest therapeutic complication, i.e., agranulocytosis, is observed in only 0.11% to 0.45% of patients. Usually agranulocytosis appears in patients suddenly, and routine examinations of the leukocyte count do not ensure an early warning.

Other drugs. Among drugs after the use of which neutropenia is observed in some patients, sulfonamides, anticonvulsant drugs, phenothiazines, cinchona alkaloids, gold salts, and phenylbutazone should be mentioned. Several chemical compounds such as DDT, hydantoin, or arsenic exert a similar effect.

CHAPTER 8

CLINICAL DEFECTS IN NEUTROPHIL PHAGOCYTOSIS AND METABOLISM

The progress in research on the biochemistry, chemotaxis, and opsonization of neutrophils as well as on the mechanism of intracellular killing of microbial agents by these cells has enabled the discovery of new clinical entities consisting in defects in the phagocytic process. Congenital defects in chemotaxis, opsonization, engulfment, and killing of bacteria have been reported (Malfatti et al., 1975; Sbarra et al., 1976). These defects depend on various mechanisms and are associated with various cellular components, from defects in the cell surface to deficiencies in particular parts of the antibacterial systems within the neutrophils. Disturbances in phagocytosis by neutrophils occurring in patients with tumors, metabolic disorders, and intoxications have also been reported.

Our knowledge of the therapy of congenital defects in phagocytosis is scanty. Probably these diseases will not receive treatment for a long time to come. Secondary defects in phagocytosis associated with the occurrence of various diseases have a greater chance for effective causal therapy. Investigations on factors stimulating phagocytosis have recently drawn attention to the low-molecular-weight peptides present in normal neutrophils, which regulate the functional state of these cells, and to thymus extracts, which increase the activity of some lysosomal enzymes in neutrophils and thus stimulate their antibacterial systems.

There are numerous conditions that diminish phagocytic activity in neutrophils. A transient decrease in the bactericidal activity of these cells may accompany states of malnutrition, iron deficiency, or severe infections, and may also be a result of the action of drugs inhibiting the cell functions.

The increased frequency of microbial infections in patients with malnutrition is a well-known phenomenon very often associated with deficiency of some proteins in the serum, e.g., of complement. It has been observed that phosphorus deficiency due to parenteral artificial nutrition may be a cause of acquired dysfunction of the phagocyte system in man (Craddock et al., 1974). This type of nutrition in experimental animals causes a decrease in the intracellular ATP content in neutrophils. In patients with hunger disease both the phagocytic activity and functional ability of neutrophils are decreased. This may be partly due to iron deficiency, causing a diminished myeloperoxidase synthesis.

There is a correlation between the degree of anemia due to iron deficiency and the depletion of the neutrophil bactericidal activity. In patients under 8 years old with a hemoglobin level below 10.0 g and an iron level in the serum below 50 micrograms per 100 ml, a lowered bactericidal activity of neutrophils against streptococci has been observed (Chandra, 1973). It has also recently been shown that a lowered iron level may reflect adaptive phenomena leading to microenvironmental alterations rendering the reproduction of microbial agents difficult (Aleksandrowicz et al., 1976). There are, however, suggestions that iron and the products of erythrocyte disintegration in patients with hemolytic anemias may have an inhibitory effect on the neutrophil functions (Quie, 1975).

A separate problem is posed by the occurrence of delayed antimicrobial activity, especially in the capacity to kill bacteria intracellularly, in neutrophils from patients with sepsis and other severe infections (Tan et al., 1971). The survival time of bacteria within the neutrophils of these patients may be significantly prolonged (Power et al., 1974). These functional alterations are usually accompanied by the presence in these cells of toxic granulations, vacuolization of the cytoplasm, diminished myeloperoxidase activity, and the appearance of younger forms (Solberg et al., 1972). In the majority of cases after treatment these functional changes in neutrophils are normalized.

In numerous experiments on animals *in vitro* and *in vivo* the inhibitory effects of phenylbutazone, the morphine analogues (levorphanol), hydrocortisone, sulfadiazine, sulfisoxazole, and the iron compounds on the bactericidal properties of neutrophils have been shown (Quie, 1975). Bactericidal activity may also be diminished by therapeutic irradiation in children suffering from acute lymphoblastic leukemia to prevent the development of leukemic infiltrations into the central nervous system (Baehner et al., 1973). It has been pointed out that in children with this leukemia a decrease in the alkaline phosphatase activity and the NBT test values is noted during remission (Pituch, 1977).

DEFECTS IN CHEMOTAXIS

Numerous defects in chemotaxis have been described in recent years. In the majority of cases reported, the defects were accompanied by increased susceptibility to infections, especially of bacterial origin. In only a few cases did an isolated defect in chemotaxis occur; much more frequently these abnormalities were accompanied by other changes in the immune system, e.g., deficiency of the complement components or hypogammaglobulinemia.

Despite the progress of biologic and clinical research on chemotaxis, the definite classification of its defects has not yet been formulated. The classification of defects in chemotaxis now presented is only preliminary and will probably be modified after further developments (Table 24). In general, defects in chemotaxis may be classified as follows: 1) primary defects; 2) defects associated with changes in the immunoglobulin system; 3) defects associated with abnormalities of the complement system; 4) defects due to the presence of inhibitors; 5) defects due to metabolic disturbances; and 6) miscellaneous defects which cannot be classified in any other subgroup (Morenz, 1977; Lisiewicz, 1978).

Primary Defects in Chemotaxis

An example of a primary defect in chemotaxis is the lazy leukocyte syndrome. The syndrome is characterized by disturbance in the nondirectional movement of neutrophils, neutropenia, abnormal mobilization of neutrophils after the injection of adrenaline or endotoxin, abnormal local mobilization in the Rebuck skin window, and, above all, abnormal chemotaxis (Miller et al., 1971, 1973; Miller, 1975). The relationship between the occurrence of defective chemotaxis and the degree of neutrophilic leukocytosis has not been fully elucidated. In patients with the syndrome, as in those with the Felty syndrome (Zikovic et al., 1972), defective chemotaxis is usually accompanied by neutropenia, though cases have been reported in which an increase in the neutrophil count was noted (Higgins et al., 1970).

The relationship between defective chemotaxis diagnosed by means of a Boyden chamber and the disturbances in the mobilization of the extramedullary neutrophil pool after the injection of epinephrine and of the bone marrow neutrophil pool after stimulation with endotoxin has also not been fully elucidated. Both the absence and the presence of relationships between the results of tests and disturbances in chemotaxis have been reported (Miller, 1971; Miller et al., 1973). In addition, in some cases there is a concordance between the occurrence of defective local migration of neutrophils in the Rebuck skin window and abnormal chemotaxis (Miller et al., 1971; Clark et al., 1973; Boxer et al., 1974); in other cases the concordance does not occur (Miller et al., 1973). In other words, there is no clear relationship between defective chemotaxis, neutrophil mobilization in the blood, and the local migration of neutrophils.

The relationship between defective chemotaxis, the state of the lysosomal apparatus, and the neutrophil capacity to reduce NBT also remains unclear. In patients with the Chediak-Higashi-Steinbrinck syndrome, the defect in chemotaxis is accompanied by abnormality in nondirectional movement, decreased

TABLE 24. Classification of defects in chemotaxis.

	References
A. Primary defects in chemotaxis	
1. Lazy leukocyte syndrome	Miller et al., 1971
2. Chediak-Higashi syndrome	Clark et al., 1971
3. Familial defect in chemotaxis	Miller et al., 1973
4. Defect in chemotaxis in newborns	Miller, 1971
5. Defect in neutrophil migration with abnormal NBT reduction	Edelson et al., 1973
B. Defects in chemotaxis associated with changes in the serum immunoglobulin level	
1. Defect in chemotaxis with deficiency of IgG, IgA, IgM	Gallin, 1975; Steerman et al., 1971
2. Defect in chemotaxis with hypergammaglobulinemia	Higgins et al., 1970
3. Defect in chemotaxis with hyperglobulinemia IgE	Hill et al., 1975; Clark et al., 1973
4. Defect in chemotaxis with disturbance of cellular immunity	Clark et al., 1973
C. Defects in chemotaxis associated with deficiency of the complement components	
1. C_{1r} deficiency	Gallin, 1975
2. C_2 deficiency	Gallin, 1975
3. C_3 deficiency	Alper et al., 1975
4. Deficiency or dysfunction of C_5	Miller, 1975
D. Defects in chemotaxis associated with the presence of inhibitors	
1. Inactivator of the chemotactic factor	Ward et al., 1974
2. Serum inhibitor of chemotaxis in children with chronic granulomatous disease	Ward et al., 1969
3. Serum inhibitor of chemotaxis in patients with cirrhosis of the liver	DeMeo et al., 1972
4. Serum inhibitor of chemotaxis in children with recurrent infections	Smith et al., 1972; Soriano et al., 1973
E. Defect in chemotaxis associated with metabolic disorders	
1. Diabetes	Hill et al., 1974; Baum, 1975; Miller, 1975
2. Uremia	Baum, 1975; Henderson et al., 1975
3. Posthemodialysis	Miller, 1975
F. Nonclassified defects in chemotaxis	
1. Severe infections	Mowat et al., 1971; McCall et al., 1971; Hill et al., 1975; Perillie et al., 1962
2. Rheumatoid arthritis	Mowat et al., 1971
3. Felty's syndrome	Zikovic et al., 1972

bactericidal activity, defective lysosomal apparatus, and chromosomal abnormality (Clark et al., 1971; Gallin, 1975). The last two defects consist in the presence of giant lysosomes in the cytoplasm and of chromosomal aberrations.

The coexistence of a defect in chemotaxis and of abnormal NBT reduction is another example of a relationship between the neutrophil capacity for directional movement and the enzymatic apparatus of these cells. This complex defect is in some cases accompanied by immunoglobulin deficiencies (Steerman et al., 1971; Gallin, 1975) or abnormal nondirectional movement (Edelson et al., 1973).

Another problem is the disturbances in chemotaxis that occur in newborns (Miller et al., 1971). According to numerous authors, the neutrophil phagocytic activity in newborns is diminished after birth and the levels of the serum complement components are decreased (Nathan et al., 1974). It is possible that there is a causal relationship between the deficiency of complement components and the defect in chemotaxis.

Defects in Chemotaxis Associated with Dysgammaglobulinemia

There have been reports on the occurrence of defects in chemotaxis both in patients with deficiency of IgG, IgA, and IgM (Steerman et al., 1971; Gallin, 1975) and in those with elevated levels of immunoglobulins (Higgins et al., 1970). Some reports concern patients with a defect in chemotaxis and an increased IgE level (Clark et al., 1973). In some of these patients a defect in cellular immunity and decreased production of MIF (migration inhibition factor) by lymphocytes also occurred (Clark et al., 1973). Other patients with a high IgE level, accompanying the Job syndrome, exhibited defective neutrophil migration *in vivo* and normal chemotaxis in the Boyden chamber (Pabst et al., 1971). In other cases the defect in chemotaxis was isolated and unaccompanied by disturbances in nondirectional movement and phagocytosis. The mechanisms of the possible relationships between the IgG, IgA, IgM, and IgE levels and defects in chemotaxis are obscure. In some patients with hyperglobulinemia of the IgE type, defects in chemotaxis are not observed at all.

Defects in Chemotaxis Associated with Deficiency of the Complement Components

The coexistence of C_{1r}, C_2, C_3, and C_5 deficiency and defects in chemotaxis has been reported in several papers (Day et al., 1972; Alper et al., 1975; Gallin,

1975; Miller, 1975). These disturbances occur together with defects in opsonization and frequent infectious complications. The mechanism of chemotactic defect in these patients has not been definitely elucidated. The clinical evaluation of the relationship between infections, on the one hand, and deficiencies in the complement components and in chemotaxis, on the other, is also difficult.

Defects in Chemotaxis Associated with the Presence of Inhibitors

Only a few patients have been described in whom a defect in chemotaxis was due to the presence of a specific inhibitor in the serum. The chemotaxis inactivator noted in patients with Hodgkin's disease indicates that the complex immune defect in these patients is also related to the neutrophil system (Ward et al., 1974). Inhibitors of chemotaxis have also been reported in patients with alcoholic cirrhosis of the liver (DeMeo et al., 1972) or chronic granulomatous disease (Ward, 1972), and in children with recurrent infections (Smith et al., 1972, Soriano et al., 1973). None of these inhibitors has been obtained in purified form, and the biochemical descriptions are unsatisfactory. The interactions between the chemotaxis activators and inactivators and the complement components still require further study.

Defective Chemotaxis Associated with Metabolic Disturbances

Defects of this type have been reported in patients with diabetes (Hill et al., 1974; Miller, 1975; Baum, 1975) or uremia (Baum, 1975; Henderson et al., 1975) and in patients after extracorporeal hemodialysis (Miller, 1975). In patients with uremia, disturbances in the multidirectional movements of neutrophils have also been observed. The mechanism of this chemotactic defect is not clear. It is known that the neutrophil phagocytic activity in patients with diabetes or uremia is decreased and the frequency of infections is elevated. In children with diabetes several cytochemical alterations of neutrophils occur, including myeloperoxidase deficiency (Pietrzyk, 1979).

Other Defects in Chemotaxis

In this group of chemotactic defects, those noted in patients with severe infections and rheumatoid arthritis should be mentioned. There have been controversial reports on chemotaxis in patients with severe infections, sometimes stating that chemotaxis was disturbed (McCall et al., 1971; Mowat et al., 1971), and sometimes that it was normal (Perillie et al., 1962; Hill et al., 1976). The reason for this controversy probably lies in differences in technique, the

selection of patients, the clinical evolution of diseases, and the sex and age of
the group studied. Little is known about the defective chemotaxis observed in
patients with rheumatoid arthritis (Mowat et al., 1971).

DEFECT OF OPSONIZATION

A child exhibiting abnormal phagocytosis of staphylococci and yeast has
been described (Miller et al., 1968). Normalization of the defect occurred after
incubation of the patient's neutrophils with the serum of a healthy subject.
It has been suggested that the defect is related to the deficiency of opsonins or
of activator of the complement system. In a patient with sickle cell anemia, an
isolated defect of opsonic activity of the serum against pneumococcus type
25 but not against *Salmonella choleraesuis* has been reported (Winkelstein et al.,
1968).

DEFECTS IN ENGULFMENT AND KILLING THE MICROBIAL AGENTS

Several patients have been described with isolated defects of phagocytosis,
i.e., engulfment of microbial agents and intracelular killing of these agents. In
some patients, however, these defects may occur simultaneously. This large
group of phagocytic defects includes those occurring in premature and full-
term infants and defects noted in patients with various proliferative and metabolic diseases, tumors, anemias, or severe infections. The functional neutrophil
defects in patients with these diseases will be discussed in detail in the next
chapters.

Phagocytosis in the Premature and the Full-Term Infant

A characteristic feature of neutrophils in newborns is the striking variability of their phagocytic activity (Forman et al., 1969). According to the opinion
of some authors, in healthy newborns the neutrophil phagocytic activity is not
significantly altered (Dossett et al., 1969), but there have also been reports on
disturbed phagocytic activity in these cells in newborns as compared with that
in adults (Iwaszko-Krawczuk, 1974; Gomez-Estrada et al., 1975). During the
first 24 hours after birth, a relatively large number of bacteria engulfed by neutrophils in newborns survive as compared with an adult control group (Coen
et al., 1969), though it has been emphasized that 2 hours after the phagocytosis

of bacteria a significant percentage is killed intracellularly in these conditions.

A decrease in this activity in a certain percentage of newborns may be a result of a deficiency of opsonizing antibodies of the IgM type. The titer of these antibodies increases in newborns after transfusion of fresh blood from adult donors. Deficiency of the complement components may also be of significance in the mechanism of lowered neutrophil phagocytic activity in newborns. In about 15% of newborns a fall in the level of proactivator C_3 of complement in the blood occurs (Stossel et al., 1974). The C_3 level in newborns represents no more than 60% of the level noted in adults. C_3 is synthesized by the fetus and does not undergo transplacental passage (Propp et al., 1968).

The phagocytic properties of neutrophils in the premature infant have not been the subject of many studies. It has been found that the killing of *Pseudomonas aeruginosa* within neutrophils in the premature infant is disturbed (Cocchi et al., 1967). The decreased total blood phagocytic activity in these subjects may also be due to a fall in the neutrophil count and its shift to the left (Toyota, 1968). Several authors, however, have reported normal neutrophil phagocytic activity in the premature infant (Forman et al., 1969; Dossett et al., 1969; Miller, 1969). The results of studies on NBT reduction in newborns are controversial (Humbert et al., 1970; Jemelin et al., 1971). Detailed analysis of the results obtained by various authors indicates that in many instances these results are in fact incomparable.

Not much work has been done on the cytochemistry of neutrophils in the premature and the full-term infant and its relationship to their metabolic and phagocytic properties. In our own investigations we have noted high indices of the neutrophil alkaline phosphatase activity in the premature infant (Bryniak et al., 1975). The acid phosphatase activity is also elevated in these conditions. The mechanism of the elevated activity of some neutrophil enzymes in the premature infant has not been elucidated. It cannot be excluded that the activity of these enzymes is influenced by some hormones capable of transplacental passage, e.g., hydrocortisone.

Defective Hydrogen Peroxide Synthesis

Defective hydrogen peroxide synthesis is known as chronic granulomatous disease (CGD), a clinical entity occurring in children and characterized by recurrent purulent infections (Berendes et al., 1957; Good et al., 1968). Clinically the disease is manifested by generalized lymphadenopathy, enlargement of the spleen and liver, symptoms of suppuration of the lymph nodes, pneumonia, and inflammatory skin lesions. The most frequent symptoms of the disease are summarized in Table 25 (according to Johnston et al., 1971).

A characteristic feature of CGD is the inability of neutrophils to kill bacteria intracellularly, despite the normal course of phagocytosis, i.e., engulfment (Quie et al., 1967). The defect is associated with intracellular depletion of hydrogen peroxide synthesis. It is inherited as a sex-linked trait occurring in males, though in some cases it may occur in females and is then inherited as

TABLE 25. Frequency of signs and symptoms in 92 patients with CGD. (According to Johnston et al., 1971)

Finding	Number of patients
Marked lymphadenopathy	87
Pneumonitis	80
Male sex	80
Suppuration of nodes	79
Hepatomegaly	77
Dermatitis	77
Onset by 1 year	72
Splenomegaly	68
Hepatic-perihepatic abscess	41
Death before 7-year-old	34
Osteomyelitis	30
Onset with dermatitis	28
Onset with lymphadenitis	28
Persistent rhinitis	23
Facial periorificial dermatitis	22
Conjunctivitis	21
Death from pneumonitis	21
Persistent diarrhea	20
Perineal abscess	17
Ulcerative stomatitis	15

a recessive autosomal trait (Koch et al., 1973). The most frequent infections in patients with CGD are caused by *Salmonella, Staphylococcus aureus,* or *Pseudomonas* (Lazarus et al., 1975). The neutrophils of these patients exhibit an abnormal glycolytic cycle, disturbed oxygen utilization, defective NBT reduction, defective hydrogen peroxide synthesis, and consequent defective iodination.

There are no differences between neutrophils from patients with CGD and those from normal subjects as far as the peroxidase, beta-glucuronidase, and alkaline phosphatase activities, as well as the localization in the granular and soluble fractions, are concerned (Baehner et al., 1967). Electron microscopic and histochemical studies as well as quantitative analysis of degranulation patterns have also failed to demonstrate the differences between normal and CGD neutrophils (Elsbach et al., 1969; Mandell et al., 1969).

Phagocytosis and killing of bacteria. Neutrophils from patients with CGD exhibit the normal capacity to engulf various objects. There is no direct relationship between enzymatic defect in CGD neutrophils and definite structural abnormalities (Douglas, 1970). A case has been reported in which neutrophils contained two different types of abnormal granules resembling those noted in patients with chronic infections; the granules had patterns different from those of toxic granulations (Egeberg et al., 1969). Among the abnormalities noted in CGD neutrophils, defective adherence of lysosomal granules to the phagocytic vacuole (Heyne et al., 1972) and delayed fusion of these granules during phagocytosis should be mentioned (Eschenbach et al., 1971).

The biologic significance of these abnormalities is not quite clear. Some authors have observed disturbances in phagocytic vacuole formation and granule lysis in neutrophils from patients with CGD (Holmes et al., 1966; Quie et al., 1967), others have not confirmed the occurrence of any degranulation defect (Baehner et al., 1969). It has been pointed out that the release of enzymes from the lysosomal granules in these neutrophils is normal. The phenomenon of the transmission of lysosomal enzymes into the phagocytic vacuole, however, should be regarded as a time-dependent process. In CGD neutrophils disturbances in the release of these enzymes during phagocytosis occur in the early stages of cell activation, between the 5th and the 15th minute after stimulation; in the subsequent period, i.e., after 30 minutes, the differences between normal and CGD cells are no longer significant (Gold et al., 1973, 1974).

CGD neutrophils exhibit no abnormalities in migration (Ward et al., 1969). These cells are characterized by defective intracellular killing of microbial agents that do not produce hydrogen peroxide, i.e., *Staphylococcus aureus*, *Serratia marcescens*, *Aerobacter aerogenes*, *Paracolon hornia*, and *Candida* (Holmes et al., 1966; Quie et al., 1967; Klebanoff et al., 1969; Lehrer et al., 1969). Microbial agents that are producers of hydrogen peroxide, e.g., *Lactobacillus acidophilus*, streptococci, or pneumococci, are normally killed by CGD neutrophils (Kaplan et al., 1968; Klebanoff et al., 1969; Mandell et al., 1969). Bacteria producing catalase but not hydrogen peroxide, e.g., *Staphylococcus aureus*, are not killed to the normal extent by the cells. The hydrogen peroxide produced by the bacteria named is used by CGD neutrophils as part of their antimicrobial systems, so that CGD may be regarded as a selective defect in the intracellular killing of microbial agents that do not produce hydrogen peroxide.

In the blood of mothers of subjects with CGD two different subpopulations of neutrophils occur, one capable and the other incapable of the iodination of engulfed *L. acidophilus* previously killed thermically (Klebanoff et al., 1969). Methimazole also inhibits the killing of *L. acidophilus* by CGD neutrophils but exerts no such effect against normal neutrophils.

Defects in the glycolysis cycle. The normal increase in the activity of enzymes involved in the pentose cycle accompanied by elevated oxygen uptake and hydrogen peroxide production does not occur in CGD neutrophils during phagocytosis. Other metabolic pathways such as the Krebs cycle, glucose utilization, lactate production, and lipid turnover are not altered in these cells. It is worth emphasizing that the content of a given enzyme must decrease to the critical point if metabolic disturbances are to appear—e.g., a decrease in the content of glucose-6-phosphate dehydrogenase in neutrophils up to 25% of the normal level does not bring about changes in the antimicrobial and metabolic functions of these cells (Rodey et al., 1970).

Among other alterations noted in CGD neutrophils, the following should be mentioned: 1) the absence of stimulation of glucose-1-^{14}C oxidation and of increased respiration during phagocytosis (Holmes et al., 1967); 2) the increase in the stimulation of glucose-1-^{14}C oxidation after adding methylene blue, which supports the concept that there is no basic defect in the pentose cycle (Baehner et al., 1967); 3) various changes in the activity of glucose-6-phosphate dehydrogenase (Bellanti et al., 1970); 4) delayed hydrogen peroxide-dependent oxidation (Holmes et al., 1967); and 5) deficiency of glutathione reductase in female patients with CGD (Holmes et al., 1970).

Reports on the content of NADH oxidase in CGD neutrophils are controversial. Both the deficiency (Baehner et al., 1968) and a normal level of this enzyme have been noted (Holmes et al., 1971). It may be assumed that these differences are due to the lack of an appropriate control group and methodologic faults, since later studies have indicated the presence of both NADH and NADPH oxidases in these cells (Hohn et al., 1975). Using an elegant isotopic technique, it was shown that in contrast to normal cells the NADPH oxidase activity in neutrophils from patients with CGD does not increase during phagocytosis; in the same conditions, the enzyme activity in normal neutrophils is more or less doubled (DeChatelet et al., 1975). These data are in accordance with the results of studies on the role of this enzyme in the initiation of the respiratory burst accompanying phagocytosis. A conclusion has been presented that a deficiency of cyanate-insensitive NADPH oxidase is a primary sex-linked metabolic defect in CGD neutrophils (Hohn et al., 1975). There is a lack of information on the molecular characteristics of the NADH and NADPH oxidases, the mechanism of the decrease in their activation, and the intracellular localization of these enzymes in CGD neutrophils.

NBT reduction. One of the main features of CGD neutrophils is the loss of the capacity to reduce NBT (Park et al., 1968). The mechanism of this defect has not been elucidated. In normal cells the reduction depends on numerous dehydrogenases. In healthy subjects about 6% to 9% of neutrophils reduce NBT; in patients with bacterial infections the percentage increases to values exceeding 10⁰/o (Matula et al., 1971). Neutrophils from patients with CGD do not reduce NBT at all. This may be associated with intracellular disturbances in activation or with a diminished availability of NBT reductase, since the content of this enzyme is within the normal range in these cells (Nathan et al., 1969).

It has been demonstrated that in CGD neutrophils the capacity to reduce cytochrome C_1 during phagocytosis is disturbed, which suggests that the super-oxide anion is not produced intracellularly (Curnutte et al., 1974). Since NBT is reduced within the phagocytic vacuoles, it may be accepted that it substitutes oxygen as acceptor of hydrogen (Baehner et al., 1968). Donors of hydrogen in this reaction in neutrophils might be the pyridine nucleotides $NADH + H^+$ and $NADPH + H^+$. Results of studies on disturbances in cytochrome C and NBT reduction in CGD neutrophils suggest that deficiency or defect of the oxidase-generating superoxide anions occurs in these cells. Recently it has been suggested that NBT reduction in neutrophils is partially associated with the generation of O_2^-, which is lacking in CGD neutrophils.

Iodination defect. CGD neutrophils are not capable of binding iodide after the phagocytosis of some bacteria such as *Serratia marcescens* and thermically killed bacteria such as *Lactobacillus acidophilus* (Klebanoff et al., 1969). This defect is related to the diminished production of hydrogen peroxide during phagocytosis.

Summing up the results of various studies on the nature of the defect in CGD neutrophils it may be accepted that the basic abnormality in this disease is the decreased production of hydrogen peroxide associated with the diminished activity of the oxidases.

Neutrophils in CGD carriers. Genetic transmission of the neutrophil defect in patients with CGD poses a separate problem. The detection of carriers of genetic defects raises some clinical problems. In CGD carriers there is a great variability in the neutrophil functional and cytochemical indices. It has been shown that in these carriers two separate populations of neutrophils exist: the first is capable of iodination of engulfed bacteria but the second is not (Klebanoff et al., 1969). In female carriers of CGD a diminished percentage of neutrophils reduce NBT (Windhorst et al., 1967). These carriers also exhibit a moderate defect in the intracellular killing of bacteria and moderate abnormalities in oxygen utilization and in the pentose cycle as compared with patients suffering from CGD and normal subjects (Quie et al., 1967).

The mode of inheritance of CGD has been established with certainty, since there are reports not only on sex-linked but also on recessive and autosomal inheritance of this trait (Baehner et al., 1968; Azimi et al., 1968). According to numerous authors the defect is chromosome X-linked. In the majority of mothers of children with CGD, moderately manifested neutrophil defects consisting in a delayed bacteria-killing capacity, abnormal NBT reduction, and abnormal iodide binding are usually ascertained (Baehner et al., 1968; Klebanoff et al., 1969; Björkstén et al., 1972). Bacterial infections, mainly of the upper respiratory tract, are more frequent in CGD carriers than in healthy subjects. Similar moderate defects in the neutrophils are also noted in the brothers and sisters of patients with CGD (Windhorst et al., 1967; Björkstén et al., 1972).

Deficiency of Myeloperoxidase

Deficiency of myeloperoxidase in neutrophils causes diminished resistance to bacterial and mycotic infections. The deficiency is easy to detect by means of a simple cytochemical method. It has been shown that in patients with this deficiency both myeloperoxidase-positive and myeloperoxidase-negative neutrophils are produced simultaneously (Lehrer, 1971). Neutrophils in these patients do not exhibit disturbances in the engulfment of *C. albicans*, but their ability to kill these fungi within the cell is strikingly diminished (Lehrer et al., 1969). The cells also have a diminished capacity to kill *Staph. aureus* and *E. coli* (Davis et al., 1971). It has been noted that *Staph. aureus* and *Serratia marcescens* are killed within neutrophils with myeloperoxidase deficiency, not during 45 to 60 minutes, but after 3 to 4 hours (Lehrer et al., 1969; Davis et al., 1971). Nevertheless, after this period more than 90% of the phagocytized bacteria are killed.

Characteristic clinical features of neutrophil myeloperoxidase deficiency are the good general state of health in the patients, the appearance of the defect in advanced periods of life, and its frequent occurrence in patients with megaloblastic anemia or leukemias, mainly myelomonocytic leukemias (Davis et al., 1971; Lehrer et al., 1972). The defect may be clinically asymptomatic. The mode of inheritance of this defect is not well known. A family has been reported in which one member exhibited infection with *C. albicans*, while others exhibited no abnormal symptoms (Lehrer et al., 1969). The occurrence of the defect in brothers and sisters argues for the autosomal and recessive inheritance of the trait (Grignaschi et al., 1963; Lehrer et al., 1969; Undritz, 1974).

Data on the biochemical composition of neutrophils with defective myeloperoxidase synthesis are relatively numerous. The normal contents of lysozyme, ribonuclease, cathepsin, and D-amino-acid oxidase have been described in one study (Lehrer et al., 1969). Cytochemical investigations on the acid and alkaline phosphatases, the glycogen and the lipid content revealed no alterations in these cells as compared with the normal. The defective neutrophils exhibit no ultrastructural changes.

Furthermore, the migration of these cells in the Rebuck skin test, the course of phagocytosis, the formation of the phagocytic vacuole, and the accompanying fusion of the lysosomal granules are also normal. The intracellular basis of myeloperoxidase deficiency is not known. Acquired myeloperoxidase deficiency has recently been reported in neutrophils from children with diabetes (Pietrzyk, 1977). These observations explain to a certain extent the increased susceptibility to bacterial infections in this group of patients.

Deficiency of 3-Phosphoglycerate Kinase

A boy aged 3 years with deficiency of 3-phosphoglycerate kinase has been described (Boivin et al., 1974). The content of the enzyme in the neutrophils was about 18% of the normal value. The patient's mother also exhibited a moderate deficiency of the enzyme, which indicates that the deficiency is not linked with chromosome X. The electrophoretic mobility of the enzyme, its action on 3-phosphoglycerate, optimum pH, resistance to heat, and preservation in neutrophils from the patient did not differ from those in normal subjects. The enzyme deficiency was not associated with defective phagocytosis of latex particles, and NBT reduction by enzyme-deficient cells was diminished only slightly.

Hitherto some cases of this deficiency have been reported in which the enzyme deficiency occurred in both neutrophils and erythrocytes (Valentine et al., 1969; Konrad et al., 1973) or additionally even in lymphocytes (Cartier et al., 1971). The neutrophil functions were studied in detail in these cases.

Deficiency of Glucose-6-Phosphate Dehydrogenase

Deficiency of glucose-6-phosphate dehydrogenase in neutrophils may be total (Cooper et al., 1970) or partial (Holmes et al., 1971). In cells with total deficiency of the enzyme the formation of H_2O_2 and activation of the pentose cycle during phagocytosis are diminished; these alterations are associated with the total loss of the intracellular bactericidal capacity. The intracellular content of the enzyme, exceeding 25% of the values in healthy subjects, is sufficient for the normal killing of bacteria. Neutrophils from patients also exhibit NADH and NADPH deficiency (Baehner et al., 1971), which indicates the mechanism of the decrease in H_2O_2 production and in the pentose cycle activation. Neutrophils with glucose-6-phosphate dehydrogenase deficiency are incapable of digesting *Staph. aureus*, *E. Coli*, and *Serratia*, though *Streptococcus faecalis* is killed normally by the cells.

The intracellular mechanism of the enzyme deficiency is not clear. The molecular description of the enzyme in patients with partial deficiency is unsatisfactory. The mode of inheritance of the enzyme deficiency has not been fully described. There are data favoring the concept that the deficiency is, like CGD, a sex-linked trait (Gray et al., 1973). Hence it has been assumed that the gene responsible for the trait is localized near the gene determining the presence of abnormal oxidase in patients with CGD. Deficiency of glucose-6-phosphate dehydrogenase may be familial. Both neutrophils and erythrocytes may be involved, and then the clinical picture of the disease corresponds to that of hemolytic anemia with mild CGD.

Alkaline Phosphatase Deficiency

Only a few cases of primary deficiency of this enzyme have been reported. In one case a defect was detected in an individual suffering from recurrent infections, eczema, and hyperglobulinemia IgE (Repine et al., 1976). The leuko-tactic, metabolic, and structural patterns of the neutrophils in this individual were normal, and the only functional abnormality was the decreased bactericidal functioning of these cells. In another patients with the deficiency, ultrastructural alterations in the specific lysosomal granules and defective formation of phagolysosomes in the neutrophils, associated with frequent infections, were reported (Strauss et al., 1974).

Defective Actin System

Studies on the locomotional apparatus of neutrophils are few in numbers. A child has been described in whom frequent bacterial infections and inability to form local pus during infections were associated with a defective actin system (Boxer et al., 1974). The neutrophils in this patient exhibited a decrease in the number of pseudopodia rich in microfilaments. The microfilaments corresponded to the actin polymers. It was shown that the neutrophil actin protein content in this patient was normal, but that the actin from the patient's neutrophils sedimented after the polymerizing action of potassium chloride was seven times less than the actin from normal subjects. It may therefore be supposed that the nature of the defects is the synthesis of actin with a lowered ability to polymerize.

The defect was manifested by abnormal locomotion and delayed engulfment and digestion of microbial agents. The concept that defects may exist in the contractile machinery of neutrophils and their "mini-muscles" requires further study (Ward, 1974).

Deficiency of Beta-Glucuronidase

We have found beta-glucuronidase deficiency in neutrophils from patients with precancerous state and from patients with cancer of the larynx (Gierek et al., 1977, 1979; Lisiewicz et al., 1977, 1978). It was expressed by a decreased enzyme activity index and the disappearance of neutrophils with high enzyme activity from the blood. The relationship between beta-glucuronidase deficiency in neutrophils and susceptibility to the action of carcinogenic agents deserves further study. The deficiency is more expressed in the patients treated by radiotherapy. Analogous deficiency of beta-glucuronidase in peripheral blood neutrophils has recently been noted in patients with chronic lymphocytic leukemia and acute hairy cell leukemia (Zeya et al., 1979). Deficiency of above enzyme in neutrophils as a possible risk factor in cancer and leukemias deserves detailed studies (Lisiewicz, 1979).

The Glutathione Redox System Deficiencies

Recently, glutathione reductase deficiency in neutrophils has been reported (Roos et al., 1979). There are suggestions that the glutathione redox system is not directly involved in the generation of bactericidal oxygen products but plays a role in the protection of phagocytic cells against oxidative injury during phagocytosis. However, patients exhibiting glutathione synthetase deficiency (Oliver et al., 1978) and glutathione peroxidase deficiency (Holmes et al., 1970) exhibit increased susceptibility to infections.

C H A P T E R 9

CELLS IN THE NEUTROPHILIC SERIES IN PATIENTS WITH LEUKEMIAS AND OTHER PROLIFERATIVE DISEASES

Leukemic proliferation of the neutrophil system occurs in various clinical forms corresponding to chronic granulocytic leukemia, promyelocytic leukemia, acute granulocytic leukemia, myelocytic leukemia, and preleukemic states. Biologic alterations of leukemic cells are of interest because of the nature of the malignant process. This problem is part of a much larger knowledge of the etiology and pathogenesis of leukemia as a whole. Progress in this field during recent years does not encourage therapeutic optimism. The leukemic process in the neutrophilic cell series brings about several changes such as delayed cell maturation, diminished phagocytic activity, and decrease in the bactericidal capacity. These alterations result in a lessened resistance of the body as far as the neutrophil system is concerned. Other cell systems involved in immunity, however, also exhibit pathologic features in leukemic patients.

Investigations on neutrophils from the peripheral blood of patients with chronic granulocytic leukemia have been very numerous. This is because it is easy to obtain these cells in quantities sufficient for biochemical studies. Progress in this field concerns mainly information on the biochemical composition of these cells. Several studies have been devoted to genetic and chromosomal equipment. Attention has also been drawn to the general ecologic conditioning of the etiology of leukemias related to the neutrophilic system. It has been hypothetized that changes in nutritional customs and of soil fertilization as well as the chemicalization of agriculture as a whole in recent years have resulted in diminishing the content of some trace elements in the food of man. This may have occasioned consequent changes in the immune system and increased leukemia and cancer morbidity (Aleksandrowicz et al., 1976). Numerous observations argue in favor of this hypothesis and further studies in this field are desirable. Only few report dealt with chronic lymphocytic leukemia with regard to neutrophilic system. Attention has been recently focused on effects of infection by etiologic agent of viral hepatitis on the clinical course of the disease and transient increase of neutrophilic leukocyte count probably due to the infection has been reported in some cases (Ważewska-Czyżewska et al., 1977).

CHRONIC GRANULOCYTIC LEUKEMIA

The basic difference between normal neutrophils and neutrophils from patients with chronic granulocytic leukemia (CGL) is closely related to the nature of the malignant proliferation. A striking feature of CGL neutrophils, in contrast to various malignant cells, is that basic physiologic properties such as the phagocytic and chemotactic activities as well as the capacity to kill bacteria intracellularly are maintained. All these activities are to a certain degree lowered in CGL neutrophils, though there are no basic qualitative differences between normal and leukemic cells in this respect. The use of CGL neutrophils for transfusion into patients with neutropenias or sepsis is based upon their ability to kill bacteria intracellularly. The cells transfused into nonleukemic subjects exhibit vigorous phagocytic activity in the blood (Shohet, 1968). Transfusions of leukemic cells, however, present a complex biologic and legislative problem, since in fact they are nothing less than transplantation of cells with malignant patterns. There are no reports on CGL occurrence in subjects who undergo transfusions of leukemic neutrophils. Despite these data, it is difficult not to mention that in practice the majority of clinicians will try to overcome infections in patients without recourse to transfusion of malignant cells. There are numerous unsolved problems as far as basic differences between normal and CGL neutrophils are concerned.

It is not known whether in the initial stage of CGL the first clones of leukemic cells are derived from normal cells. In other words, it is not known whether in CGL patients only one type of neutrophilic cell, i.e., the leukemic, is produced or whether there is a simultaneous but separate production of leukemic and normal cells in the neutrophilic series. This basic question despite studies on leukemic twins (Goh et al., 1967) still remains unanswered.

Light microscopic examination reveals only small differences between normal and CGL neutrophils. In CGL patients neutrophils more frequently exhibit numerous toxic granulations and atypical lysosomes. Few differences between normal and CGL neutrophils have been found by using the transmission and the scanning electron microscopes; the majority of mature leukemic neutrophils exhibit no differences as compared with the normal (Ullyot et al., 1974). The numbers of azurophilic and specific granules in CGL neutrophils remain within the normal range. In some of these leukemic cells large granules bizarre in shape have been noted. In some of the cells rough endoplasmic reticulum corresponding to Döhle bodies and aggregates of smooth endoplasmic reticulum are observed, though these patterns are also seen in the neutrophils of nonleukemic patients with severe infections.

Many more abnormal features occur in CGL neutrophil precursors. The main abnormality in CGL myeloblasts and promyelocytes is the presence of increased numbers of nucleosomes and microfilaments (Ullyot et al., 1974). Similar bundles of microfilaments are also present in the promonocytes and monocytes of CGL patients. Attention has been called to the occurrence in these patients of three abnormal neutrophil populations: 1) peroxidase-negative, 2) exhibiting the presence of normal peroxidase-positive granules, and 3) containing granules that morphologically correspond to azurophilic granules but are devoid of peroxidase (Ullyot et al., 1974). In CGL patients the absence of specific granules within the neutrophils may occur despite the normal development of the cell nucleus.

Changes in the cell karyotype and chromatin structure and the occurrence of chromosome Ph_1 in CGL neutrophils should also be mentioned. Several variants of chromosomal aberrations in these cells are well known (Sandberg, 1971; Horland et al., 1976). These changes are not specific for CGL, since they are also noted in patients with acute myeloblastic leukemia. Chromosome Ph_1, belonging to group G of chromosomes (No. 21), characterized by the absence of about half of the big arm, is present in almost 90% of CGL neutrophils, and as a rule is not observed in patients with other myeloproliferative diseases (Whang et al., 1963; Goh et al., 1964). Morphologic abnormalities of chromosome Ph_1 may also consist in chromosomal breakages and varying localization (Baikie, 1966). Some CGL patients, however, do not show chromosome Ph_1. A striking feature is the presence of this chromosome not only in neutrophils but also in cells of the megakaryocytic and erythrocytic series. This indicates the genetic relationship between these cell series and is an argument in favor of the neounitarian theory of blood cell cytogenesis (Aleksandrowicz et al., 1976). Chromosome Ph_1 is of an acquired character. It occurs, e.g., only in one twin in whom CGL has developed. The chromosome does not disappear during remission and is also present in the neutrophil precursors; its appearance might be caused by irradiation (Tough, 1965). Chromosome Ph_1 is noted in patients with mongolism, who are especially prone to leukemias.

It is only recently that more has been learned about the clinical significance of the presence or absence of chromosome Ph_1. In a group of 230 CGL patients, only 20 did not exhibit the chromosome (Canellos et al., 1976). The chromosome Ph_1-negative patients had higher mean values of age, the platelet and leukocyte counts were lower, and their mean survival time was only 15 months as compared with 44 months in the chromosome Ph_1-positive patients. These observations agree with data indicating that the chromosome Ph_1-positive patients are more sensitive to therapy than those without the chromosome (Tijo et al., 1966). The clinical use of the results of these studies for the differentiation of particular forms of leukemias of the neutrophilic series requires further observations (Brière et al., 1975; Michaux et al., 1975). It was previously assumed that the presence of chromosome Ph_1 was a cause of diminished alkaline phosphatase activity in neutrophils; it was later demonstrated

that the activity of the enzyme and the presence of the chromosome are not
closely related (Winkelstein et al., 1967). There is a report on a patient with
chronic lymphocytic leukemia exhibiting chromosome Ph_1 in whom CGL developed (Whang-Peng et al., 1974). Chromosomal abnormalities in juvenile
CGL lack specificity so far as the Ph_1 chromosome is concerned (Inoue et al.,
1977).

Several differences in the biochemical composition of normal and of leukemic neutrophils have been demonstrated. Of course, the basic nature of the
biochemical changes determining the malignant patterns of CGL neutrophils is
not known. The differences so far known will be briefly summarized.

Relatively numerous studies have been devoted to the nucleic acids of leukemic cells in the neutrophilic series. Most of these studies have shown an increase in the DNA content in these cells. Sometimes this increase corresponds
to the multiplication of the normal diploidal number of chromosomes. It is of
interest that the pathologic chromosome Ph_1 of CGL patients from the 21st
chromosome pair may contain only 61% of DNA in comparison with the
DNA content in the second chromosome of this pair. There are no data
on the differences in the nucleotide composition of DNA in normal and CGL
neutrophils; the differences discovered refer to the molecular weight and
physical characteristics of DNA in these cells.

Numerous authors have reported an increase in the total RNA content in
homogenates of CGL neutrophils. This probably corresponds to the increased
numbers of immature cells, which contain more RNA. In the general consensus,
RNA metabolism is enhanced in both mature and immature CGL neutrophils.
There are a number of observations on the increased incorporation of ^{14}C into
the thymidine of these cells. The increase in the incorporation of labeled thymidine into DNA and RNA is to a certain extent proportional to the degree of
immaturity of the leukemic cell population in the blood.

In CGL neutrophils there is also a tendency toward an increase in the activity of enzymes participating in the synthesis of nucleic acids, such as thymidine kinase, thymidilate synthetase, DNA polymerase, or other enzymes in the
purine and pyrimidine syntheses. No conclusive evidence of disturbed feedback
control of the nucleic acid synthesis in these cells has been presented, however,
except for experimental data on the abnormal synthesis of pyrimidine.

The metabolism of proteins and amino acids is enhanced in cells of the neutrophilic series from CGL patients. This was shown in investigations on the enhanced incorporation of labeled *l*-valine and *l*-methionine in these cells. Analogous observations have been made on the incorporation of *l*-alanine, *l*-cystine,
and *l*-methionine in cells of acute myeloblastic leukemia. In CGL cells, increased
utilization of ^{35}S-*l*-cysteine has also been noted (Sznajd et al., 1971). Information
on the activity of enzymes taking part in the protein metabolism in CGL cells
is controversial. According to some authors the cells exhibit elevated glutamin-

182

acetate aminotransferase, arginase, and glutaminic dehydrogenase activities; others have not confirmed these data.

New information has been collected from studies on the isozymic proteins in CGL neutrophils. Biologic immaturity and capacity to divide mitotically are associated in the cells with a high content of lactic acid dehydrogenase (LDH), its isozyme LDH_1, and the isozyme of malonic acid dehydrogenase, MDH_2. In CGL myeloblasts the total LDH and H-LDH contents (heart type of LDH) are elevated but in mature cells of this leukemia are lowered. There are also observations on the increased activity of the nonspecific esterase fraction in CGL neutrophils. Basing on studies on isoenzymes of glucose-6-phosphate dehydrogenase it has been suggested that CGL is a disease of clonal origin (Fialkow et al., 1977).

It should also be mentioned that leukemic neutrophils have an antiheparin activity associated with cationic proteins (Lisiewicz et al., 1966; Sznajd et al., 1969). The antithrombin and fibrinolytic activities of these cells are also associated with several proteins; this has been the subject of a more recent review (Lisiewicz, 1976).

The carbohydrate metabolism in cells of the neutrophilic series from CGL patients exhibits the following differences in comparison with normal neutrophils (Seitz, 1965; Sznajd et al., 1971):

1. Decreased glycogen content; enhanced metabolism and resynthesis of glycogen.

2. Lowering of the respiratory process and enhancement of the glycolytic process (decreased oxygen utilization, elevated rate of lactic acid production).

3. Lowering of the hexokinase activity controlling the production of glucose-6-phosphate and of a number of various enzymes in the Embden-Meyerhof pathway, e.g., lactic acid dehydrogenase, phosphofructokinase, pyruvic kinase, or 3-phosphoglyceraldehyde dehydrogenase.

4. Decreased production of ATP with accompanying ADP deficiency.

Lipid metabolism is enhanced in CGL neutrophils. This is reflected in the increased incorporation of precursors of free fatty acids, cholesterol esters, and phospholipids (Cline, 1975). The total lipid content in CGL neutrophils is a subject of controversy. According to the majority of authors the phospholipid content increases in these cells. Phospholipids are mainly localized in the granular fraction. However, there are also data indicating a decreased lipid content due to a diminished triglyceride, diglyceride, cholesterol ester and sphingomyelin level in above cells (Gola, 1976). Metabolism of gangliosides in leukemic neutrophils deserves further studies (Dacremont et al., 1976).

Among more recent data on differences between normal and CGL neutrophils, the following should be mentioned:

1. CGL neutrophils exhibit a decreased ability for the surface binding of

pyroantimonate osmium (PAO) (Ackerman, 1975). This defect occurs only in mature neutrophils and is not detectable in their precursors. The reaction of PAO binding is conditioned by the presence of some cations, such as calcium, magnesium, and sodium, on the cell surface. Defective PAO binding does not occur in cells from patients with myelomonocytic leukemia, myelofibrosis, or acute myelocytic leukemia.

2. CGL neutrophils exhibit a decreased alkaline phosphatase content. We have called attention to the fact that, as in non-leukemic persons, in CGL patients the injection of testosterone results in an increase in enzyme activity

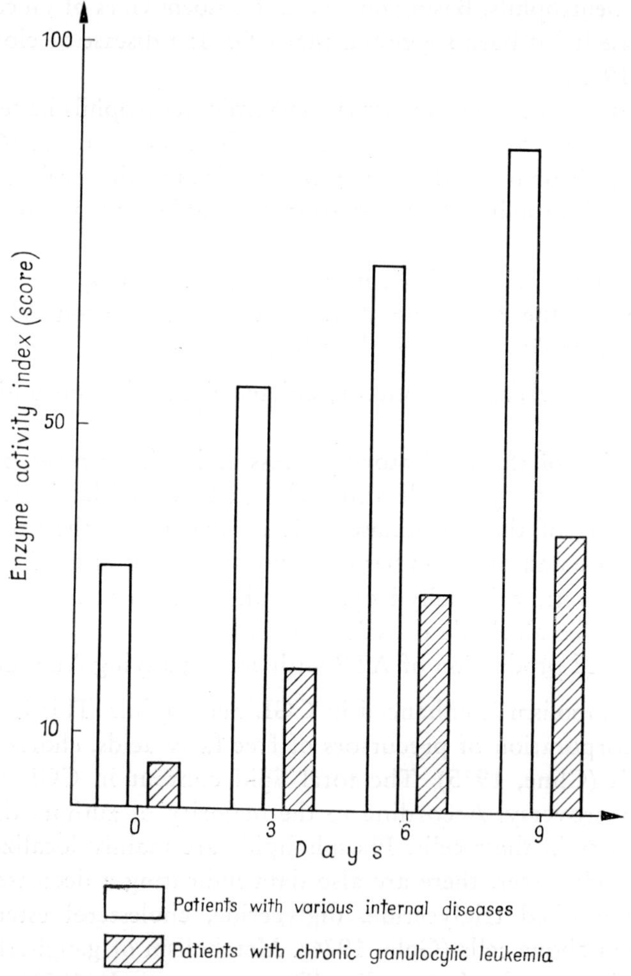

Fig. 18. Effect of testosterone on alkaline phosphatase activity in the neutrophils of 20 patients with various nonproliferative internal diseases and of 20 patients with chronic granulocytic leukemia. Both groups of patients observed exhibited an increase in enzyme activity after 7 and 9 injections of 25 and 50 mg of testosterone, respectively. (According to Lisiewicz et al., 1975; Janicki et al., 1977)

(Fig. 18) (Lisiewicz et al., 1975; Janicki et al., 1977). This favors the concept that the basic apparatus of the enzyme synthesis is not irreversibly altered within the cells (Chikkappa et al., 1973). In other studies no immunologic or chromatographic differences were found between normal and CGL neutrophils. There are also no differences as far as the number and distribution of enzyme-positive granules are concerned (Rosenblum et al., 1975). These data indicate that CGL cells synthesize a probably molecularly normal enzyme. In pregnant women suffering from CGL there is a correlation between the degree of the enzyme activity, which is elevated, and the severity of the clinical course of the disease (Grozdea et al., 1975). An increase of the enzyme activity has also been noted in *in vitro* soft agar culture of bone marrow cells from CGL patients (Chiyoda et al., 1977).

3. During a phase of myeloblastic exacerbation, CGL blasts show increased terminal deoxynucleotide transferase activity (Sarin et al., 1976). Hence a suggesion has been made that a phase of exacerbation of the disease may be accompanied by the appearance in the blood not only of myeloblasts but also of lymphoblasts, in which the characteristic pattern is a high activity of this enzyme.

4. Glycogen synthetase activity is decreased in cells of the neutrophilic series in patients with CGL (Custo et al., 1975) although the rate of glycogen synthesis is elevated in these cells (Gahrton et al., 1972). It has just been mentioned that the total glycogen content in CGL cells is lowered.

5. Investigations on the isozymic composition of CGL neutrophil acid phosphatase (Pajdak et al., 1972), the physicochemical properties of arginases (Reyero et al., 1975) and the characteristics of the vitamin B_{12} and folic acid carriers of these cells (Gullberg et al., 1975; Fischer et al., 1975) indicate new horizons for further research in this field.

6. Colony-stimulating activity (CSA) is significantly diminished in leukemic neutrophils despite the fact that there is a high content of the colony-stimulating factor (CSF) in the urine of patients (Brunelli et al., 1976).

Data on the phagocytic properties of CGL neutrophils are controversial, since several authors have observed both a normal (Sbarra et al., 1965) and an abnormal phagocytic capacity (Rosner et al., 1970; Raichs et al., 1972). CGL patients treated by chemotherapy and having normal values for leukocyte count do not show abnormalities in the phagocytosis of intracellular killing of *Candida albicans* (Goldman et al., 1973). In the same circumstances, a neutrophil phagocytic activity even higher than normal has been noted in CGL patients (Serafińska, 1970).

Phagocytosis of yeast by CGL neutrophils is also disturbed and normalizes during remission (Rosner et al., 1970). CGL patients show a lower percentage of neutrophils phagocytizing *Staph. aureus* than normal subjects (Szmigiel et al.,

1957). Similar results were obtained in studies of phagocytosis of *Staph. epidermidis*, *Pseudomonas aeruginosa*, and *E. coli* (Serafińska, 1970), but the numbers of bacteria phagocytized by individual cells were increased. Vigorous phagocytic activity is observed in CGL neutrophils after their transfusion into nonleukemic patients suffering from sepsis due to streptococcal infection (Shohet, 1968). The relationship between the adhesive and phagocytic properties of CGL neutrophils is not clear. In CGL patients the adhesive properties of these cells are diminished (Zittoun et al., 1973). Comparison of phagocytic activity in neutrophils from patients with CGL and from patients with chronic lymphocytic leukemia indicates that CGL cells are less active than cells from patients with lymphocytic leukemia (Szmigiel et al., 1957; Serafińska, 1970).

Disturbances in the metabolic functioning of CGL neutrophils (Selvaraj et al., 1967) and abnormal fusion of primary lysosomes during the formation of phagocytic vacuoles (El-Haalem et al., 1976) have been proposed as possible bases for the inefficient phagocytosis in CGL patients. A degranulation defect accompanying by a decreased iodination has been reported with this regard (Cramer et al., 1977).

A comparison of the phagocytic activity in CGL and normal neutrophils should include not only the properties of individual cells but also the neutrophil population as a whole, since it is known that a certain percentage of leukemic neutrophils do not phagocytize foreign objects. The phagocytic activity of these cells does not change evidently during subsequent periods of the clinical evolution of the disease, nor is it correlated with the serum levels of properdin and complement (Serafińska et al., 1973). The bacteriolytic activity of the serum in CGL patients is even higher than that in normal subjects (Prużanski et al., 1973). Adhesion of leukemic neutrophils to a glass surface and their pinocytic capacity are lessened (Bölling et al., 1973). Knowledge of the mechanism of these abnormalities is scanty.

Despite numerous studies, the differences between the rates of neutrophil productions in patients with CGL and normal subjects have not been elucidated. In CGL patients the neutrophil survival time is prolonged, which results in an accumulation of cells in the circulating blood (Galbraith et al., 1972). Hence it may be accepted that the normal mechanism of balance between the neutrophil production and destruction rates does not function efficiently. The significance of the cyclic variations in the neutrophil count in the peripheral blood observed every 53 to 69 days in patients with CGL is not clear (Chikkappa et al., 1976). Oscillations in the circulating white blood cell counts in the patients are related to larger problem of physiological control systems which are a subject of intensive studies during last years (Mackey et al., 1977).

It seems that further trials of the mathematical approach in CGL patients by means of computer analysis of the relationship between the production and destruction of leukemic cells will enable a deeper insight into this complex problem (Wheldon et al., 1974). It should be made clear, however, that simulated systems of correlation between various parameters in the living body cannot include all the factors involved in the leukemic process.

*

In evaluating the biologic differences between normal and CGL neutrophils, the effects induced by antileukemic therapy should also be taken into consideration. Cytostatic drugs, radiotherapy, and corticoids have a significant influence on the biochemical composition and functions of CGL neutrophils. Therapy with busulfan results in the normalization of the indices of mobilization and NBT reduction, but has no effect on the indices of phagocytosis (Whittaker et al., 1974). The phagocytic efficiency of the neutrophil system as a whole changes, owing to the decreased neutrophil count in the blood after antileukemic therapy. Several antimetabolic drugs induce such an effect.

It has been reported that clofazimine (B 663) induces a double effect on neutrophils in the blood — on the one hand, it decreases the numbers of these cells and, on the other, it increases their phagocytic capacity (Brandt, 1972). Hydroxyurea causes elevation of the free nucleotide pool in neutrophils, probably as a result of the increased synthesis of these nucleotides and their less intensive utilization in the synthesis of nucleic acids (Maj et al., 1975).

PROMYELOCYTIC LEUKEMIA

Promyelocytic leukemia represents a separate cytologic type of acute leukemia (Hillestad, 1957; Didisheim et al., 1964). The frequent occurrence of local or generalized thrombi at autopsy in patients who have died of this leukemia has suggested the involvement of an intravascular clotting mechanism in the pathogenesis of the hemorrhagic diathesis. Attention was turned to leukemic myelocytes as a source of thromboplastic substances to be released into the circulating blood, where the induction of the coagulation mechanism and consumption of blood coagulation factors take place (Quigley, 1967). It was later demonstrated, however, that disseminated intravascular coagulation as a mechanism of the hemorrhagic diathesis occurs in patients with various types of leukemia, and not only the promyelocytic; it has also been shown that thromboplastic substances are present in all types of leukemic white blood cells (Lisiewicz, 1976).

Lukemic promyelocytes differ in numerous respects from normal cells as far as structure is concerned (Goldman, 1974). In leukemic promyelocytes there are nucleoli with nonspecific patterns within the nuclear chromatin; the nucleus is bilobed, dense, often double; the cytoplasm contains numerous azurophilic granules which are larger, denser, and exhibit more intensive staining than normal promyelocytes. Many leukemic promyelocytes contain elongated crystalline splinter-shaped cytoplasmic inclusions staining for acid phosphatase and peroxidase. Electron microscopic examination has revealed that these inclusions differ from Auer bodies and show a hexagonal arrangement of tubes. The scanning electron microscope reveals narrow ridgelike profiles on the surface of leukemic promyelocytes (Polliack et al., 1975). These profiles occur in 55% to 60% of cells. Less than 10% of cells contain ruffled membranes or microvilli. A greatly dilated cisternae of endoplasmic reticulum resulting in flaming in the peripheral parts of promyelocytes have also been reported (Stavem et al., 1977).

The cytochemical characterization of leukemic promyelocytes makes possible the differential diagnosis between acute promyelocytic, acute myelomonocytic, and both chronic and acute monocytic leukemia. Leukemic promyelocytes are characterized by strongly positive cytochemical reactions to peroxidase, Sudan black B, and naphthol-AS-D-chloroacetate esterase (Liso et al., 1975). Naphthol-AS-LC-acetate esterase and acid phosphatase are also present in these cells. Details of the differentiation between leukemic promyelocytes and other types of leukemic blasts are given in Table 8. It should be emphasized that despite numerous methods and trials, the cytochemical diagnostics of leukemic promyelocytes is still far from satisfactory, hence the significance of biochemical studies of these cells.

The thromboplastic activity of leukemic promyelocytes resembles that of brain thromboplastin (Quigley, 1967). The cells also exhibit a fibrinolytic activity (Cattan et al., 1966) which varies greatly in individual cases (Gralnick et al., 1973). It has been suggested that in patients with promyelocytic leukemia there may occur a lack of equilibrium between the blood coagulation and the fibrinolytic system, which is due to the intracellular equipment of the promyelocytes. It is not known whether leukemic promyelocytes are able to phagocytize fibrin fragments. A preliminary report on this subject (Matsuoka et al., 1969) has not yet been confirmed. The problem of whether leukemic promyelocytes are able to release into the blood other substances influencing blood coagulation or the fibrinolytic system has also not been solved. Suggestions that these cells may release a trypsinlike substance (Hillestad, 1957) or a plasminogen activator (Gupta et al., 1969) require confirmation.

There are few studies on the promyelocyte functions in patients with promyelocytic leukemia. Some reports present data on the phagocytic properties of these cells. The role of leukemic promyelocytes in the total body metabolism, consumption, and turnover of fibrinogen and fibrin and in the possible digestion of other substances present in the blood is not known in detail.

ACUTE MYELOBLASTIC LEUKEMIA

Acute myeloblastic leukemia (AML) is a clinically and cytochemically well-defined disease. The differential diagnosis of AML and other forms of acute leukemia is of prognostic and therapeutic importance. The diagnosis is mainly based on the results of cytochemical studies of leukemic cells (see Table 1).

In scanning electron microscopic examinations, AML blasts exhibit acute ridgelike profiles, and some of these cells are characterized by wrinkled membranes and microvilli (Polliack et al., 1975). A certain percentage of these cells exhibit spherical structures and a smooth surface. Blasts from the blood of patients with acute promyelocytic leukemia have a similar surface structure. Correlated electron microscopic and cytochemical studies made it possible to subtype cells of the neutrophilic series from the blood of patients with AML into the following three subgroups (Bainton, 1975): 1) neutrophils in which there are no specific granules but only peroxidase-positive azurophilic granules, showing that the development of the cytoplasmic organelles has been inhibited at the myelocyte stage; 2) neutrophils containing no azurophilic granules but only specific granules; this shows inhibition of the neutrophil development at the promyelocyte stage or the presence of numerous mitoses resulting in a striking fall in the azurophilic granule count; and 3) neutrophils containing two types of granules, i.e., azurophilic and specific, but the azurophilic granules have no peroxidase activity. These last cells are especially frequent in patients with AML. These results indicate the simultaneous presence of various subpopulations of neutrophils in the blood of patients with AML and the specific "mosaicism" of cells characteristic of leukemias. There have been numerous reports on the presence of unusual inclusions in AML blasts; these possibly correspond to viruslike particles (Brunning et al., 1974).

Biochemical and cytochemical studies of cells in the neutrophilic series in patients with AML deal, above all, with the differential diagnosis of young blastic cells. Blasts from the blood of patients with various types of leukemia are difficult to differentiate on the grounds of morphologic patterns only, and it is very often impossible to establish the cytologic type of leukemia when using only the light microscope. Hence cytochemical methods of differentiation between particular types of acute leukemia blasts have been developed—i.e., for myeloblasts, promyelocytes, monocytes, lymphoblasts, and leukemic cells in patients with erythremic myeloses and plasma cell leukemia. Details of cytochemical findings in patients with acute leukemias are summarized in Chapter 2.

The basic difficulty lies in the differentiation between leukemic myeloblasts and lymphoblasts. The cytochemical examination of these cells using staining for peroxidase, glycogen, lipids, and esterases is of practical importance. Cells in the monocytic series, i.e., promonocytes and monoblasts, are characterized by electron-dense lysosomal granules staining intensively for alpha-naphthyl-acetate esterase (Glick et al., 1974). In these studies typical promyelocytes and myelocytes were stained for the presence of naphthol-AS-D-chloroacetate esterase. N-AS-A esterase in monocytic leukemia cells is strongly inhibited by NaF (Morimoto, 1975). In AML cells this inhibition is much less evident.

The value of cytochemical examination in the differential diagnosis of acute leukemias is still a subject of controversy. It seems of importance that the blastic cells appearing in the blood of patients with chronic granulocytic leukemia during myeloblastic exacerbation may be PAS-positive and thus correspond to the lymphoblasts of acute lymphoblastic leukemia (Litwin et al., 1974). This observation emphasizes the difficulties of classifying leukemia merely on the basis of cytochemical findings. There are also striking individual variations in the cytochemical composition of leukemic cells. In a single subject the simultaneous presence of various subpopulations of leukemic cells may be noted. The PAS reaction varies greatly in different leukemias, and the presence of PAS-positive blasts is not explicitly of diagnostic significance (Malaskova, 1975). Staining for peroxidase has a more established importance in practice (Hennekeuser et al., 1974). Recently, the fluorescence method for identification of lysosomes has been proposed for diagnosis of acute leukemia (Mdzewski et al., 1977). Among more recent advances in biochemical studies of blasts from patients with AML the following should be mentioned:

1. The electrophoretic patterns of histones isolated from AML blasts, blasts of myelomonocytic leukemia, and cells of chronic granulocytic leukemia are similar (Kass, 1975). It has hence been concluded that myelomonocytic leukemia is a variant of AML.

2. The presence of ferritin has been found in AML blasts, blasts of chronic granulocytic leukemia during the exacerbation phase, and blasts of acute lymphoblastic leukemia, but not in mature neutrophils of chronic granulocytic leukemia (Mori et al., 1975).

3. In leukemic cells the presence of at least three different DNA polymerases has been ascertained (Rainer et al., 1974).

4. The content and composition of lipids does not differ in normal and in leukemic neutrophils (Bleiber et al., 1976).

5. The results of the NBT test vary in acute leukemias, and no correlation between the number of NBT-positive cells and the occurrence of fever of bacterial origin has been found (Wantzin et al., 1975).

There is still a lack of more detailed data on the possible correlation between the results of cytochemical examination and the survival time of patients. It has been noted that remissions are more frequent in children with acute leukemia in whom the percentage of PAS-positive cells is equal to 100%/o (Kruse, 1975). There are suggestions concerning the possible relationship between alkaline phosphatase activity and C or G chromosome in patients with the disease (Kamada et al., 1976).

The lysozyme content in mature neutrophils isolated from the blood of patients with AML is significantly lowered (Hansen et al., 1974). During remissions the lysozyme content increases both in these cells and in the plasma. In contrast to normal myeloblasts, AML myeloblasts exhibit a relatively high lysozyme content, which is frequently associated with a high activity in the serum (Karle et al., 1974). In some cases of AML circulating neutrophils deficient in lactoferrin were reported (Mason, 1977).

The phagocytic properties of neutrophils in patients with AML have been the subject of more numerous reports. It has been observed that the capacity of these cells *in vitro* to phagocytize and kill *Candida albicans* is diminished during the acute period of the disease and normalizes after cytostatic therapy (Wilkinson et al., 1975). In nontreated AML patients who are not in full remission, neutrophils phagocytize *Candida albicans* normally, but the intracellular killing of these agents is defective (Goldman et al., 1973). Plasma of the patients inhibits the phagocytic activity of normal neutrophils; the nature of this phenomenon has not been elucidated. Cytostatic therapy may not affect the capacity of neutrophils from AML patients to phagocytize *Brucella* (Silver et al., 1957). Some authors have observed decreased neutrophil phagocytic function in patients with AML before the clinical manifestation of the disease (Solberg et al., 1975). It has also been shown that AML blasts exhibit stronger phagocytic activity than those from patients with acute lymphoblastic leukemia (Neuwirtová et al., 1975). Blasts of myelomonocytic leukemia also have phagocytic properties. It is not known whether neutrophils from patients with AML are capable of phagocytizing autologous myeloblasts. Such a phenomenon has been observed in patients treated immunologically by means of autologous leukemic cells (Gomez-Estrada et al., 1976). In nonimmunized patients, neutrophils do not exhibit phagocytosis.

Disturbances in the maturation of leukemic cells are reflected in the prolongation of the myelocyte-to-tissue transit time in patients with AML (Galbraith et al., 1972). This symptom is a result of abnormalities in the final stages of neutrophil production (dysgranulopoiesis) occurring in patients treated with cytostatic drugs and in patients in remission. There are preliminary reports on chalone-induced complete remission of AML, however, details of biochemical mechanism of this effect are still not known (Rytömaa et al., 1977).

ACUTE LYMPHOBLASTIC LEUKEMIA

The functions of neutrophils in children suffering from acute lymphoblastic leukemia (ALL) represent a separate problem which has become a subject of interest only recently. The functional state of the neutrophils is of special significance during remission of the disease when the main danger to patients comes from infections. Neutrophils from these patients exhibit several cytochemical abnormalities, consisting in increased alkaline phosphatase activity and a rise in the NBT test values as well as diminished myeloperoxidase activity and a decrease in the lipid content (Pituch, 1977). In some patients during relapse the reduction of NBT may be diminished (Humbert et al., 1976). It has been emphasized that elevated values of the NBT test in children with acute leukemia might render the diagnosis of infections and inflammatory states difficult (Pilgrim et al., 1974). It is of interest that high neutrophil alkaline phosphatase activity occurred most frequently in patients with a low neutrophil count, which suggests the reactive intracellular mobilization of the enzyme. In contrast, an elevated neutrophil count was accompanied by high indices of acid phosphatase activity, and in subjects with a lowered neutrophil count a low activity of the enzyme has been noted. Data on the cytochemical differences between the cells in healthy children and those with ALL are summarized in Table 26 (according to Pituch, 1977).

TABLE 26. Cytochemical characteristics of the peripheral blood neutrophils in children with acute lymphoblastic leukemia during remission. (According to Pituch, 1977)

Test	Children with acute lymphoblastic leukemia	Control group of healthy children
	arithmetic mean (26 cases)	arithmetic mean (20 subjects)
Myeloperoxidase (score)	193.2*	248.8
NBT test (%)	22.4*	11.2
Alkaline phosphatase (score)	154.9*	114.7
Acid phosphatase (score)	39.6	48.6
Glycogen (score)	264.2	250.8
Lipids (Sudan Black B) (score)	195.3*	233.5

* Statistically significant differences.

Methods: myeloperoxidase — Graham-Knoll; NBT — Park; alkaline phosphatase — Kaplow; acid phosphatase — Barka and Anderson; glycogen — McManus; lipids — Sheehan.

It is worth noting that the NBT test shows different results in children with ALL and in those with Hodgkin's disease or lymphosarcoma. In children with Hodgkin's disease an increase in the NBT test values is always associated with the active stage of the disease, whereas in subjects with ALL the test values are low during relapses and high during remissions (Zajączkowski et al., 1976). In children with lymphosarcoma no significant alterations have been noted in this respect. It has been shown that treatment of ALL children with L-asparaginase results in a transient decrease in the NBT test values, the myeloperoxidase activity, and the glycogen content in neutrophils (Zajączkowski, 1977). In contrast, the treatment induces elevation of the neutrophil alkaline phosphatase activity. These cytochemical alterations are accompanied by an increase in the IgG, IgM, and IgA levels (Zajączkowski et al., 1975, 1976). The complex relationships between enzymatic changes in the neutrophil system and other indices of the immune system found in children with ALL during treatment have been the subject of recent reviews (Zajączkowski, 1976, 1977). Infectious complications of ALL result in an increase in the activity of some enzymes within neutrophils, such as the alkaline and acid phosphatases and alpha-naphthyl esterase (Kruse, 1975). The lysozyme content in these cells is evidently diminished during relapses and normalized during remissions of ALL (Hansen, 1974). The serum lysozyme level is also diminished in these patients.

Enzymatic alterations of neutrophils in patients with ALL are related to functional disturbances. Half of these patients show disturbances in the bactericidal activity of these cells during relapses, but this activity is normalized during remissions (Humbert et al., 1976). The phagoctyic activity of neutrophils does not change. In patients with abnormal neutrophil bactericidal activity, infections are more frequent than in others. The information on neutrophils in patients with chronic lymphocytic leukemia is scanty. The only data are on disturbances in phagocytosis and the killing of *P. aeruginosa* (McRipley et al., 1967). It has been shown that in patients with ALL the colony forming potential is significantly reduced in early remission (Morris et al., 1977).

MYELOMONOCYTIC LEUKEMIA

The myelomonocytic syndrome is more often observed in children than in adults. The syndrome consists in the simultaneous proliferation of monocytes and cells in the neutrophilic series. Ultrastructural studies do not enable monocytic leukemia to be differentiated from myelomonocytic leukemia (Freeman et al., 1971). The neutrophil system in these syndromes, as in monocytic leukemias, has never been the subject of major studies. The cytogenetic relationship between myelomonocytic lukemia and acute myeloblastic leukemia has not been fully elucidated. The leukemic cells of both types of leukemia are similar as far as the electrophoretic patterns of its histones, rich in arginine and lysine, are concerned (Kass, 1975). Despite this fact, the concept that acute myelomonocytic leukemia is a variant of acute myeloblastic leukemia deserves further study. Blast cells from patients with myelomonocytic leukemia are capable of phagocytizing ferrioxidsaccharate, in contrast to leukemic cells of the lymphoblastic series (Neuwirtová et al., 1975).

In scanning electron microscopic examination these cells are characterized by ridgelike profiles and ruffled membranes (Polliack et al., 1975). These patterns occur in 59% to 92% of the cells. The differentiation between myelomonocytic cells with a smooth surface and lymphocytes is difficult in these patients.

PRELEUKEMIA

The term preleukemia refers to states preceding the development of the clinical picture of leukemia. It has been pointed out that preleukemic states are frequently accompanied by changes in the neutrophil system. In many patients acute leukemia is preceded by neutropenia. The fact that agranulocytosis may precede leukemia has long been known (Schaefer, 1926; Borchardt, 1930; Burkens, 1931; Strumia, 1934). Reports indicating that neutropenia may be an expression of preleukemic states have also been published during the past 20 years (Marchal et al., 1944; André et al., 1953; Block et al., 1953; Blair et al., 1966; Heimpel et al., 1972), but this concept needs confirmation. Population studies to show that leukemias occur more frequently in subjects with neutropenias have not yet been carried out. Observation of single cases of such types may reflect the fact that a leukemogenic factor acting in the body has induced the initial phase of neutropenia. Hence neutropenia may also be regarded not as a preleukemic state but as a part of the leukemic process.

Since there is also a lack of studies on the action of the known leukemogenic factors of chemical, physical, or biologic origin in animals in which neutropenia has been artificially provoked, it is not known whether neutropenia facilitates the effect of these factors. A case has been reported in which acute myeloblastic leukemia was preceded by disturbances in the neutrophil bactericidal functions, characterized by the presence of skin granulomas (Schreiner et al., 1976). In another case this type of leukemia was preceded by the occurrence of a myeloperoxidase deficiency in about 36% of the neutrophils in the peripheral blood (Breton-Gorius et al., 1975). These neutrophils showed defective bactericidal activity against *Staph. aureus*, defective fusion of myeloperoxidase-positive granules, and defective formation of the phagocytic vacuole accompanied by abnormal degranulation. One of the symptoms of preleukemia is the increased number of myeloblasts in the bone marrow (Takahashi et al., 1975). Cytochemical examination of neutrophils from patients with preleukemia reveals no characteristic patterns (Heller et al., 1974). These neutrophils exhibit a varying response to the colony-stimulating factor *in vitro* (Ricci et al., 1975). Defects in neutrophil function consisting of reduced phagocytosis, impaired ability to kill *Staph. aureus*, and abnormal chemotaxis were noted in several patients with preleukemia (Ruutu et al., 1977).

PRIMARY POLYCYTHEMIA

Studies on neutrophils in patients with primary polycythemia have been few in number and have dealt with increased phagocytic activity, enhanced NBT reduction, and increased metabolic activity in the pentose cycle (Cooper et al., 1972). The neutrophil alkaline phosphatase activity is also increased and does not change under the influence of treatment with busulfan (Szczepkowska et al., 1973). Electron microscopic studies reveal no alterations in the number or localization of granules containing the enzyme (Rosenblum et al., 1975).

HODGKIN'S DISEASE

Few investigations have been made on neutrophils in patients with Hodgkin's disease. In studies *in vitro* it has been found that the formation of neutrophil colonies is abnormal in these patients (Bull et al., 1975). Patients with a generalized malignant process show several alterations in the neutrophils, including an increase in the acid and alkaline phosphatases, chloracetate esterase, and the glycogen content, accompanied by a decrease both in the phospholipid content and in the peroxidase activity (Sarnitski et al., 1975). All these indices were normalized in patients in whom an amelioration of the general state due to therapy was noted. The neutrophil fungicidal activity against *Candida albicans* is lowered in subjects with the disease (Lehrer et al., 1971), but the bactericidal activity of these cells against *Staph. aureus* is not altered (Vildé, 1974). In patients with lymphosarcoma or reticulosarcoma, an increase of the neutrophil alkaline phosphatase activity is not noted (Loginsky et al., 1975).

Infections are frequently the main complication in patients with plasma cell myeloma. The neutrophil functions in these patients are not well known. It has been reported that the lysozyme content is significantly diminished in their neutrophils (Karle et al., 1976). The mechanism of this phenomenon is not known; it does not occur in patients with lymphoma. The fungicidal activity of the neutrophils is normal in these patients (Lehrer et al., 1971).

EFFECT OF ANTIPROLIFERATIVE DRUGS ON THE NEUTROPHIL SYSTEM

It is well known that the majority of antileukemic drugs, with the exception of the corticosteroids, have a depressive action on the neutrophilic cell line. Neutropenia and agranulocytosis are inherent risks associated with antiproliferative therapy. What is more, in the majority of patients with acute leukemias, severe leukopenia is one of the conditions for inducing remission. Numerous drugs act by inhibiting normal proliferation and interfering with the mitotic cycles in the neutrophil precursors. Therapy with corticosteroids, in contrast, stimulates the neutrophil system and increases the number of normal precursors in the bone marrow. In patients treated with prednisone, a decrease is noted in the neutrophil bactericidal activity, in NBT reduction, and in lysozyme content (Clemmensen et al., 1976). The phagocytic functions of neutrophils are depressed by daunorubicin and arabinoside cytosine (Davies et al., 1976). A similar action is induced by vincristine and vinblastine (Whittaker et al., 1975). Some indices of the neutrophil functions—e.g., mobilization, phagocytosis, and NBT reduction—are normalized in patients treated with busulfan (Whittaker et al., 1974). Colchicine may cause structural alterations in neutrophils. In a woman who took a large dose of this drug in order to commit suicide, the presence of large, darkly staining inclusions in the neutrophil cytoplasm was observed (Powell et al., 1976). The mechanism of these changes is unknown.

The antiinflammatory drugs frequently administered to patients with leukemias may also affect the neutrophils. Phenylbutazone and acetylsalicylic acid induce *in vitro* an inhibitory effect on neutrophil phagocytic activity (Whittaker et al., 1975). Perorally administered aspirin, in contrast, does not cause a similar effect.

The following observations should also be mentioned in discussing the effect of therapy on the neutrophilic system in leukemia patients:

1. The changes in the PAS reaction during the therapy of chronic granulocytic leukemia may resemble those seen in patients with acute lymphoblastic leukemia (Litwin et al., 1974).

2. The deoxycytidine kinase and cytidine deaminase activities in leukemic cells do not change to an extent enabling the mechanism of resistance to antileukemic drugs to be elucidated (Coleman et al., 1975).

3. It has been suggested that resistance to 6-mercaptopurine therapy might be associated with both the supply and availability of phosphorylpyrophosphate (Higushi, 1975).

4. Proresid does not change the peptidaselike activity in neutrophils; the changes in the alkaline phosphatase activity in these cells during therapy with this drug are not characteristic (Kotlarek-Haus et al., 1971). Cyclophosphamide increases the activity of this enzyme (Moszczyński, 1976).

CHAPTER 10

NEUTROPHILS IN PATIENTS WITH METABOLIC DISEASES

Recently, remarkable progress in the knowledge of the mechanisms of metabolic disorders has been made. A significant percentage of these disorders are congenital, but the clinical manifestation of a given defect may take place in various periods of life. Genetic studies on the regulation of enzyme synthesis are important for the understanding of the mechanisms of these disorders. The concept that all biochemical processes in the body are under genetic control is especially fruitful. These processes represent a series of individual reactions forming definite chains. Each single reaction is under the final control of individual single genes, so that the mutation of a single gene may cause only a change in the cell capacity to regulate a single primary chemical reaction.

Recently, the hypothesis that one gene controls the synthesis of only one enzyme has been advanced. This hypothesis accepts the view that one cistron controls the synthesis of one polypeptide. The term cistron is used of a functional unit of DNA controlling the structure of a single polypeptide chain. Metabolic disturbances might result from the mutation of structural genes or control genes. Mutation of a structural gene causes changes in the specific protein structure. Mutation of a control gene causes a change in the intensity of action of one or more structural genes and induces quantitative alterations in one or more proteins without affecting the structure. The limited scope of this book does not permit a wider discussion of the genetic basis of metabolic disorders, which has been the subject of various monographs (Stanbury et al., 1972).

The first result of the disturbed synthesis of a given enzyme is its deficiency in various cells, tissues, and body fluids in comparison with normal healthy subjects. The list of enzymatic deficiencies of this type is very long and includes a number of enzymes with various metabolic pathways, including those of carbohydrates, amino acids, lipids, purines and pyrimidines, metals, porphyrins, etc. Independently of the genetic mechanism of the abnormal synthesis of a given enzyme, the general result of enzymatic deficiencies is the defective formation of the specific product of a given enzymatic reaction. The simultaneous deficiency of a metabolite directly deriving from a given product of reaction is also noted. There are pathologic states in which the disturbed formation of a specific product of a given reaction represents the main symptom deciding the diagnosis. This may be exemplified by the deficiency of glucose-6-phosphate in patients with von Gierke's disease, resulting in hypoglycemia during fasting, or by the absence of melanin formation in patients with the type of albinism due to tyrosinase deficiency.

The second result of the deficiency of a given enzyme is the accumulation of precursors of blocked reaction. This process may be accompanied by an increased production of substances deriving from those precursors via alternative metabolic pathways. If the accumulated metabolites are soluble, their concentration in the body fluids and excretion in the urine increase. An example of this type of disturbance, consisting in the accumulation of precursors of blocked reaction, is the excessive storage of glycogen in the cells of patients with glycogenoses. The separate mechanism involved in the overproduction of particular metabolites is due to an increase in the activity of the regulatory enzyme.

The diagnosis of metabolic defects is based on the determination of the content of abnormal metabolites, direct examination of the activity of a given enzyme, identification of variants of abnormal proteins, and results of cell cultures. The direct examination of a given enzyme may be performed in the blood as a whole, in particular blood components such as the white blood cells, or in tissue samples taken by biopsy. The technique of examining the enzyme content in the white blood cells is especially useful. The cells are easy to obtain in the form of concentrated suspensions and may serve for the diagnosis of several metabolic diseases such as glycogenoses, orotic aciduria, or methylmalonic aciduria. Enzymatic or phenotypic abnormalities in leukocytes are known as a cause of at least 35 various diseases (Hsia, 1970). A number of congenital errors in metabolism may be detected by examining erythrocytes.

From the point of view of the knowledge of human neutrophils, it should be emphasized that most investigations on congenital and acquired metabolic defects have been carried out by authors who used leukocyte samples of a mixture of neutrophils, lymphocytes, eosinophils, monocytes, and basophils. Few studies have been made using purified neutrophil samples. In a number of publications the term leukocytes is used, which in a given publication means a mixture of white blood cells or neutrophilic leukocytes without further specification. The reason for this lies in the fact that many centers of research on metabolic errors are not particularly experienced in isolating neutrophils from other white blood cells. Conversely, hematologic centers, with routine experience in this respect, only rarely undertake major studies on the alterations in neutrophils accompanying metabolic defects. Hence, numerous morbid entities included among metabolic defects have not been intensively studied with regard to neutrophils.

In a number of cases the biologic significance of observations on neutrophils from patients with metabolic disorders is not fully clear—e.g., the observation that the serum from patients with cystic fibrosis enhances the release of myeloperoxidase and beta-glucuronidase from neutrophils (Conod et al., 1975) is not well understood. Several clinical entities have been studied in detail as far as lymphocytes and monocytes are concerned, but neutrophils have not been the object of such interest. In other entities, e.g., Niemann-Pick disease, the neutrophils do not show the structural abnormalities or the presence of cytosomes which characterize the lymphocytes from patients with the disease (Lazarus et al., 1967). For these reasons, in the present monograph only those clinical entities due to metabolic defects and known better from the standpoint of knowledge of alterations in neutrophils will be discussed.

DISEASES OF CARBOHYDRATE METABOLISM

Diabetes Mellitus

It is well known that diabetic patients are prone to bacterial and fungal infections. The mechanism involved in this phenomenon is related to the neutrophil system. The neutrophil phagocytic activity may be diminished in patients with various types of diabetes (Rohmann, 1966). This defect in phagocytosis is especially marked in patients with ketoacidosis, though it is not associated with changes in the blood pH, since a suspension of neutrophils from these patients in the serum of healthy subjects does not result in normalization of phagocytosis (Bybee et al., 1964). Disturbances in phagocytosis occur in about half the patients with diabetes, and are accompanied by defective intracellular killing of bacteria in about 10% of these patients (Tan et al., 1975). The simultaneous occurrence of defects in both phagocytosis and killing might be the cause of severe infectious complications in a given patient.

Not much is known of the mechanisms of diminished neutrophil phagocytic activity in patients with diabetes. Probably the mechanism are associated *inter alia* with decreased chemotactic activity in the cells (Mowat et al., 1971). The relationship between the chemotactic reactivity of neutrophils and their capability of ameboid movement is not clear, since the latter shows no abnormality in treated patients (Lapin et al., 1956). The degree of the defect in phagocytosis is not correlated with the glucose level in the serum, and incubation of the neutrophils in the serum of healthy subjects does not lead to correction of the defect.

There have been attempts to elucidate the disturbances in neutrophil phagocytic functioning in diabetic patients by demonstrating intracellular metabolic defects in these cells. The following observations should be mentioned:

1. The decrease in the neutrophil glycogen content (Esmann, 1972) is associated with a low level of glycogen synthetase (Williams et al., 1968). In patients treated with insulin of tolbutamide, the content of the enzyme increases.

2. The contents of glucose-6-phosphate and fructose-6-phosphate increase in the neutrophils, which suggests a lowered phosphofructokinase content (Esmann, 1972). These alterations are accompanied by a moderate decrease in glucose utilization and a slight increase in the pentose cycle activity during phagocytosis (Esmann, 1968).

3. The effect of insulin on glucose utilization in neutrophils has been the subject of experimental studies. Most of the data are in favor of the increased utilization of glucose by the neutrophils during the treatment of patients with insulin (Esmann, 1972).

4. Uptake of oxygen by the neutrophils does not differ from that in healthy patients (Esmann, 1972). Similarly, the Crabtree effect in these cells is identical both in patients with diabetes and in normal subjects. It indicates the absence of respiratory disturbances in neutrophils from these patients.

5. Neutrophils from diabetic patients exhibit an increased synthesis of intracellular proteins, reflected in the increased incorporation of glycine and cystine (Tokodi et al., 1967).

6. The most important contribution to our understanding of diminished neutrophil phagocytic activity in diabetic patients is the observation that the intracellular myeloperoxidase activity in these cells is evidently diminished both in diabetic children and adults (Palimąka, 1979 (personal communication); Pietrzyk, 1979; Pietrzyk et al., 1979). The more evident the enzyme deficiency is, the more frequent are infectious complications in the patients. Myeloperoxidase is an important component of the neutrophil intracellular antimicrobial systems, and its deficiency is critical for the appearance of complications due to bacterial infection, very frequent in patients with diabetes.

Glycogen Storage Diseases

At least eight different clinical entities due to abnormal excessive glycogen storage are known. A knowledge of the enzymatic alterations in the leukocytes in the peripheral blood is of diagnostic importance in patients with these diseases (Table 27). The data hitherto available are, however, not satisfactory. Case reports on glycogenoses frequently contain only partial or controversial data. In numerous cases reported, the results of examinations refer to "leukocytes" and not to neutrophils.

Glycogenosis type I (von Gierke's disease) has never been studied in detail from the standpoint of enzymatic disturbances in neutrophils. Normal glycogen phosphorylase content in leukocytes has been reported in a single publication

(Williams et al., 1963). In patients with glycogenosis type III, the leukocyte glycogen content varies, and is elevated only in some patients (Williams et al., 1963; Brandt et al., 1966; van Creveld et al., 1964). Similar variations in the debrancher enzyme have been observed in the leukocytes of some patients. In patients with glycogenosis type III, however, both decreased (Williams et al.,

TABLE 27. Classification of the glycogen storage disease.

Type of disease	Enzyme deficient	Synonyms	Alterations in neutrophils
Type I	glucose-6-phosphatase	von Gierke's disease	
Type II	alpha-1,4-glucosidase	Pompe's disease	
Type III	amylo-1,6-glucosidase (debrancher)	Cori's disease (dextrinosis)	deficiency of the enzyme or its normal content
Type IV	alpha-1,4-glucan 6-glucosyl transferase (brancher)	Andersen's disease	
Type V	muscle phosphorylase	McArdle's disease	
Type VI	glycogen phosphorylase	Hers' disease	deficiency of the enzyme in some patients
Type VII	muscle phosphofructo-kinase		
Type VIII	liver phosphorylase kinase		deficiency of the enzyme

1963; Steinitz et al., 1963; Williams et al., 1968) and normal contents of this enzyme (Huijing et al., 1968) have been reported. An elevated activity of the enzyme has also been noted in some patients (Brandt et al., 1966; Williams et al., 1968). Hence the estimation of the enzyme activity in patients with this glycogenosis is not of much diagnostic value.

Glycogenosis type IV is characterized by glycogen phosphorylase deficiency only in some patients (Williams et al., 1963; Ockerman et al., 1966). The activity of this enzyme varies in different members of a family and does not exhibit any direct relationship with the mode of inheritance. Phosphorylase deficiency has also been found in patients with glycogenosis type IV (Huijing, 1967). The enzyme was less stable than in healthy subjects, and the defect showed a sex-linked mode of inheritance. In some patients, however, activity of the enzyme was normal, which indicates that at least two variants of the disease may occur, one characterized by simultaneous deficiency of both glycogen phosphorylase and phosphorylase kinase and the other by deficiency only of the first enzyme.

In patients with glycogenosis type VIII, phosphorylase deficiency occurs both in neutrophils and in the liver cells (Huijing, 1967). The degree of enzyme deficiency in the neutrophils corresponds to that in the liver cells (Huijing et al., 1970).

DISORDERS IN LIPID METABOLISM

Diseases related to disturbances in the lipid metabolism include numerous clinical entities consisting in the excessive accumulation of lipids in various cells and body tissues. The main group of these disorders is represented by the neurologic diseases of childhood. These degenerative brain diseases are characterized by the presence of abnormal granules in the neutrophils and other cells of the peripheral blood. The granules correspond to the lipid material stored in the cells. Little is known about metabolic alterations in neutrophils from patients with lipomucopolysaccharidoses, which are disorders intermediate between sphingolipidoses and mucopolysaccharidoses.

Familial Amaurotic Idiocy

The classification of the diseases in this group has not been finally established. The following clinical entities within this group of disorders should be cited: congenital familial amaurotic idiocy (Normann-Wood disease), infantile familial amaurotic idiocy (Tay-Sachs disease), late infantile familial amaurotic idiocy (Jansky-Bielschowsky disease), juvenile familial amaurotic idiocy (Spielmeyer-Vogt disease), and adult amaurotic idiocy (Kufs' disease). Only some of these disorders have been studied from the point of view of alterations in the neutrophils.

It has been stated that in patients with familial amaurotic idiocy several changes in neutrophils occur, including hypersegmentation of the nucleus and the presence of cytoplasmic vacuoles, varying in size, and of abnormal granules (Strouth et al., 1966). The granules vary in diameter from 0.5 to 2 microns and differ from toxic granulations, since they do not stain with neutral red. Morphologically the granules resemble Alder-Reilly granules.

Evaluation of the patterns of these granules does not permit the diagnosis of a given type of lipidosis, but studies of this type in the members of a family enable carriers of the disease to be detected (heterozygotes). About one third of the siblings of patients exhibit these abnormal granules. No detailed genetic studies have yet been made.

204

G_{M2} Gangliosidose (Tay-Sachs Disease)

It has been pointed out that in patients with this metabolic disorder characteristic granules occur in the peripheral blood neutrophils (Strouth et al., 1966). The granules are basophilic rather than azurophilic and are less numerous but larger than those in patients with Jansky-Bielschowsky disease. The significance of these granules is difficult to evaluate, especially in the light of the fact that other authors do not confirm their occurrence (Rosner et al., 1968).

Jansky-Bielschowsky Disease

An increase in the number of azurophilic granules in the neutrophils was reported in a patient with this disease (Rosner et al., 1968). A simultaneous increase in the neutrophil alkaline phosphatase activity was also noted in this patient, but it was not established whether the granules contained the enzyme. There are few cytochemical studies on neutrophils from patients with this disease.

Glucosylceramide Lipidosis (Gaucher's Disease)

Information on neutrophils from patients with Gaucher's disease is scanty. The presence of neutrophils and other leukocytes as well as of erythrocytes within the Gaucher cells has frequently been noted; hence it has been suggested that the cerebroside in the Gaucher cells derives from normal neutrophils. The source of glucosylceramide in Gaucher cells is not known. Attention has been drawn to the fact that in patients with chronic granulocytic leukemia, the cells in the neutrophilic series show an increase in the activity of the cerebrosidases (Kampine et al., 1967; Kattlove et al., 1969). At the same time it was stated that in these patients cells morphologically resembling Gaucher cells frequently appear in the bone marrow (Smith et al., 1968; Rosner et al., 1968). Hence the hypothesis has been advanced that cells in the neutrophilic series in patients with this leukemia cause excessive utilization of the glucocerebroside-cleaving enzyme, which subsequntly results in the storage of glucocerebrosides in the cells of the reticuloendothelial system and the appearance of cells morphologically resembling Gaucher cells (Smith et al., 1968). This hypothesis, however, has been severely criticized (Rosner et al., 1970).

Galactosylceramide Lipidosis (Krabbe's Disease)

A galactocerebroside beta-galactosidase deficiency has been noted in the neutrophils, serum, and cultured fibroblasts of patients with this disease (Suzuki et al., 1971). The activity of this enzyme was also lower in the respective parenteral cells. Striking individual variations in enzyme activity were observed.

DISORDERS OF PURINE AND PYRIMIDINE METABOLISM

Gout

The neutrophils play an important role in the mechanism of local inflammatory changes in patients with gout. In dogs with experimental gout and inflammations induced by sodium urate, the injection of antineutrophilic serum or administration of vinblastine, causing neutropenia, resulted in a significant decrease in the local inflammatory reaction (Chang et al., 1968; Phelps et al., 1966).

Characteristic morphologic changes within neutrophils of patients with gout may be observed by means of phase-contrast microscopy. The neutrophils present in the joint exudates show areas of light transmission which cause a mottled or "honeycomb" appearance (Riddle et al., 1967). The mechanism of these changes has not yet been elucidated. It has been demonstrated that the neutrophils of these patients are capable of engulfing urate crystals (Howell et al., 1962). The crystals may be released by cell disruption and engulfed once more by other neutrophils (McCarty, 1964). The crystals are visible in 7% to 100% of these cells. In most cells the crystals have no delineation membrane and seem to lie loosely within the cytoplasm (Riddle et al., 1967). In some cells the crystals have an electron-dense delineation membrane varying in continuity. Only rarely are the crystals seen within the phagosomes. The occurrence of free crystals without a delineation membrane suggests that they are formed within the cell. Several ultrastructural patterns of these neutrophils, however, indicate intensive pinocytosis and micropinocytosis.

The effect of colchicine on neutrophils of patients with gout is a different problem. Colchicine exerts an antiinflammatory effect. There have been suggestions that the influence of colchicine is associated with its action on the biologic properties of neutrophils, since it inhibits adhesion, ameboid movements, mobilization, and chemotaxis in these cells (Fruhman, 1960; Malawista, 1964; Wechsler et al., 1965; Phelps, 1970). Colchicine also diminishes the degranulation of the neutrophil lysosomes (Rajan, 1966; Malawista et al., 1967) and inhibits its metabolism during phagocytosis (Melmon et al., 1968). Conclusive evidence has not yet been brought forward that the beneficial therapeutic effect of colchicine in patients with gout is solely due to its action on neutrophils. It is known that colchicine does not change the level of the serum uric acid or its renal excretion. The effect of another therapeutically active agent, allopurinol, widely used in the treatment of gout, on neutrophils is also scantily documented.

The Lesch-Nyhan Syndrome

This syndrome represents a congenital defect consisting in a total deficiency of hypoxantin-guanin phosphorybosil transferase, one of the enzymes involved in purine metabolism. The deficiency of the enzyme has been found not only in neutrophils but also in erythrocytes, skin fibroblasts, the liver, and the brain tissue (Rosenbloom et al., 1967; Kelley 1968).

PHOSPHOGLYCERATE KINASE DEFICIENCY

The deficiency has been reported in both neutrophils and erythrocytes (Valentine et al., 1969). Mothers of children suffering from this deficiency also exhibit significant decrease in the neutrophil enzyme activity.

DEFICIENCIES OF ENZYMES AND PROTEINS IN THE BLOOD

Hereditary Diseases of Hemostasis

The most frequent cause of death in patients with hemophilia is infection. The basis of that often fatal complications has not been studied, at least as far as neutrophils are concerned. It has been reported that leukocytes isolated from the blood of a patient with hemophilia A exhibit a thromboplastic activity similar to that in normal cells (Eiseman et al., 1954).

Acatalasemia

The cases of acatalasemia hitherto reported have been characterized by the absence of catalase in various cells, including the neutrophils. The functional state of these cells has not been the subject of any detailed studies.

OTHER DISORDERS

Uremia

The infections frequently noted in patients with uremia are mainly due to defects of the lymphocyte system (Astaldi et al., 1971). Neutrophils from healthy subjects suspended in the serum of patients with uremia do not show any significant alteration or glucose oxidation during phagocytosis (Davidson et al., 1976). Other authors, however, have reported diminished neutrophil phagocytic activity in these patients (Brogan, 1967). The spreading of these cells on a glass surface is more intensive in patients than in healthy subjects; this gives the impression that the neutrophils from patients are larger. The cells from patients are also characterized by greater numbers of vacuoles, longer pseudopodia, and more visible cytoplasmic granules. Hypersegmentation of the nucleus is another characteristic pattern of these neutrophils (Hattersley et al., 1974). Reinfusion of the blood in circumstances resembling those of extraperitoneal dialysis results in transient neutropenia (Jensen et al., 1973).

Alcoholism

There are few data on the neutrophil functions in patients intoxicated with ethyl alcohol. It is known from practice that severe intoxications of this type are accompanied by elevated neutrophilic leukocytosis. In some of our own cases we have observed an increased neutrophil alkaline phosphatase activity.

Toxicoses

Reports on neutrophil functions in patients with toxicoses are few. In experimental intoxication of mice by sodium selenate, we have noted a decreased neutrophil acid phosphatase activity. Sodium selenate administered to patients with chronic lymphocytic leukemia in small doses did not change the count or the neutrophil acid phosphatase activity. Increased numbers of neutrophils have been noted in workers in contact with zinc or zinc dyes (Jeremin, 1973).

CHAPTER 11

NEUTROPHILS IN PREGNANT WOMEN, PATIENTS AFTER SURGERY, AND THOSE WITH ANEMIAS, TUMORS, PRECANCEROUS STATES, AND OTHER PATHOLOGIC SYNDROMES

It is surprising that diseases as frequent as malignant tumors, anemias of various origin, postoperative states, and even infections have only rarely been a subject of interest from the point of view of alterations in neutrophils. The biologic role of these cells in the majority of these conditions needs no emphasis. The reason for this neglect is that physicians working in various branches of medicine have not any great interest in hematology as a whole, and their technical possibilities for research on particular functions of various white blood cells are limited; hence their attention is focused on other subjects of interest. Conversely, hematologists only rarely have opportunities to cooperate with researchers in other branches, who work for patients differing from those in hematologic divisions. The majority of such studies on neutrophils are therefore incomplete, and not very sophisticated. Some of these studies have been carried out by means of simple cytochemical methods, especially those for the estimation of the activity of both alkaline phosphatase and peroxidase and of glycogen content. Biochemical methods have only rarely been used, and there have been few functional studies of neutrophils in patients with the syndromes mentioned.

PREGNANCY AND THE PUERPERAL PERIOD

Alterations in the neutrophil cell system in women during pregnancy and the puerperal period reflect the antiinfectious and antiinflammatory mobilization of these cells. During the third trimester of pregnancy, about 18% of women exhibit leukocytosis higher than 10,000 per cu mm (Diamant et al., 1970). The leukocytosis corresponds to an increase in the absolute neutrophil count. Simultaneously neutrophil precursors appear in the peripheral blood, i.e., metamyelocytes and myelocytes; this indicates the stimulation of the neutrophilic cell series in the bone marrow (Kuvin et al., 1962). A transient increase in neutrophilic leukocytosis is noted for 2 to 3 days after delivery (Lisiewicz et al., 1974). Normalization of the leukocyte count usually occurs in 1 or 2 days. Little is known of the biochemical alterations in neutrophils from pregnant women. It has been shown that the glycogen content increases in these cells (Kowalczyk, 1969). The mechanism of this increase is not known; it may be due to a transient decrease in the content of the enzymes involved in glycogen utilization.

Enzymatic neutrophil mobilization is reflected by an increase in alkaline phosphatase activity, which gradually reaches higher values during the subsequent months of pregnancy (Pritchard, 1957; Cardinali et al., 1970). Maximum enzyme activtiy is observed just before delivery. For 2 to 3 weeks after delivery the enzyme activity normalizes. We have noted that a transient increase in neutrophilic leukocytosis on the second day after delivery is accompanied by an additional transient peak of neutrophil alkaline phosphatase activity (Lisiewicz et al., 1974). The clinical significance of these changes has not been finally established. It has been noted that preeclamptic states, hypertension, and dead fetuses are more frequent in women with low activity of neutrophil alkaline phosphatase than in women with normal activity of this enzyme (Zuckerman et al., 1969; Elder et al., 1971). It is, however, difficult to predict these complications by the enzyme activity index. Evidence has also been advanced that the neutrophil alkaline phosphatase in pregnant women does not differ from that in nonpregnant women as far as thermostability, sensitivity to phenylalanine, and the patterns of distribution on acrylamide gel are concerned (Diamant et al., 1970). Elevated activity of the enzyme in women in advanced pregnancy has been observed by numerous authors (Quigley et al., 1960; Zuckerman et al., 1969; Lisiewicz et al., 1974). The increase in the activity of the enzyme in the neutrophils of pregnant women is due to the thermolabile fraction (Wawryk et al., 1971). Alterations in the activity of the two fractions are not reciprocal.

Mobilization of the intracellular enzymatic apparatus of neutrophils in pregnant women is also reflected in an elevation of the acid phosphatase activity. We have found that the activity of the enzyme is higher in pregnant than in nonpregnant women (Lisiewicz et al., 1977). This increase is significant as soon as during the first months of pregnancy, and later there are no greater changes in the activity of the enzyme. In women with serologic Rh-incompatibility, the activity of the enzyme does not differ from that in other groups of pregnant women (Fig. 19). It may hence be concluded that this type of immune response, due to fetomaternal antigenic incompatibility, the lysosomal apparatus of only lymphocytes and not that of neutrophils is involved (Piotrowski et al., 1977).

Recently attention has been drawn to the diagnostic value of the presence of large numbers of neutrophils in the amniotic fluid. Women with elevated counts of these cells more frequently undergo fever complications (Larsen et al., 1976).

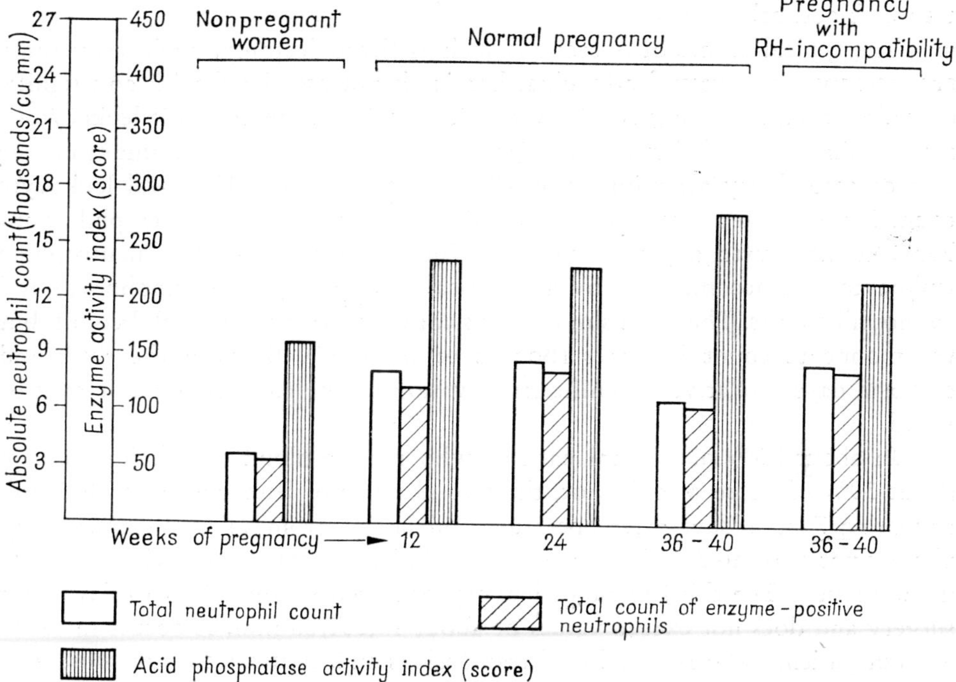

FIG. 19. Alterations in the acid phosphatase activity in peripheral blood neutrophils in women in various periods of pregnancy and in women with fetomaternal Rh-incompatibility. In pregnant women, a significant increase in the enzyme activity is noted, especially during the final stage of pregnancy. In women with fetomaternal Rh-incompatibility, a similar phenomenon is observed. (According to Lisiewicz et al., 1977)

POSTOPERATIVE STATES

In patients after surgery the most frequent change in the neutrophil system is the neutrophilic leukocytosis. The mechanism of this elevation is complex, since several factors—e.g., surgical trauma, basic diseases, the anatomic region of the operation, transfusions or drugs, and anethesia—may be involved. Reactive increase in the neutrophilic leukocytosis is associated with the removal of the tissue remnants from the site of operation, the reaction to the presence of local inflammatory lesions, infections, and pyrogens of various origin.

Surgery influencing the neutrophil system may be exemplified by splenectomy. In many patients this operation results in an increase in the leukocyte count, as well as in the erythrocyte and platelet counts. These changes are associated with the functions of the spleen, such as sequestration and destruction of blood cells.

The typical course of operations such as thyroidectomy, cholecystectomy, gastrectomy, or surgery for inguinal hernias is not associated with any significant alterations in the neutrophil system. In these cases neutrophilic leukocytosis may attain values of about 22,000 per cu mm, reaching the maximum on the first or second day after operation (Bogusz et al., 1967). The total leukocyte count is normalized after one or two days, and the absolute neutrophil count between the fourth and seventh days. The maximal increase in neutrophilic leukocytosis is accompanied by a significant decrease in the lymphocyte and eosinophil counts. There is a similar transient decrease in the basophil count, but the monocyte count increases (Bogusz et al., 1967). Between the sixth and eleventh days a relatively significant elevation of the eosinophil count may be noted.

In about 70% of surgical patients who receive blood transfusions and in about 30% of those who do not, the second phase of leukocytosis is observed, appearing 7 or 8 days after operation and lasting from 24 to 48 hours. This phase is not associated with any detectable clinical alterations, especially fever or inflammation. The third phase of leukocytosis occurs from 10 to 13 days after surgery and does not exceed values of about 14,000/cu mm. It occurs in about 64% of patients who receive blood transfusions and in about 20% of those who do not. As in the second phase, no clinical symptoms explaining the leukocytosis are noted.

There is an almost complete absence of cytokinetic studies elucidating the mechanisms of the variations in neutrophilic leukocytosis in patients after surgery. Despite the fact that the bone marrow contains from 20 to 70 times greater amounts of mature neutrophils than the circulating blood, the tissue neutrophil resources cannot be omitted when these mechanisms are considered (Aleksandrowicz et al., 1976).

A transient neutrophilic leukocytosis in patients after surgery is not *per se* an index of the presence of severe infection or thrombophlebitis, but the inflammatory character of this leukocytosis is unquestionable.

The inflammatory character of postsurgery neutrophilic leukocytosis has also been shown in our studies on the changes in some enzymes in neutrophils. We have demonstrated a significant increase in the neutrophil alkaline phosphatase characterizing inflammations, appearing during the first day after thyroidectomy, reaching its peak on the third day, and gradually normalizing by the end of the first week (Bogusz et al., 1967). A characteristic feature of this increase was that its maximal values were reached after the maximal count in neutrophilic leukocytosis. These observations have been confirmed by other authors (Lyulka et al., 1974). The increase in the neutrophil alkaline phosphatase activity was accompanied by enhanced phagocytic activity and raised glycogen content.

A similar increase in activity in neutrophils from patients after surgical treatment for hyperthyroidism or inguinal hernia is exhibited by acid phosphatase and beta-glucuronidase (Cichocki et al., 1968). In contrast to alkaline phosphatase, the increase in the activity of these two enzymes is maintained on

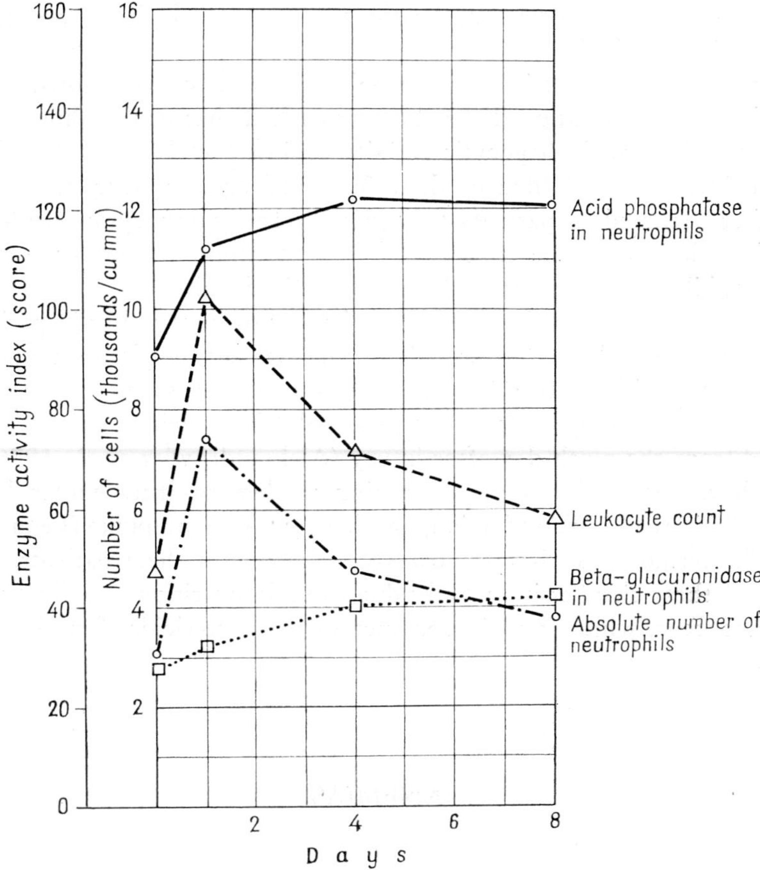

FIG. 20. Changes in the neutrophil acid phosphatase and beta-glucuronidase activities in patients with reactive leukocytosis after surgical operations. (According to Cichocki et al., 1968)

a high level for 8 days after operation despite the normalization of leukocyte and the neutrophil count (Fig. 20). Hence the evolution of activity in the acid and alkaline phosphatases in neutrophils after surgery is not identical.

The mechanisms of increase in the activity of neutrophil lysosomal enzymes in these circumstances are very probably associated with fever and inflammatory reactions, as well as with the release of tissue pyrogens into the blood. The increased neutrophil phagocytic activity reflect attempts to remove the damaged tissue remnants, fibrin, and fragments of connective tissue. It has been stressed that the transient lowering of neutrophil bactericidal activity noted in some patients after surgery might be related to periodic undernutrition (Dhillon et al., 1975). In the patients observed, hypoalbuminemia was not rare. A knowledge of the evolution of changes in the neutrophil system after surgery is of practical importance, since it enables an early diagnosis of inflammatory, hemorrhagic, or thrombotic complications in cases in which the normal course of changes is disturbed.

Significant alterations in the neutrophil system have been noted in patients after kidney transplantation. It has been remarked that neutrophils from these patients exhibit normal phagocytic activity against *Pseudomonas aeruginosa* but abnormal intracellular killing of these microbial agents (Grogan et al., 1975). This defect occurred in patients treated with antilymphocytic serum or high doses of methylprednisone. The effect of these immunosuppressive agents on the neutrophil system has not yet been studied in detail.

Few reports concern the functional changes of neutrophils in patients suffering from burns, who represent a significant percentage of patients hospitalized in surgical divisions. In a 72-year-old woman with severe burns involving about 40% of the body surface, the neutrophil bactericidal activity gradually decreased from the ninth day after injury (Aleksandrowicz et al., 1976). Other authors have reported changes consisting in delayed intracellular killing of bacteria, diminished NBT reduction, and lowered oxygen uptake (Lennard et al., 1974). The phagocytosis index, however, increases in these patients. The mechanism of these changes is partially due to undernutrition and fluctuations in the zinc content, which is of importance in the bactericidal functions of neutrophils.

ANEMIAS

Studies on the structure and functions of neutrophils in patients with various types of anemia have been scanty. This subject, however, is of interest from the standpoint of mechanisms influencing the diminished immunologic response of patients with anemias. It is well known that infectious diseases occur more often in patietns with anemia than in those not showing this condition (Aleksandrowicz et al., 1976). The mechanisms of this phenomenon are not known. The possible relationship between the degree of anemia and of the diminution in the neutrophil functions is not clear. It is not known whether patients with more advanced anemia exhibit a more severe functional defect in the neutrophils, and statistical investigations should be made. Only a few data refer to the effect of anemia on the production and survival time of neutrophils. It is also not known whether the type of anemia is critical for the occurrence of alterations in the neutrophil system.

These problems are directly related to the effect of malnutrition on cells in the neutrophilic series. Children with clinical patterns of undernutrition exhibit a lower count of neutrophils capable of NBT reduction (DeBuse, 1974). The lowered phagocytic activity of neutrophils in patients with burns is probably due to undernutrition and zinc deficiency (Lennard et al., 1974). The effect of protein-calorie malnutrition on neutrophil functions is a problem that has recently been the subject of large population studies. The problem is of special importance in the underdeveloped countries of the "Third World." The results of these studies may be summarized as follows:

1. The chemotactic properties of neutrophils do not undergo any major alterations in protein-calorie undernourished children (Douglas et al., 1977). In 1- to 4-year-old severely malnourished Ghanaian children enhancement of neutrophil chemotaxis has even been noted in some of the subjects studied (Rich et al., 1977).

2. Studies on the early exudative cellular response in skin abrasion sites in undernourished children with kwashiorkor showed no differences as compared with normal healthy children, and it has been concluded that the mobilization of neutrophils in the inflammatory exudate is not diminished in these subjects (Edelman et al., 1977; Leitzmann et al., 1977).

3. The engulfment of particles, polystyrene latex, *Staph. aureus*, *Candida albicans*, and antibody-coated erythrocytes is not altered in undernourished children (Douglas et al., 1977).

4. Intracellular killing of bacteria within the neutrophils is impaired in malnourished children (Douglas et al., 1977). This impairment is especially significant in children with kwashiorkor suffering from various infections, while noninfected children may have normal bactericidal activity.

5. Neutrophils from malnourished children show a quantitative defect in the hexose monophosphate shunt during chronic granulomatous disease (Keusch et al., 1977). In subjects with protein-calorie malnutrition, defective NBT reduction may be concurrent with normal NADPH oxidase activity. A decreased content of some metabolites—e.g., lactate, pyruvate, oxaloacetate, ADP, and ATP—has been found in the neutrophils of undernourished children (Douglas et al., 1977).

It should, however, be emphasized that many reports on the functional and biochemical state of neutrophils in children with protein-calorie malnutrition are controversial, especially as far as the chemotactic activity of these cells is concerned.

In patients with sickle cell anemia the neutrophils show a lowered oxygen uptake, low oxidation of formate, and abnormal NBT reduction during phagocytosis (Dimitrov et al., 1972). These changes do not occur in patients with the sickle cell trait, after splenectomy, or in healthy subjects. It has also been stated that the neutrophil alkaline phosphatase activity in patients with sickle cell anemia showed periodic increases due to vascular crises and hemolysis (Janis et al., 1976). The increases are accompanied by the appearance of abdominal pain. Increased enzyme activity cannot, therefore, be an index of inflammatory processes in every case. Moderate neutrophilia in patients with anemia is due to an increase in the circulating neutrophil pool and reflects, at least to a certain degree, the transition of cells from the marginal to the circulating pool (Boggs et al., 1973). The neutrophil turnover index in these patients indicates a shortened turnover, an unusual feature in neutrophilia for which the mechanism has not yet been fully clarified. The interaction between neutrophils and erythrocytes in patients with hemolytic anemias is not fully understood. The formation of erythrocyte-neutrophil rosettes observed in subjects with autoimmune anemias and the presence of IgG and IgM antibodies is closely related to the same problem (Marmont et al., 1976).

In children with iron deficiency anemia the bactericidal activity of neutrophils may be lowered, while the chemotactic activity of these cells is increased (Chandra, 1974; Kulapongs et al., 1974; MacDougall et al., 1975). Abnormal phagocytic and bactericidal activity in neutrophils is observed relatively rarely. The reduction of NBT may also be diminished in some of these cases. It is interesting that these abnormalities may appear in a subject with latent iron deficiency before the onset of clinical symptoms. The treatment of iron deficiency anemia results in the normalization of the neutrophil function indices within 2–3 months. Other indices of the state of the immune system, such as the immunoglobulin and complement levels, as well as changes in lymphocyte functions, are also normalized during this period. Iron deficiency anemia may be accompanied by hypersegmentation of neutrophils (Doscherholmen et al., 1974).

In patients with acquired refractory anemia a decreased ability of neutrophils to reduce NBT has been noted (Hakim et al., 1974), but a major degree of this abnormality is seldom encountered. Defective iodination occurs in over one fifth of these patients. At the same time, the neutrophils exhibit diminished myeloperoxidase and pyruvic kinase activities; in contrast an increased activity is shown by aldolase, phosphofructokinase, and phosphoglycerate kinase; the activities of glucose-6-phosphate dehydrogenase, 6-phosphogluconate, and NADPH-glutathione reductase are not changed significantly. The mechanism of these enzymatic alterations is not yet known.

216

Alterations in the neutrophil system in patients with anemias due to deficiency of vitamin B_{12} and folates have not often been studied. The most important feature of these anemias is the appearance of neutrophil giant metamyelocytes in the peripheral blood. Some authors have considered these abnormal cells to be degenerating cells which die in the marrow (Tempka et al., 1932). This opinion has recently been confirmed by means of electron microscopic and autoradiographic studies. It has been shown that these cells are characterized by the presence of intracytoplasmic vacuoles and a marked depression of RNA and protein synthesis; they represent cells corresponding to promyelocytes and myelocytes arrested or retarded in their progress through the cell cycle (Wickramasinghe et al., 1977).

The occurrence of hypersegmentation of the nucleus in neutrophils is another aspect of a deficiency of vitamin B_{12} and folate (Hattersley et al., 1974) which may accompany beta-thalassemia E and hemoglobinopathy H (Liyamaswas et al., 1975). There have also been reports on disturbed NBT reduction in neutrophils from patients with megaloblastic anemia (Dreyfus, 1973).

TUMORS

It is known from clinical practice that the terminal phases of malignant processes are accompanied by frequent infections. The mechanism of decreased immune response in patients with malignancies varies, but a certain role is played by disturbances in the neutrophil functions (McRipley et al., 1971; Merkiel et al., 1977). Some data have recently been presented on the role of neutrophils in antitumor immunity. These cells induce a cytotoxic effect on mammalian tumor cells by a mechanism associated with the antimicrobial system composed of myeloperoxidase, hydrogen peroxide, and halide (Clark et al., 1975). It has been shown that neutrophils may exhibit an inhibitory effect on leukemic cells of C57BL/6 mice (Gale et al., 1974). A cytolytic effect is exerted on leukemic cells covered by specific antibodies. The antitumor activity of neutrophils may be inhibited by colchicine and factors interfering with the release of the enzymatic content of the lysosomal granules.

It is not known whether the neutrophil antitumor activity due to the myeloperoxidase-H_2O_2-halide system is identical with that exerted against antibody-coated cells (Gale et al., 1975). Since the lymphoid system produces antibodies to tumor-specific antigens (TSA), these observations on neutrophil action against tumor cells emphasize the link between the neutrophil and the lymphocyte systems in the body response to a malignant process. These data are related to more general problem of mechanisms of the malignant cell killing by hemic cells studied recently (Karpas, 1977).

Diminished neutrophil phagocytic activity has been noted in patients with melanoma (Sander et al., 1976). During the terminal stages of this disease this abnormality was more significantly expressed. The mechanism involved in the decrease in neutrophil phagocytic ability in these cases has not been elucidated. Attention has been called to the fact that the sera of about 50% of melanoma patients inhibit the migration of autologous neutrophils (Cochran et al., 1976). It has recently been demonstrated that decreased bactericidal activity of neutrophils in patients with tumors of digestive tract recovers after its surgical removal (Prokopowicz et al., 1977). Analogously, after the surgical treatment of the tumors normalizes the diminished serum level of lysozyme (Merkiel et al., 1977).

In our own investigations we have ascertained several alterations of the neutrophil lysosomal enzymes in patients with cancer of the larynx. The absolute count of acid phoshpatase-positive and N-acetyl-beta-glucosaminidase-positive neutrophils is elevated in these patients (Gierek et al., 1977, 1979; Lisiewicz et al., 1977), though the intracellular activity of the enzymes, expressed in terms of score index, is not changed significantly (Table 28). A characteristic feature is the diminished beta-glucuronidase activity (Fig. 21). A similar finding has been noted in patients with precancerous states predisposing to cancer of the larynx (Lisiewicz et al., 1978). It is not known whether intracellular neutrophil beta-glucuronidase deficiency in these patients is a primary or secondary phenomenon. It is possible that congenital or acquired deficiency of the enzyme may be a cause of the diminished reactivity of the cells involved in the immune response to tumor tissue. The participation of neutrophils in this response has recently been demonstrated (Clark et al., 1975). Hence it cannot be excluded that deficiencies of some enzymes in neutrophils may result in greater susceptibility to cancerogenic agents. Recently, we have demonstrated that intracellular deficiency of beta-glucuronidase and N-acetyl-beta-glucosaminidase in neutrophils is more expressed in patients underwent radiotherapy and reexamined after 6 to 9 years from the onset of the disease when compared with untreated ones (Gierek et al., 1979; Lisiewicz et al., 1979). Moreover, activity of neutrophil alkaline phosphatase is slightly elevated in irradiated patients whereas activity of myeloperoxidase and the glycogen and the lipid content do not change significantly (Table 28). The diminished resistance of irradiated patients to infections is probably related to above enzymatic deficiencies of neutrophils.

Differentiation between changes in neutrophils caused by inflammatory reaction in the tissues surrounding tumors and those reflecting the cell response to tumor components is difficult. It has been shown that NBT reduction in

TABLE 28. Enzymatic patterns of peripheral blood neutrophils in patients with precancerous states and cancer of the larynx. (According to Lisiewicz et al., 1977, 1978,; Gierek et al., 1979)

Cytochemistry of neutrophils (Methods)		Healthy subjects (20 men)	Patients with precancerous states (24 men)	Patients with cancer of the larynx untreated (20 men)	Patients with cancer of the larynx after radiotherapy (30 men)
		Enzyme activity index (score)			
Beta-glucuronidase	$\overline{X}$	210.1	114.0*	114.5*	84.0**
(Hayashi et al., 1964)	SD	68.7	25.8	46.7	23.8
N-acetyl-beta-glucosami-	$\overline{X}$	133.9	128.2	150.7	73.5**
nidase (Hayashi, 1965)	SD	44.1	39.2	32.3	32.4
Acid phosphatase (Barka	$\overline{X}$	289.3	281.4	287.7	295.4
et al., 1962)	SD	51.0	41.3	48.8	64.8
Alkaline phosphatase	$\overline{X}$	46.8	105.6*	52.7	87.4**
(Kaplow, 1955)	SD	16.2	52.7	23.0	53.2

* Statistically significant differences in comparison to healthy subjects.
** Statistically significant differences in comparison to untreated patients.

neutrophils increases only in these patients with lung cancer in whom infectious complications are concurrent with the malignant process.

Neutropenia and fever are serious clinical problems in patients with malignancies. In many cases the cause of the fever remains obscure, while neutropenia may be a result of antitumor therapy (Rodriguez et al., 1973). The admin-

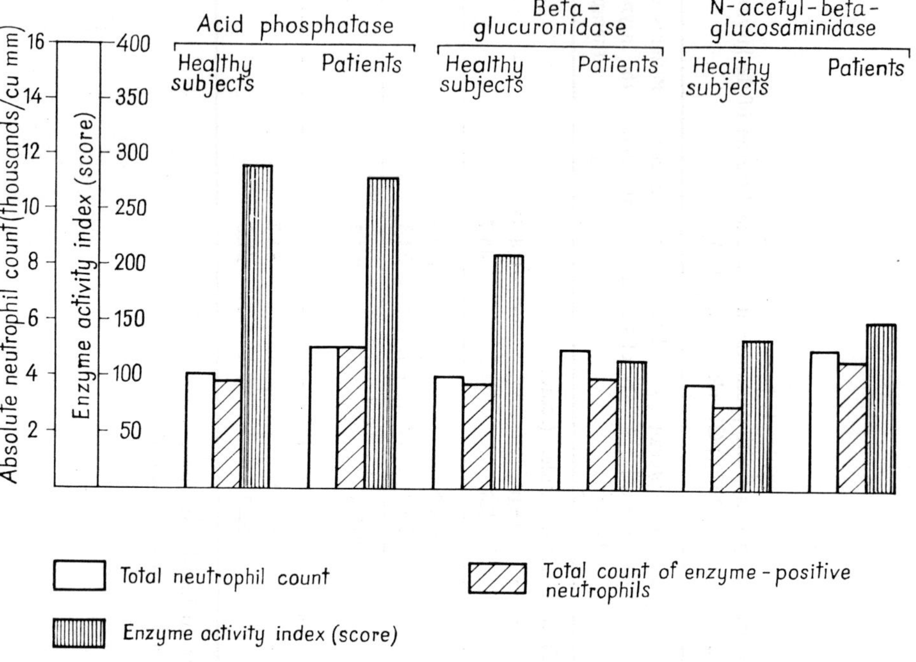

Fig. 21. Acid phosphatase, beta-glucuronidase, and N-acetyl-beta-glucosaminidase activities in peripheral blood neutrophils from healthy subjects and patients with cancer of the larynx. The beta-glucuronidase activity index (score) is significantly diminished in the patients, while the activities of other enzymes are not significantly altered. (According to Lisiewicz et al., 1977; Gierek et al., 1979)

istration of antibiotics like carbenicillin or cephalothin is justified in these patients; the lack of appropriate response for some days is an indication for the use of gentamicin. This therapy diminished the morbidity due to infections in patients with neoplasms. The chemotherapy of malignancies also has an influence on the functional state of neutrophils; in patients treated for metastases in the course of melanomas, sarcomas, cancers of the lung, uterus, testes, breast, etc., neutrophil fungicidal activity is diminished, in contrast to untreated patients (Lehrer et al., 1971). Recently, we have observed diminished activity of N-acetyl-beta-glucosaminidase and myeloperoxidase in neutrophils from women with malignant tumors of reproductive organs (Lisiewicz et al., 1980, unpublished data).

A concept that neutrophils may take part in the immunologic response to tumor tissue (Clark et al., 1975) has initiated our studies on the enzymatic components of these cells in patients with precancerous states of the larynx, i.e., leukoplakia, papillomas, or pachyderma. Numerous alterations have been noted, such as 1) a significant decrease in the beta-glucuronidase-positive neutrophil count; 2) the total absence from the blood of neutrophils with a high activity of this enzyme; the majority of cells contain only traces of the activity of this enzyme; 3) a significant decrease in the enzyme activity index (score) values (Table 29) (Lisiewicz et al., 1978; Gierek et al., 1979).

A decrease in the lipid content and increased alkaline phosphatase activity have also been noted in neutrophils (Table 29). Neither the acid phosphatase and N-acetyl-beta-glucosaminidase activities nor the glycogen content show any changes in these patients. These observations suggest that the metabolic processes related to beta-glucuronidase, with oligosaccharide degradation in the first place, may be depressed in the neutrophils of patients with precancerous states. It is not known whether the energy supply in the cells of these patients is normal. If not, a biologically lowered cell efficiency may be expected. Beta-glucuronidase deficiency in the neutrophils of the patients may be an intracellular defect causing lowered resistance to malignant transformation. This concept, however, requires further study. It should be mentioned that in several women with myomas of the uterus, another precancerous state, we have noted a decrease in the activity of N-acetyl-beta-glucosaminidase and myeloperoxidase in peripheral blood neutrophils (Lisiewicz, 1980, unpublished data).

RHEUMATOID ARTHRITIS

This disease is accompanied by proliferation of the synovial lining and of the stromal cells as well as by infiltrations of neutrophils within the connective tissue of the flexible joints (Zvaifler, 1971). The destruction of the collagenous connective tissue of the articular cartilage is the main alteration accompanying the pathologic process. Several papers on the role of neutrophils in the mechanism of articular lesions in patients with rheumatoid arthritis have recently been published. First of all it has been pointed out that neutrophils possess an enzymatic apparatus which enables them to digest the connective tissue components in the joints. Among the enzymes which have been a subject of interest

TABLE 29. Cytochemistry of neutrophils in patients with precancerous states of the larynx.*
(According to Lisiewicz et al., 1978)

Cytochemical pattern (Methods)	Beta-glucuronidase (Hayashi et al., 1964)	Alkaline phosphatase (Kaplow, 1955)	Acid phosphatase (Barka et al., 1962)	N-acetyl-beta-glucosaminidase (Hayashi, 1965)	Glycogen content (PAS reaction) (Lillie et al., 1953)	Lipids (Sheehan et al., 1947)
Healthy subjects (20 men)						
$\overline{X}$	210.1	52.6	289.3	133.9	296.1	288.4
SD	69.0	23.0	51.0	44.1	2.7	12.5
Patients with precancerous states (24 cases)						
$\overline{X}$	114.0**	105.6**	281.4	128.2	290.8	257.1**
SD	25.8	52.7	41.3	39.3	9.9	43.9

* Results expressed in score values.
** Statistically significant difference.

in this regard collagenase, elastase, and cathepsin G (chymotrypsin) should be mentioned.

Collagenase. This enzyme has now been adequately described in human neutrophils (Lazarus et al., 1968). Two distinct forms of collagenase which can be inactivated by alpha$_1$-antitrypsin are known (Ohlsson et al., 1973). This enzyme acts on cartilage collagen and tendon collagen. According to some suggestions collagenase also degrades proteoglycans.

Elastase. The physicochemical and other properties of this enzyme are well known (Janoff, 1973). The enzyme degrades cartilage matrix proteoglycan, participates in the formation of kinins, and induces increased vascular permeability, which results in swelling and local pain in the joints. The molecular details of the enzyme action on proteoglycans are not known. The esterolytic activity of neutrophil elastase on a synthetic substrate may be inhibited by incubation of a cell granule extract with gold sodium thiomalate (Malemud et al., 1975). It is well known that this agent is efficacious in the therapy of rheumatoid arthritis.

Cathepsin G. This enzyme has been isolated from an extract of neutrophil granules exhibiting properties corresponding to those of the chymotrypsinlike esterases (Rindler et al., 1974; Gerber et al., 1974). Since the enzyme hydrolyzes only some substrates of chymotrypsin, it is usually known as cathepsin G rather than chymotrypsin. Studies of the enzyme action on various substrates suggest that it plays a part in the mechanism of inflammatory changes in the joints (Janoff et al., 1971). The identity of cathepsin G (chymotrypsin) is a subject of discussion (Malemud et al., 1975).

Enzymes degrading components of the connective tissue in the joints may originate not only in neutrophils but also in the rheumatoid synovial tissue. It is not known whether degradation of the substrates mentioned is the only action of neutrophils as far as pathologic articular changes are concerned. The possibility that the neutral proteases in neutrophils might convert bradykininogen into bradykinin and cause increased vascular permeability and consequent swelling of the joint has also been discussed (Movat et al., 1973). It has been suggested that the neutrophil proteases after the degradation and solubilization of the proteoglycans of the articular matrix may release antigenic material, change the antigenic structure of the matrix, and cause an autoimmunologic inflammatory process (Malemud et al., 1975).

Neutropenia is a serious complication in the treatment of rheumatoid arthritis. The mechanism of this neutropenia is currently being studied. The presence of neutrophil-specific antinuclear factors in the serum of patients with the disease has been shown (Wiik et al., 1974). The factors belong to three main

immunoglobulin classes. They are capable of binding with the third component
of the complement system (C_3) and hence are named complement-fixing neutrophil-specific antinuclear factors (NS-ANF). The factors have been detected
in patients who have no symptoms of rheumatoid arthritis but have positive
Waaler-Rose test results and neutropenia. These factors are probably the main
cause of neutropenia in the patients; an autoaggressive mechanism of the neutropenia is highly probable. Rheumatoid complex factor (RCF) may be detected
within the neutrophils by electron microscopic technique (Hoffstein et al.,
1976).

RADIATION INJURY

Irradiation with gamma rays may induce severe depletion of the hematopoietic tissue, resulting in leukopenia and secondary infections. One of the main

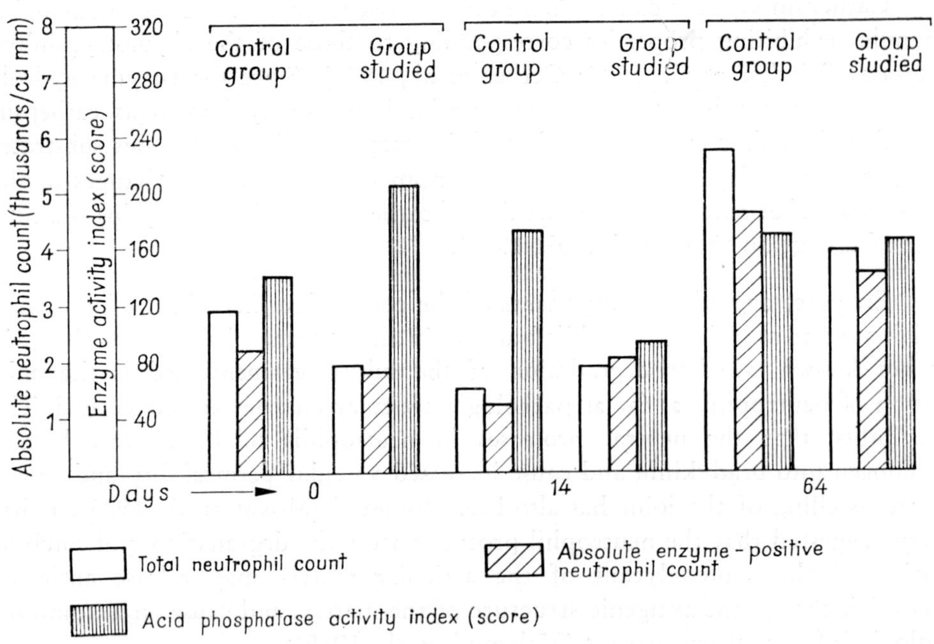

FIG. 22. Effect of irradiation with 450 r on acid phosphatase activity in neutrophils from
Albino-Swiss mice. A decrease in the numbers of both enzyme-negative and enzyme-positive cells
is noted on the 14th day after irradiation, accompanied by a slight rise in enzyme activity. On
the 64th day a reactive increase in the enzyme-positive cell count occurs. (According to Aleksandrowicz et al., 1976)

symptoms of radiation injury is a fall in the neutrophil count. Human neutrophils are relatively resistant to irradiation *in vitro* (Holley et al., 1974). Irradiation causes structural alterations consisting in increased numbers of cytoplasmic vacuoles and diminished density of both nucleus and cytoplasm. It is striking that these alterations are to a certain degree dose-independent. High doses of irradiation may totally arrest chemotactic activity and cause cell death. Neutrophil phagocytic activity is also diminished after irradiation. Experimental irradiation of mice provokes a decrease in the numbers of both acid-phosphatase-positive and acid-phosphatase-negative neutrophils, noted on the 14th day after irradiation (Aleksandrowicz et al., 1976). After about 60 days a reactive increase in the enzyme-positive cell count is noted (Fig. 22).

HYPOGAMMAGLOBULINEMIA

The phagocytic activity of neutrophils from patients with IgG, IgM, and IgA deficiency against *Staph. albus*, *E. coli*, and *Staph. aureus* is normal when the cells are suspended in the serum of healthy subjects (Mickenberg et al., 1970). Incubation of neutrophils from healthy subjects and patients with the foregoing deficiencies in sera of the patients results in diminishing its phagocytic activity. This phenomenon is dependent on opsonizing action of normal serum.

MISCELLANEA

There have been some reports on alterations of the neutrophil system in patients with various diseases which are a subject of interest to dermatologists, allergists, and pulmonologists. The classification of these reports is rather difficult.

In patients with the Sweet syndrome, a type of neutrophilic dermatosis characterized by a specific histologic appearance and an acute clinical course, neutrophilia is less frequently noted than an accelerated erythrocyte sedimentation rate and skin infections (Gunawardena et al., 1975). The edema and articular pains accompanying the syndrome are probably due to the increased numbers of neutrophils in the joint exudate and the presence of large phagocytic cells (Krauser et al., 1975).

Knowledge of neutrophils in patients with lupus erythematosus is scanty. The suppressive action of the patients' sera on the phagocytic properties of these cells has been noted (Zurier, 1976). It is accompanied by a diminished release of lysosomal enzymes within the neutrophils during phagocytosis. This inhibitory effect has not yet found an explanation. It is more marked in patients treated with corticosteroids.

Several dermatologic diseases are characterized by the appearance of pustules, blisters, and eczematous changes in the skin. The neutrophils frequently present within these changes have seldom been studied. The exudative fluid from patients with dermatitis herpetiformis exerts a strong chemotactic effect on neutrophils (Bork, 1975). A patient has been reported in whom generalized pustular psoriasis was accompanied by neutrophil myeloperoxidase deficiency (Stendahl et al., 1976).

In patients with focal and systemic sclerodermia, the neutrophils may exhibit deficiency of acid and alkaline phosphatase (Shapiro et al., 1971). Recurrent defective neutrophil phagocytosis has been observed in a patient with sarcoidosis (Drutz et al., 1975). The defect appeared during periods of complications such as hypercalcemia, erythema nodosum, and pneumococcal pneumonia. The neutrophils from this patient showed a periodic decrease in the alkaline phosphatase content.

In patients with allergic syndromes the neutrophil functions have been studied only occasionally. It has been stated that in patients with rhinitis allergica, specific antiallergic treatment causes a transient decrease in cell phagocytic activity which normalizes after therapy (Nilzen, 1975). In patients with occupational dust bronchitis and an asthmatic component, an increased neutrophil lysosomal enzyme activity has been observed (Ivanova et al., 1975). Patients with ulcerative colitis during exacerbation show an almost threefold increase in the count of neutrophils undergoing damage in the leukocytolysis test (Shakhabazian, 1975). Similar alterations have been noted in patients with rheumatic fever or recurrent tonsillitis (Kustova, 1974).

The neutrophil system in patients with psychoses has not often been investigated. Several ultrastructural alterations have been observed in neutrophils from the blood of patients with schizophrenia. Among the alterations, the appearance of coarse-grained chromatin, indicating elevated numbers of dense helical chromosomes, diminution of the endoplasmic reticulum, and enlarged glycogen granules should be noted (Nanoishvilli et al., 1976). The swelling of the mitochondria, spherical and less compact in structure, intensive breakage of the mitochondrial cristae, an increase in the azurophilic granule count and a decrease of the specific granule count, and an increased amount of granular endoplasmic reticulum, as well as other changes, have been observed. In other studies the greater accessibility of the arginine-rich histones of the neutrophils from schizophrenic patients to the anionic phosphotungstic acid-hematoxylin staining reagent has been demonstrated (Issidorides et al., 1975). These changes reflect ultrastructural alterations in the nuclear chromatin and the altered genome expression. Discussion on the significance of these observations is difficult because

226

of the total absence of other biochemical data on neutrophils from these patients. It may be mentioned that lymphocytes from schizophrenic patients also show define alterations as compared with those from normal subjects (Astaldi et al., 1971).

The biology of neutrophils from patients with congenital hormonal defects and malformations is also known inadequately. Some patients with the Turner syndrome exhibit abnormalities in neutrophil phagocytosis of *Candida albicans* accompanied by disturbances in intracellular killing (Costello, 1975).

Complex cytochemical alterations have been found in neutrophils from patients with the Down syndrome. The alterations consisted in increased alkaline phosphatase activity and decreased activities of ATPase, acid phosphatase, and 5-nucleotidase (Ostojska, 1972). In children with this syndrome complicated by infections, the activities of these enzymes increased. The number of phagocytizing neutrophils in the children was lower than normal, though the phagocytosis index was not altered significantly. Furthermore, the content of pyridoxal phosphate was lowered in the cells (Mahuren et al., 1974). It has been assumed that the turnover of this compound is enhanced in these patients.

In children with proliferative glomerulonephritis, a complex interaction between neutrophils and the glomerular capillary basement membrane has been shown by means of electron microscopy (Morita et al., 1971). The interaction is probably part of a pathogenic process leading to damage of the capillaries.

CHAPTER 12

NEUTROPHILS IN PATIENTS WITH INFECTIOUS DISEASES

Despite the progress of clinical research, numerous infectious diseases have not been studied systematically as far as neutrophil functions are concerned (Aleksandrowicz et al., 1976). The percentage of patients with infectious diseases exhibiting functional defects in the neutrophils prior to patent infection is not known. In children suffering from infections of the urinary tract a decline in the neutrophil ability to reduce NBT is frequently noted (Wolfish et al., 1975). It cannot be excluded that in a number of these cases a congenital or acquired defect in NBT reduction forms the basis for a diminished resistance to infections. Knowledge of the differences in the biologic reactions of neutrophils in relation to the type of microbial causative agent of a given infection is also scanty (Graham, 1975). The results of the NBT test reveal no differences between patients with streptococcal pharyngitis and pharyngitis due to other agents (Shapera et al., 1973). In patients with liver abscesses in the course of amebiasis, the NBT test shows no alterations (Garcia-Tamayo et al., 1974). Significant differences have been noted between the degree of neutrophilic leukocytosis in patients with acute endocarditis, pneumonia, sepses, or local suppurative lesions due to anaerobic infections and in patients with subacute bacterial endocarditis (Frottier et al., 1975). Patients with severe bacterial infections, in contrast to those with viral infections, exhibit a transient defect in the killing of the bacteria after phagocytosis by neutrophils (Solberg et al., 1972; Koch, 1974). The nature of this defect has not been elucidated, but there have been suggestions that bacterial toxins induce a pluridirectional effect on the neutrophil locomotional and enzymatic systems. The bactericidal abilities of neutrophils in patients with severe infections vary on account of various factors. In many cases treatment with antibiotics results in the normalization of previously abnormal bactericidal functions (Copeland et al., 1971). The intracellular content of cathepsin D increases in the neutrophils of these cases. Patients with meningoencephalitis of bacterial origin exhibit more intensive changes in the neutrophil phagocytic activity, as well as more pronounced alterations in the alkaline phosphatase and myeloperoxidase activities, than those with viral meningoencephalitis (Rastuntsev, 1973). In general, neutrophil reactivity is higher in patients with bacterial infections than in those with viral infections.

There are general relationships between the neutrophilic leukocytosis, monocytosis, lymphocytosis, and the immunoglobulin levels, on the one hand, and the clinical stage and evolution of infection, on the other. Neutrophilic leukocytosis is only a small part of the complex immune process occurring in the peripheral blood in the course of infections and inflammations of microbial origin. The first phase of this immune process consists in the mobilization of the phagocyte system, i.e., of the neutrophils and monocytes, resulting in phagocytosis and the intracellular killing of microbial agents. The second phase of the process is accompanied by the mobilization of the lymphocyte and plasma cell system and the synthesis of specific antibodies. The dynamics of this process vary greatly, depending on the type of causative agent, its localization, and individual immunologic patterns (Aleksandrowicz et al., 1976).

The neutrophil reactions in subjects with infections consists in the activation of the lysosomal apparatus and increase in the activity of myeloperoxidase, lysozyme, acid phosphatase, etc. The degree of fluorescence in neutrophils after supravital staining with acridine orange is greater in patients with infections than in healthy volunteers (Melamed et al., 1974). It seems possible that this phenomenon is connected with an increased uptake of dye by the activated lysosomal apparatus of the cells. In patients with chronic inflammatory states of the gut, neutrophil sensitivity to damage increases (Kryshen et al., 1975). The index values of this sensitivity are parallel to the extent of the clinical symptoms. In children with infectious diarrhea, the neutrophil alkaline phosphatase activity is elevated, especially in subjects with toxic forms of the diarrhea (Czauderna, 1973).

As we have recently published a monograph on the alterations in the neutrophil system of patients with infectious diseases, the present chapter will include only general data on substantial changes, especially those concomitant with the infectious diseases that are better known from the point of view of knowledge of neutrophils (Aleksandrowicz et al., 1976). The alterations noted in the neutrophils of patients with various infectious diseases refer to the overall biologic activities of these cells. The general mechanisms of phagocytosis and the intracellular killing of microbial agents engulfed by neutrophils were discussed in detail in previous chapters. Here only the main facts on the response of the neutrophil system in particular infectious diseases will be presented.

DISEASES CAUSED BY VIRUSES

The response of the neutrophil system to infection by viruses depends on the nature of the causative agent, its virulence, the extent of infection, the general state of the patient, and the bone marrow neutrophil reserve. In a number of patients decreased neutrophil and increased lymphocyte counts occur relatively frequently. The evolution of these alterations varies in relation to the nature of the infection.

Infectious Mononucleosis

Absolute neutropenia is noted in about 80% of patients (Cantow et al., 1966). The number of neutrophils in the blood increases during the first 1–2 days but later diminishes significantly (Lou, 1959). By the end of the first week after the onset of illness, leukopenia may occur. About 95% of neutrophils exhibit toxic granulations and Döhle bodies. In individual patients the appearance of 1%–3% of myelocytes and metamyelocytes may be noted. A shift to the right, i.e., an increase in the number of neutrophils with 4, 5, or 6 lobes, is observed in about 45% of patients. The suggestion has been made that this phenomenon is due to a deficiency of folic acid.

Viral Hepatitis

The shift to the left in the neutrophil system is sometimes marked. Neutrophil alkaline phosphatase activity is lowered in the majority of patients (Boll et al., 1969). Increase in the enzyme activity suggests the presence of additional bacterial infection in the body. Leukocyte leukergy is increased (Kowalewski et al., 1953). Few investigations on the kinetics of neutrophils in these patients have been made. Transient disturbances in the migratory capabilities of the cells have been reported (Lorenz et al., 1972). The numbers of neutrophils and their precursors in the bone marrow diminish. Several cases of aplastic and hypoplastic changes in the marrow have been reported as a complication of the disease (Kędrowa, 1966; Rohde et al., 1967; Stieglitz et al., 1968). In some cases diminished numbers of neutrophil precursors, erythroblasts, and megakaryocytes and increased numbers of plasma cells and reticular cells have been observed in the bone marrow (Spatz et al., 1968). An increase in the neutrophil count in the blood and bone marrow in patients with pancytopenia complicating infectious mononucleosis is rare.

Smallpox

The initial period of the disease is characterized by leukopenia (Herrlich et al., 1960). In patients with acute forms of the disease severe neutropenia may be observed, and fragments of neutrophil nuclei appear in the peripheral blood. The progress of the disease is accompanied by a gradual increase in leukocytosis, which may reach values of 12,000 to 15,000/cu mm by the third or fourth day. In patients with additional bacterial infection the leukocyte count in the blood may exceed 50,000/cu mm. A characteristic feature of the leukocyte differential count is the presence of 2% to 15% of myelocytes and metamyelocytes. Myeloblasts and cells classified as hemohistioblasts and hemohistiocytes appear in the blood less frequently (Baugé, 1953). The neutrophils show toxic granulations and vacuolization. Cases have been reported in which the clinical symptoms, the blood and bone marrow pictures, and the autopsy findings resembled those observed in patients suffering from acute leukemia of the paramyeloblastic type.

Dengue

Leukopenia appears between the third and eighth days of illness. In about half the patients with the acute form of the process, the leukocyte count rises above 12,000. In many patients in this group, leukocytosis may reach values within the range of 20,000 to 40,000 per cu mm. Leukocytosis is usually accompanied by absolute neutrophilia. The presence of antileukocyte agglutinins in the serum has not been found in these patients. The neutrophils may exhibit toxic alterations in the nucleus and toxic granulations. The differential leukocyte count is characterized by an increased percentage of stabs and monocytes and the appearance of metamyelocytes.

Influenza

An increase in the leukocyte count exceeding 10,000 per cu mm is observed mainly in cases complicated by pneumonia (Burch et al., 1959). Agranulocytosis is a rare complication of influenza (Dąbski, 1959). The presence of the causative agent of the disease may induce structural changes in the neutrophil nuclear chromatin (Elliot et al., 1958). The acute stage of the disease caused by virus A_2 may be accompanied by diminished phagocytosis of *Staphylococcus epidermidis* by the neutrophils; this normalizes after about a fortnight (Ruutu et al., 1971).

Viral Pneumonia

The hematologic changes in patients with viral pneumonia due to various causative agents are similar. Leukocytosis is usually within the range of 10,000 to 12,000 per cu mm and exceeds these values only in cases with other complications. The first days of illness are accompanied by neutropenia and lymphocytosis, which gradually increase for several days. A shift to the left is noted. Neutrophils may show toxic granulations, but these are not so numerous as in pneumonia of bacterial origin. The leukocyte count may even reach values of about 40,000 per cu mm in patients in whom pneumonia is complicated by hemolytic anemia. In these cases the majority of white blood cells are neutrophils; a shift to the left is also frequently noted, and myelocytes may appear in the circulating blood (Dacie, 1960, 1962).

Measles

It has been demonstrated that neutrophils in the blood of patients with measles exhibit a transient defect in chemotaxis (Anderson et al., 1974). The mechanism of this phenomenon is not known, but it is probably associated with intracellular changes due to the presence of the virus. There is concurrent leukopenia in the majority of cases. The effect of infection by the causative agent of measles on the white blood cell system is especially interesting in patients with concomitant whooping cough. Measles in the early period of whooping cough (second to fourth week) is accompanied by leukopenia (Szczepańska, 1961). Before the appearance of the measles eruption, leukocytosis is high, but during the eruptive period markedly decreases. After the eruptive period leukocytosis again increases but does not attain the previous level. In addition to leukocytosis, the percentage of lymphocytes in the differential blood count is reduced. These observations indicate that the leukopenic effect of measles is also manifested in patients suffering from whooping cough with high leukocytosis. It should be emphasized that measles has an effect on leukocytosis and the differential picture of leukocytes in whooping cough patients differing from that in patients with other infections. Scarlet fever, typhoid fever, viral hepatitis, diphtheria, and mumps concurrent with whooping cough do not influence the white blood cell picture, which remains characteristic of *Bordetella pertussis* infection (Szczepańska, 1961).

DISEASES CAUSED BY RICKETTSIAE

Epidemic Typhus

The febrile period of the disease is characterized by increased leukocytosis with a shift to the left and the appearance of giant promyelocytes. Leukocyte count increases proportionally to the severity of the disease and ranges from 2000 to 26,000 per cu mm (Rosnay, 1947). Leukopenia is usually observed in patients in whom the disease takes a severe course. Neutrophils may exhibit toxic granulations. Convalescence is characterized by neutropenia, monocytosis, and lymphocytosis (Elkeles, 1917). During relapses of the disease the leukocyte count is usually normal, but an increased percentage of stabs may be noted (Kostrzewski, 1956).

Q Fever

The leukocyte count is normal or moderately diminished. The differential leukocyte count is shifted to the left (Oleś et al., 1956). Convalescence is characterized by normalization of the differential leukocyte count, a decrease in the stab numbers, and the appearance of eosinophils; a slow increase in the lymphocyte count may also be observed (Lutyński et al., 1957). The neutrophil alkaline phosphatase activity increases parallel to the increase in the neutrophil count, especially in the early stage of the disease (Beisel, 1966). The maximal increase in enzyme activity is noted on the fifth day of illness, i.e., after the maximal manifestation of the clinical symptoms of the disease, normalization of fever and leukocytosis.

Tsutsugamushi Fever

In the majority of typical cases of the disease leukopenia, neutropenia, and lymphocytosis occur. A characteristic feature is the appearance in the blood of giant mononuclear cells resembling those seen in patients with infectious mononucleosis. Cases have been reported, however, with leukocytosis up to 20,000 per cu mm. The diminished leukocyte count may be due to a decrease in both the neutrophil and lymphocyte count. Occasionally the first attack of the fever may be accompanied by a shift to the left and the disappearance of eosinophils from the blood.

Rocky Mountain Spotted Fever

Leukopenia and neutropenia are noted from the onset of illness, and after about 2 weeks neutrophilic leukocytosis from 10,000 to 15,000 per cu mm occurs, as well as a shift to the left (Phillips et al., 1960; Rubio et al., 1968).

DISEASES CAUSED BY BACTERIA

Pulmonary Tuberculosis

In most patients suffering from pulmonary tuberculosis there are only slight or no alterations in the white blood cell system during the initial stage

(Burgess, 1968; Skotnicki, 1975). Exacerbation of the tuberculous process is usually accompanied by an increase in leukocytes up to 15,000–20,000 per cu mm. In the differential leukocyte count the neutrophil percentage may reach a value of about 80%. The glycogen content within these cells increases (Mecheva et al., 1968). It was long since noted that the increase in the neutrophil count in these patients is an expression of the formation of an abscess or a tuberculous cavity in the lungs (Fenczyn, 1948). In severe cases and in periods of exacerbation neutrophilia is more significant (Lisiewicz, 1963; Sanchez Yllades, 1964). The mechanism of this neutrophilia is not clear. It is known that tuberculin induces a strong chemotactic effect in neutrophils (Boyden, 1962).

The neutrophil alkaline phosphatase (NAP) activity is higher in patients with tuberculosis and a concurrent nonspecific inflammatory process (Godes, 1969). Nonspecific antiinflammatory treatment causes an initial decrease in the NAP activity in this group of patients, and subsequently the normalization of the activity is noted. In patients with focal or disseminated pulmonary tuberculosis, specific treatment may be associated with high NAP activity. In patients with tuberculous meningitis, a high NAP activity is noted for 3 to 4 weeks despite specific treatment. This observation is of importance for the differential diagnosis of various types of meningitis, since patients with meningitis of viral origin exhibit normal activity of the enzyme. Suppurative meningitis due to bacterial infection may also be accompanied by high NAP activity.

An increase in NAP activity may appear in patients prior to the clinical manifestation of the morbid symptoms. In untreated patients with initial asymptomatic pulmonary tuberculosis, the NAP activity is elevated (Lisiewicz et al., 1972). In individual patients we have noted even a fourfold increase in the enzyme activity in comparison with a control group of healthy subjects. In light of these observations, a high NAP activity may serve as an additional indicator of the presence of a tuberculous process. In patients with the infiltrative, focal, or fibrocavernous form of pulmonary tuberculosis, neutrophils also exhibit an increase in cytochrome oxidase activity (Khodyaeva, 1975). In patients with either of the first two forms of the disease, the specific therapy causes normalization of this enzyme's activity, but patients with the third form do not respond in this manner to therapy. Elevation of the cytochrome oxidase activity in the neutrophils persists longer than the pulmonary lesion in the patients treated.

Patients suffering from infiltrative pulmonary tuberculosis exhibit an increae in neutrophil NBT reduction (Ryden et al., 1974; Szczepaniec et al., 1976). Tuberculostatic drugs administered to these patients normalize the NBT test results (Mandell et al., 1972).

There are data indicating that tuberculin may be absorbed on the surface of the neutrophils. In the presence of complement and the respective antibodies, the antigen-antibody reaction takes place on the surface of the neutrophils, and secondary damage of these cells is noted (Kitaev et al., 1975).

Leprosy

An increase in leukocyte count and a shift to the left occur in about 15% of patients (Lechat et al., 1968). The neutrophil alkaline phosphatase activity is not changed significantly (Avila et al., 1970). NBT reduction is also normal (Lim et al., 1974; Goihman-Yahr et al., 1975). Only patients with reactive leprosy exhibit an increase in the number of neutrophils reducing NBT. In a certain percentage of leprotic patients in whom secondary amyloidosis appears, a correlation is observed between the elevated neutrophil count and the serum protein content (SAA), which antigenically is associated with the amyloid fibril protein AA in the serum (McAdam et al., 1975). The suggestion that neutrophils take part in SAA production needs confirmation.

Brucellosis

In about 87% of patients the leukocyte count is normal (Mathur, 1955). The mean values of leukocytes in a group of 308 patients with brucellosis during the first 10 days of the disease were lower than in the next 20 days (Brussolati et al., 1965). In patients with the acute form of the disease without complications, leukocyte count does not usually exceed 10,000 per cu mm. Some authors have noted increased leukocyte counts in about 10% of patients (Giudice, 1956), and others in about one third of patients (Trever et al., 1959). Only a few of the cases reported showed leukocytosis ranging from 14,000 to 19,000 per cu mm. The frequency of occurrence of leukopenia is not high. Only exceptionally has a leukocyte count below 3000 per cu mm been noted. In patients with enlargement of the spleen, leukopenia may be more marked (Civeira et al., 1953).

Individual cases of agranulocytosis have been described. Agranulocytosis may be a result of treatment with chloramphenicol. Leukemoid reactions have been reported in a few cases (Mikułowski et al., 1956).

Some striking features of the phagocytosis of *Brucella* by neutrophils should be emphasized. After engulfment of these microbial agents they do not undergo intracellular killing within the neutrophils *in vitro*, and remain alive for several days (McCullough, 1970). After damage to the neutrophils the *Brucella* microorganisms pass into the surrounding areas. The bacteria are also capable of growth in monocytes. *Brucella* microorganisms are also able to survive in several cells of the body. The presence of these bacteria has been reported in tissue microphages and cells of the reticuloendothelial system. Those properties of *Brucella* which determine their capacity to survive intracellularly are not fully known. The bacteria produce catalase and urease, but do not produce toxins or lytic enzymes, so that the survival of *Brucella* within various cells is possible.

Plague

The bubonic form of the disease is characterized by local swelling of the lymph nodes and bacteremia or septicemia by invasion of the causative agent through the lymphatic vessels. A primary pneumonia is another form of the disease. In both forms of plague, the total leukocyte count is moderately elevated, with a predominance of neutrophils in the differential leukocyte count. In severe cases leukopenia and toxic damage to the bone marrow may be observed (Reed et al., 1970).

Cholera

Neutrophilic leukocytosis is a characteristic feature of the disease. The leukocytosis may reach values of 50,000 to 80,000 per cu mm. Only rarely have cases with neutropenia been reported; these cases have often a fatal prognosis (Chatterjee et al., 1958).

Dysentery

In many patients leukocytosis is significant. Maximal values of leukocytosis are noted at the end of the second week after the onset of illness. The increase in leukocytes is associated mainly with an increase in the neutrophil and neutrophilic stab counts. The phagocytic activity of these cells and their intracellular content of alkaline phosphatase increase (Belogurova, 1971). Leukemoid reactions have been reported in the course of the disease.

Typhoid Fever

During the first one or two weeks the leukocyte count may remain within the normal range. The characteristic leukopenia does not develop before the end of the first or second week (Kostrzewski, 1947). The lower the leukocyte count, the more severe the clinical state of the patients. Usually leukocyte count varies from 3000 to 6000 per cu mm. Leukopenia, however, is not a constant pattern in the patients with typhoid fever. Some authors have observed leukopenia in 68% of cases. Leukocytosis suggests the presence of additional complications. The mechanism of leukopenia in these patients has not been elucidated despite numerous studies.

An autoimmune mechanism with an increased level of antileukocytic antibodies has been suggested (Timina, 1967). The differential leukocyte count usually exhibits an increase in the neutrophil count, a decrease in the lymphocyte count, and the absence of eosinophils from the blood. Patients with normal total leukocyte counts, however, may show no changes in the differential leukocyte count (Kostrzewski, 1947).

Syphilis

Little is known of the alterations in the neutrophil system of patients with primary syphilis. Patients with secondary syphilis show increased leukocyte counts in about half the cases; leukocytosis in these cases does not exceed 12,000 to 15,000 per cu mm. Relative neutropenia is noted in about 71% of patients; it is accompanied by a shift to the left. Leukopenia and neutropenia due to treatment with arsenicals, bismuth, and mercurial preparations were frequently observed in syphilis patients during the early years of this century. Agranulocytosis after treatment has also often been reported. Modern antisyphilitic therapy does not usually cause these complications. Leukopenic reactions after penicillin administration are relatively rare. In patients with the Jarisch-Herxheimer reaction, an increase in neutrophilic leukocytosis is noted (Davis et al., 1969; Warrell et al., 1971). Pyrogens released from the neutrophils very probably play a role in the mechanism of the reaction. There are few cyto-chemical changes in the neutrophils of patients with this reaction. It has long been known that neutrophils accumulate at the site of syphilitic lesions (Lejman, 1952). This is connected with the destruction of the treponemas by these cells. In patients with the Jarisch-Herxheimer reaction, accumulations of neutrophils in the lymph nodes reflect intensive local phagocytosis of the agent causing the disease.

In patients with congenital syphilis leukocytosis varies from 5000 to 30,000 per cu mm, depending on concomitant additional infections. The increase in leukocyte count is not parallel to the severity of the disease (Whittaker et al., 1965). Only on rare occasions does the high leukocytosis resemble a leukemoid reaction with the appearance of young blastic forms. The differential leukocyte count varies greatly; in particular patients an increase in the neutrophil percentage is noted, though in many cases no abnormal values are noted with respect to this. Sometimes neutrophil vacuolization is noted.

Leptospirosis

A leukocyte count ranging from 10,000 to 30,000 per cu mm is a characteristic sign in patients with this disease. Severe cases are characterized by extremely high leukocytosis (Kennedy, 1958). The differential leukocyte count is

238

characterized by an increase in the neutrophil percentage accompanied by a decrease in the lymphocyte and eosinophil percentages. Toxic granulations are often noted in the neutrophils. A shift to the left is observed in many cases.

Whooping Cough

Neutropenia, an elevated total leukocyte count, and lymphocytosis are characteristic changes. Cases have been reported in which leukocytosis up to 110,000, 160,000, 195,000, or 236,000 per cu mm and even more have occurred (Bogdanowicz, 1954; Szczepańska, 1961). According to the general consensus, the lowest level of leukocytosis in patients with whooping cough is at least 10,000 to 15,000 per cu mm. In almost half the patients with complications of this disease, leukocytosis was within the range of 15,000 to 30,000 per cu mm (Szczepańska, 1961). Leukocytosis higher than 60,000 is noted in about $5^0/0$ of cases. In contrast, only $1^0/0$ of patients with uncomplicated whooping cough show such high values of leukocytosis.

Leukocytosis varies depending on the stage of the disease. High leukocytosis persists during the first 4 weeks, and returns to normal values between the fifth and seventh weeks (Szczepańska, 1961). Chloramphenicol therapy causes a lower level of leukocytosis from the beginning of the disease and a more rapid return to normal values. The differential leukocyte count undergoes characteristic changes. First of all there is a significant fall in the percentage of neutrophils while that of lymphocytes rises. In complicated cases neutrophils represent about $20^0/0$ of the white blood cells (Szczepańska, 1961). The lowest neutrophil count is observed during the first 4 weeks of illness, and in the next period the neutrophil count increases gradually. In patients treated with chloramphenicol, the neutrophil count is usually higher than in others. It has been noted that during the first 3 weeks of illness the number of stabs diminishes, but normalizes during the next 2 or 3 weeks (Hansen, et al., 1954).

The mechanism of leukocytosis in whooping cough patients has been the subject of numerous studies and speculations (Fichtelius et al., 1957). It has been suggested that the increase in the lymphocyte count may result from the mechanical removal of cells from the lung tissue or mediastinal lymph nodes. According to one hypothesis, the damaged lungs, where the lymphocytes are destroyed, are unable to remove the cells from the blood, which leads to their accumulation in the circulating blood (Hansen et al., 1954). An allergen isolated from *Bordetella pertussis* causes an increase in the neutrophil count in the blood. A test using this allergen is employed to evaluation of the extent of immunization in children with whooping cough and children vaccinated with ADPT (Pryadkina et al., 1975). It has not been pointed out that the absolute neutrophil count in patients with leukocytosis of about 200,000 per cu mm and a percentage of neutrophils within the range of 10% to 20% is, in fact, significantly elevated. The mechanism of this increase has not been studied as yet.

Diphtheria

In patients with a mild form of the disease leukocytosis is about 11,000 per cu mm; severe cases are characterized by leukocytosis up to 16,000 (Gajda, 1962). In fatal cases prior to death leukocytosis within the range of 20,000 to 56,000 has been reported. The increase in the neutrophil percentage in the differential leukocyte count is proportional to the severity of the disease. In more severe cases a shift to the left and the appearance of myelocytes and metamyelocytes in the circulating blood are observed. Hyperplasia of cells in the neutrophilic series in the bone marrow is a specific pattern of the disease. Toxic granulations frequently occur in the neutrophil cytoplasm (Oye, 1952).

Tetanus

In patients in whom the disease takes a severe course there is a significant neutrophilic leukocytosis (Okulski et al., 1969). We have demonstrated that neutrophils from patients with tetanus show an increase in alkaline phosphatase activity (Caban et al., 1970). The activity of this enzyme is especially high during the full manifestation of the clinical symptoms in patients in whom the disease takes a severe course (Fig. 23). Convalescence is accompanied by normalization of the enzyme activity. The increase in neutrophil alkaline phosphatase activity may be considered an additional prognostic index for the disease. There are few objective indices of the severity of tetanus; hence these observations seem to be of clinical importance. The activity of the neutrophil alkaline phosphatase is not correlated with the activity of the enzyme in the serum (Okulski et al., 1969).

Streptococcal Pneumonia

The number of neutrophils in the blood increases significantly during the first days of illness. In patients treated with antibiotics, the evolution of the total leukocyte and of the neutrophil count is probably parallel. After 10–20 days from the onset of illness, normalization of leukocyte values is observed. Fulminant forms of the disease may result in leukopenia, which has a bad prognostic significance. We have shown that there is a significant increase in neutrophil alkaline phosphatase activity from the onset of clinical symptoms (Mirecka et al., 1970). The increase in enzyme activity was of shorter duration than that in the neutrophil count (Fig. 24). Toxic granulations are numerous in the neutrophils.

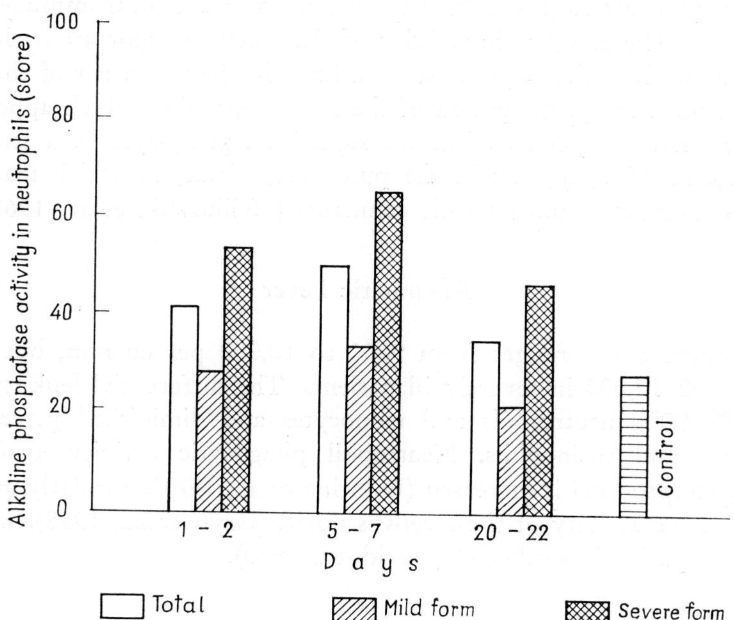

Fig. 23. Changes in alkaline phosphatase activity of neutrophils in patients with tetanus. The highest activity of the enzyme in the group of patients studied was noted between the fifth and seventh days of hospitalization. Patients with a mild clinical form of the disease exhibited lower mean values of the enzyme activity as compared with those in whom the form was severe. (According to Caban et al., 1970)

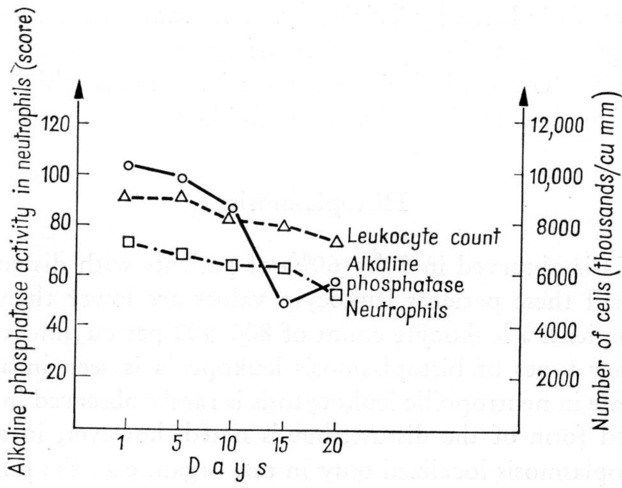

Fig. 24. Changes in neutrophil alkaline phosphatase activity, leukocyte count, and the neutrophil count in streptococcal pneumonia. (According to Mirecka et al., 1970)

Neutrophils are involved in the mechanism of the local immune response in lung tissue. The phagocytic activity of these cells is vigorous at the sites of inflammation. They phagocytize bacteria fixed in the fibrin net of the alveolar exudate without the participation of the serum opsonins, which appear in the blood later. After a period of active superficial phagocytosis, a strong local macrophage reaction appears in the pulmonary tissue, in which macrophages remove inflammatory and necrotic remnants (Halikowski et al., 1968).

Rheumatic Fever

Leukocyte count ranges from 9000 to 10,000 per cu mm, but does not exceed 15,000–19,000 in severely ill patients. The differential leukocyte count shows 70%–90% neutrophils and monocytes and diminished percentages of lymphocytes and eosinophils. Neutrophil phagocytic activity against beta-hemolytic streptococci is increased (Bolotina et al., 1971). Similarly an increase in the leukergic activity of these cells is noted (Grybowska, 1958), while their migratory capacity is weakened (Davidova, 1970).

MYCOSES

There is a lack of systematic studies of the neutrophil system in patients with mycoses. Incubation of neutrophils from the blood of patients suffering from mycosis induced by *Trichophyton rubrum* with an antigen isolated from this fungus causes the appearance of numerous damaged neutrophils (Stepanova, 1975). The clinical significance of the neutrophil sensitivity test against the antigen has not been finally established.

Histoplasmosis

Leukopenia is observed in 50%–60% of patients with disseminated histoplasmosis. In half these patients leukocyte values are lower than 3000 per cu mm. In some patients a leukocyte count of 800–900 per cu mm is noted. In patients with other types of histoplasmosis leukopenia is seen in about 30% of cases. An increase in neutrophilic leukocytosis is rarely observed in patients with the disseminated form of the disease, but is noted, however, in a third of the cases with histoplasmosis localized only in one organ, e.g., the lungs or tongue. A shift to the left and variations in the absolute neutrophil count may also be encountered. Toxic granulations seldom appear.

Candidiasis

Leukocytosis and toxic granulations in neutrophils are seen in some patients (Hulewicz-Grabowska, 1957). Leukocyte count exhibits variations ranging from 8000 to 18,000 per cu mm and is higher in patients with additional bacterial infections (Chlebowski, 1955). In some cases, however, leukopenia is also observed. A case of myeloblastic reaction and thrombocytopenia has been reported (Hański, 1956). In patients with the pleural form of the disease, the evaluation of the hemogram may by difficult owing to other simultaneous infections. An elevated neutrophil count has been noted in cases of pulmonary abscesses. Probably infection with *C. albicans* is easier in a subject with intracellular neutrophil defects. In a 12-year-old boy with candidiasis both the chemotactic and phagocytic neutrophil functions were found to be defective (Bork et al., 1975). The fungicidal properties of these cells are not changed by antibiotics (Kernbaum, 1974).

DISEASES CAUSED BY PROTOZOA

Malaria

During a paroxysm the leukocyte count increases, but in the majority of patients does not exceed 10,000–20,000 per cu mm. Neutrophilia and a shift to the left accompany this increase. According to some authors the neutrophilia denotes an attempt to phagocytize the parasites before the proper phagocytic response of the reticuloendothelial system (Brumpt et al., 1953). The increased biologic activity of the neutrophils is also reflected in enhanced NBT reduction (Anderson, 1971). The neutrophilic leukocytosis is of diagnostic significance during an acute paroxysm, especially in children (Coutellier, 1956). The failure of neutrophilic leukocytosis to decline after the administration of antimalarial drugs casts doubt on the diagnosis. In adults, this phenomenon is less reliable. Toward the end of the febrile period, neutrophilic leukocytosis usually drops and the eosinophil count increases. The neutrophils may contain toxic granulations. Agranulocytosis as a complication of malaria is rare and may be provoked by the therapeutic use of atabrine (Fretland, 1958).

Kala-Azar

Leukopenia is one of the most characteristic features of the disease and is observed in about 90% of patients. It results from a decrease in the neutrophil count. It appears in the early period of the disease and remains within the range of 3000–3500 per cu mm. A normal or increased leukocyte count is usually associated with additional infections. The migratory capacity of neutrophils examined in the Rebuck skin window is lowered (Fernandez et al., 1967). Agranulocytosis is observed in about 3.8% of patients (Kuang-Li, 1959); sometimes it is a result of the morbid process itself, and sometimes it is induced by treatment with antimony preparations (Brachmachari et al., 1955).

DISEASES CAUSED BY WORMS

Hitherto the majority of studies on immunologic alterations in patients infested by worms have been concerned with the lymphocyte system. There have been few publications on the part played by neutrophils. The characteristic pattern of severe infestation by worms is neutrophilic leukocytosis and eosinophilia. In patients with fascioliasis, leukocytosis may reach 20,000–40,000 per cu mm. These changes are not pathognomonic, since patients with normal leukocyte counts or leukopenia have also been reported (Guichard et al., 1959). There are important individual variations in the patient's response to a given worm infestation. The mechanism of this variability is not clear. In some cases the decrease in the neutrophil count may be due to the enlargement and hyperactivity of the spleen. Defective neutrophil NBT reduction has been seen in patients with schistosomiasis in whom hepatosplenomegaly is present (Bagneid et al., 1975). Lowered phagocytic and bactericidal activities have also been noted in the cells of these patients. The morphology of the local inflammatory and infiltrative lesions near the area of the parasite location is another problem. The cellular composition of such lesions is complex, since they consist of various cells involved in the immune response—i.e., neutrophils, lymphocytes, macrophages, etc. There is an almost total lack of data on the functional state and biochemistry of the neutrophils in these inflammatory areas.

The neutrophil cytochemistry in patients infested by worms has seldom been studied. Patients with ancylostomiasis show a decrease in the polysaccharide content in these cells (Nunziante et al., 1956). Knowledge of the state of the antimicrobial machinery of the neutrophils is also very scanty. It may be supposed that the neutrophilic leukocytosis in the majority of patients is associated with an increase in the intracellular content of various enzymes, especially those in the lysosomes. Kinetic studies on neutrophils in patients infested by worms are also inadequate.

FINAL REMARKS

The prospects of research on human neutrophils are closely related to the main biologic activities of these cells, i.e., the phagocytic and the antitumor activities. It has been a striking finding that these activities operate through the same intracellular machinery, the myeloperoxidase-H_2O_2-halide system. Lysosomal enzymes, antibacterial cationic proteins, lysozyme, and other components are also involved in the killing of microbial agents within the cells. The discovery of congenital and acquired deficiencies in the individual components of this antimicrobial machinery of neutrophils, resulting in abnormalities in phagocytosis and the intracellular killing of engulfed microbial agents, and corresponding to definite clinical entities, has been the most important advance in the field. The frequency of these deficiencies and their extent in the human population in various geographic regions are not known and should be the subject of major statistical studies. Prophylaxis with regard to selected subjects with various neutrophil defects who are at high risk of infection should be the target of separate studies and social efforts. Another line of research on neutrophils is investigation of congenital enzymatic deficiencies of these cells which are not known as yet. Several inherited deficiencies in the enzymes involved in the glycolytic pathway have recently been reported in erythrocytes, and it is highly probable that analogous defects will also be demonstrated in neutrophils. Some examples of congenital deficiencies of various enzymes in neutrophils are known and have been discussed in this book.

It should be kept in mind that some intracellular enzymatic deficiencies may represent a secondary effect of biochemical events within a cell; for instance, the diminished activity of pyruvate kinase may be a simple result of a congenital defect in enzyme synthesis but may also be a result of primary ATPase deficiency, causing the accumulation of ATP and secondary feedback-regulated inhibition of pyruvate kinase synthesis, with a consequent decrease in the content of this enzyme in the cell studied. The clinical significance of this phenomenon has recently been demonstrated in erythrocytes.

Human neutrophils are also involved in antitumor immunity through their cytotoxic effect on tumor cells. There is a possibility that deficiencies of various enzymes in neutrophils, congenital or acquired, are critical for the efficacious effect of these cells in antitumor response. We have shown that patients with precancerous states of the larynx—i.e., leukoplakia, papillomas, and pachyderma—and patients with cancer of the larynx exhibit beta-glucuronidase deficiency in the neutrophils. It is difficult to establish the significance of this observation definitively, but a program of further studies to detect subjects with intracellular enzymatic deficiencies in the neutrophils and consequent defective antitumor immunity seems well founded. The cytotoxic effects of neutrophils on human tumor cells should also be the subject of detailed biochemical and biologic studies, since so far the data on this are still scanty.

The next subject for future research on neutrophils is the effects of environmental conditions and nutritional factors on neutrophil function. An excess of chemicals of industrial origin, toxic to neutrophils, has appeared in the human environment in recent years; and the deficiency of various components in food and water, including proteins and trace elements, may result in manifold alterations diminishing the reactivity and vitality of neutrophils. A large-scale program of research in this field has recently been proposed in our division.

The author is free from the illusion that this book comprises to a satisfactory degree the total scope of knowledge on human neutrophils, but if students in the field find in this text information not easily available in the sources at their command, or the impetus to undertake investigations on hitherto unanswered questions, the author will have realized his aim.

REFERENCES

Ackerman BD: Dysgammaglobulinemia: report of a case with a family history of a congenital gamma globulin disorder. Pediatrics, 1964, 34, 211–219

Ackerman GA: Ultrastructural histochemical alteration of the plasma membrane in chronic myelocytic leukemia. Blood, 1975, 46, 869–881

Ageikin VA, Filin VA, Khalidova RR: Functional condition of neutrophils of the blood in neutropenias of children. Pediatriya, 1973, 8, 33–37

Albarracin NS, Haust MD: Intravascular coagulation in promyelocytic leukemia. Ann J Clin Pathol, 1971, 55, 677–685

Alder A: Über Konstitutionell bedingte Granulationsberänderungen der Leukozyten. Deutsch Arch Klin Med, 1939, 183, 372–378

Aleksandrowicz J (ed): Diseases of the Blood and Blood Forming Organs (in Polish). Polish Medical Publishers, Warsaw, 1969

Aleksandrowicz J: Micotoxinas, bioelementos y perspectivas de la profilaxis ecológica délla leukemia. Rev Esp Oncol, 1975, 22, 311–334

Aleksandrowicz J, Blicharski J, Lisiewicz J, Dzigowska A: Leuko- and oncogenesis in the light of studies on the metabolism of magnesium and its turnover in biocenosis. Acta Med Pol, 1970, 11, 289–302

Aleksandrowicz J, Lisiewicz J: The cytogenesis of the white blood cells in the light of the neounitarian theory. Acta Med Pol, 1970, 11, 43–57

Aleksandrowicz J, Lisiewicz J: Hematology of Infectious Diseases. Polish Medical Publishers, Warsaw, 1976

Aleksandrowicz J, Ważewska-Czyżewska M, Szybiński Z, Bodzoń A, Sąsiadek U, Lisiewicz J: Effect of irradiation on activity of lysosomal acid phosphatase in peripheral blood granulocytes of mice (in Polish). Post Fiz Med, 1976, 11, 113–118

Allen RC, Steele RH: The functional generation of electronic excitation states by myeloperoxidase. Fed Proc, 1973, 32, 478–482

Allen RC, Stjernholm RL, Steele RH: Evidence for the generation of an electronic excitation state(s) in human polymorphonuclear leukocytes and its participation in bactericidal activity. Biochem Biophys Res Commun, 1972, 47, 679–684

Allison F, Lancaster MG: Studies on factors which influence the adhesiveness of leukocytes in vitro. Ann NY Acad Sci, 1964, 116, 936–944

Allison F, Lancaster MG: Pathogenesis of acute inflammation. VI. Influence of osmolarity and certain metabolic antagonists upon phagocytosis and adhesiveness by leukocytes recovered from man. Proc Soc Exp Biol Med, 1965, 119, 56–61

Alnikov GP: On the problem of influence of the formed blood elements on blood coagulation in acute leukemia (in Russian). Probl Gematol, 1973, 18, 38–41

Alper CA, Stossel TP, Rosen FS: Complement disease in man. In Bellanti JA, Dayton DH (eds): The Phagocytic Cell in Host Resistance. National Institute of Child Health, New York, Raven Press, 1975, pp 127–143

Alpidovskii VK: On procoagulant and fibrinolytic properties of hemocytoblasts and their effect on the expression of hemorrhagic syndrome in patients with acute leukemia (in Russian). Probl Gematol, 1967, 11, 24–28

Altman AJ, Stossel TP: Functional immaturity of bone marrow bands and polymorphonuclear leukocytes. Br J Haematol, 1974, 27, 241–245

Altman PL, Dittmer DS: Blood and Other Body Fluids. Federation of American Societies for Experimental Biology, Washington, 1961

Andarzhanov FK, Nikolaeva LD, Makareva LM: Characteristics of the hemogram and cytochemical indices of peripheral blood neutrophils in children living in the region of the discharges from petrochemical industry enterprises (in Russian). Gig Sanit, 1974, 10, 117–118

Anderson BR: Ultrastructure of normal and leukemic leukocytes in human peripheral blood. Ultrastruct Res, Suppl, 1966, 9, 6–42

Anderson BR: NBT test in malaria. Lancet, 1971, 2, 317

Anderson BR, Sher R, Rabson AR, Kornhof HJ: Defective chemotaxis in measles patients. S Afr Med J, 1974, 48, 1819–1920

Anderson BR, Van Epps DE: Suppression of chemotactic activity of human neutrophils by streptolysin O. J Infact Dis, 1972, 125, 353–359

André L, Marty J, Rispe R: Sur un cas de leucémic aiguë précédée de neutropénic pendant dix-huit mois. Bull Soc Med Hop Paris, 1953, 69, 419

Arrowsmith D, Morin RJ: Oral contraceptives and the NBT test. Lancet, 1973, 1, 148–149

Asamer H, Schmazl F, Braunsteiner H: Der Immunzytologische Lysozymnachweis in menschlichen Blutzellen. Acta Haematol, 1969, 41, 49–54

Asghar SS, Cormane RH: Some properties of proteolysis by polymorphonuclear leukocyte-granule extracts. J Invest Dermatol, 1976, 66, 93–98

Ashkenazi YE, Ramot B, Brok-Simoni F, Holtzman F: Blood leukocyte enzyme activities. I. Diurnal rhythm in normal individuals. J Interdiscipl Cycle Res, 1973, 4, 193–205

Astaldi G, Lisiewicz J: Lymphocytes: Structure, Production, Functions. Casa Editrice Idelson, Naples, 1971

Aster RH, Euright SE: A platelet and granulocyte membrane defect in paroxysmal nocturnal hemoglobinuria: usefulness for the detection of platelet antibodies. J Clin Invest, 1969, 48, 1199–1210

Astrup T, Henrichen J, Kwaan HC: Protease content and fibrinolytic activity of human leukocytes. Blood, 1967, 29, 134–138

Athens JW: Leukocyte physiology. JAMA, 1966, 198, 38–42

Athens JW, Haab OP, Raab SO, Mauer AM, Ashenbrucker H, Cartwright GE, Wintrobe MM: Leukokinetic studies. IV. The total blood, circulating and marginal granulocyte pools and the granulocyte turnover rate in normal subjects. J Clin Invest, 1961, 40, 989–991

Avila JL, Convit J: Studies of cellular immunity in leprosy. I. Lysosomal enzymes. Int J Lepr, 1970, 38, 359–364

Azimi P, Bodenbender JG, Hintz RL, Kontras SB: Chronic granulomatous disease in three sisters. Lancet, 1968, 1, 208–209

Babior BM, Kipnes RS, Curnutte JT: Biological defense mechanisms. The production by leukocytes of superoxide, a potential bactericidal agent. J Clin Invest, 1973, 52, 741–744

Bacz A, Borkowski W, Lisiewicz J, Paradysz A: The neutrophil alkaline phosphatase activity in women with the hypothalamosis syndrome (in Polish). Ginekol Pol, 1974, 55, 961–964

Baehner RL: Microbe ingestion and killing by neutrophils: normal mechanism and abnormalities. Clin Haematol, 1975, 4, 609–633

Baehner RL, Johnston RB, Nathan DG: Reduced pyridine nucleotide (RPN) content in G-6-PD deficient granulocytes (PMN): an explanation for their defective bactericidal function. Proc Am Soc Clin Invest, 1975, 13, 4–8

Baehner RL, Karnovsky ML: Deficiency of reduced nicotinamide-adenine dinucleotide oxidase in chronic granulomatous disease. Science, 1968, 162, 1277–1280

Baehner RL, Karnovsky MJ, Karnovsky ML: Degranulation of leukocytes in chronic granulomatous disease. J Clin Invest, 1969, 48, 187–190

Baehner RL, Nathan DG: Leukocyte oxidase: defective activity in chronic granulomatous disease. Science, 1967, 155, 835–837

Baehner RL, Nathan DG: Quantitative nitroblue tetrazolium test in chronic granulomatous disease. N Engl J Med, 1968, 278, 971–976

Baehner RL, Neiburger RG, Johnson DE: Bactericidal defect in blood of children with acute lymphoblastic leukemia. N Engl J Med, 1973, 289, 1209–1212

Baggiolini M, deDuve C, Masson PL, Heremans JF: Association of lactoferrin with specific granules in rabbit heterophil leukocytes, J Exp Med, 1970, 131, 559–570

Baggiolini M, Feigenson ME, Schnebli HP: Ricin- and concanavalin A-binding sites on the surface of polymorphonuclear leukocytes have no receptor function in phagocytosis. Schweiz Med Wschr, 1976, 106, 1371–1372

Bagneid M, Kamel MS, Shaker A: Effectiveness of the nitroblue tetrazolium test in demonstrating reduced bactericidal activity of polymorphonuclear neutrophils in schistosomal hepatosplenomegaly and ascites. Am J Clin Pathol, 1975 63, 921–926

Baikie AG: Chromosomes and leukemia. Acta Haematol, 1966, 36, 157

Bainton DF: Sequential degranulation of the two types of polymorphonuclear leukocyte granules during phagocytosis of microorganisms. J Cell Biol, 1973, 58, 249–264

Bainton DF: Abnormal neutrophils in acute myelogenous leukemia: identification of subpopulations based on analysis of azurophil and specific granules. Blood Cells, 1975, 1, 191–199

Bainton DF: Differentiation of human neutrophilic granulocytes: normal and abnormal. In Greenwalt TI, Jamieson GA (eds): The Granulocyte: Function and Clinical Utilization. Alan R Liss, Inc, New York, 1977, pp 1–27

Bainton DF, Farquhar MG: Nature of human neutrophilic leukocyte granules (PMN). Fed Proc, 1969, 28, 617–620

Bainton DF, Ullyot JL, Farquhar MG: The development of neutrophilic polymorphonuclear leukocytes in human bone marrow. Origin and content of azurophil and specific granules. J Exp Med, 1971, 134, 907–1001

Ban A, Nagy M: A granulocyták alkilus phosphatase aktivitásának és osmotikus resistentiájának változása bakteriális lipopolysaccharida hatására. Haematol Hung, 1966, 6, 153–162

Banerjee TK, Senn HJ, Holland FJ: Comparative studies on localized leukocyte mobilization in patients with chronic myelocytic leukemia. Cancer, 1972, 29, 637–640

Barkve H: Cyclic neutropenia. Report of a case treated with high doses of testosterone. Acta Med Scand, 1967, 182, 503–507

Barnhart MI: Importance of neutrophilic leukocytes in the resolution of fibrin. Fed Proc, 1965, 24, 846–853

Baugé E: L'hémogramme dans la variole en Nord-Viet-Nam. Sang, 1953, 24, 23–37

Baum J: Chemotaxis in human disease. In Bellanti JA, Dayton DH (eds): The Phagocytic Cell in Host Resistance. National Institute of Child Health, New York, Raven Press, 1975

Beaver DL, Dummit ES: "Leukocyte emigrating factor" of mouse uterus. Arch Pathol, 1963, 75, 543–548.

Beck WS: The control of leukocyte glycolysis. J Biol Chem, 1958, 232, 251–254

Becker EL, Davis AT, Estensen RD, Quie PG: Cytochalasin B. IV. Inhibition and stimulation of chemotaxis of rabbit and human polymorphonuclear leukocytes. J Immunol, 1972, 108, 396–402

Beckmann A: Über die Beteiligung von Neutrophilen, Eosinophilen und Basophilen granulozyten an immunologischen Prozessen. Folia Haematol (Leipz), 1974, 101, 889–898

Beisel WR: Neutrophil alkaline phosphatase changes in tularemia, sandfly fever, Q fever and non-infectious fevers. Blood, 1966, 29, 257–268

Belding ME, Klebanoff SJ, Ray CG: Peroxidase-mediated virucidal systems. Science, 1970, 167, 195–196

Běleš P, Sova J: Immunofluorescence of neutrophil leukocytes as evidence of phagocytosis of fibrinogen, fibrin or their metabolites. Cas Lek Cesk, 1972, 111, 224–225

Bellanti JA, Cantz BE, Schlegel RJ: Accelerated decay of glucose-6-phosphate dehydrogenase activity in chronic granulomatous disease. Pediatr Res, 1970, 4, 405–409

Berendes H, Bridges RA, Good RA: Fatal granulomatous disease of childhood. Clinical study of a new syndrome. Minn Med, 1957, 40, 309–312

Berlin RD: Effect on concanavalin A on phagocytosis. Nature (Lond), 1972, 235, 44–45

Bernard J, Lasneret J, Choma J, Levy JP, Boiron M: A cytological and histological study of acute promyelocytic leukaemia. J Clin Pathol, 1963, 16, 319–324

Bertino JR, Dilber R, Freedman M, Alenty A, Albrecht M, Gabrio MW, Huennekens FM: Studies on normal and leukemic leukocytes. IV. Tetrahydrofolate-dependent enzyme systems and dihydrofolic reductase. J Clin Invest, 1963, 42, 1899–1904

Bessis M: Living Cells and Their Ultrastructure. Springer-Verlag, Berlin–Heidelberg–New York, 1973, pp 284–323

Belogurova AF: Phagocytic and phosphatase activities of leukocytes in acute dysentery (in Russian). Sov Med, 1971, 34, 130–131

Bierman HR, Hood JE: Study of a granulopoietic factor from endotoxin-stimulated mouse plasma. Br J Haematol, 1972, 22, 145–153

Bierman HR, Kelly KH, Byron RL Jr, Marshall GJ: Leukapheresis in man. I. Haematological observations following leukocyte withdrawal in patients with non-haematological disorders. Br J Haematol, 1961, 7, 51–63

Bierman HR, Marshall GJ, Kelly KH, Byron RL: Leukapheresis in man. III. Hematological observations in patients with leukemia and myeloid metaplasia. Blood, 1963, 21, 164–182

Bishop CR: Leukokinetic studies. XIV. Blood neutrophil kinetics in chronic, steady-state neutropenia. J Clin Invest, 1971, 50, 1678–1680

Björkstén B, Lundmark KM: Abnormal nitroblue tetrazolium test in relatives of a female with chronic granulomatous disease. Scand J Infect Dis, 1972, 4, 167–169

Bjure N, Nilsson LR, Plum CM: Familial neutropenia possibly caused by deficiency of a plasma factor. Acta Pediatr, 1962, 51, 497–498

Blair TR, Bayrd ED, Pease GL: Atypical leukemia. JAMA, 1966, 198, 21–24

Bleiber R, Kunze D, Reichmann G: Leukocyte lipids in mature cell leukemias. Acta Haematol, 1976, 55, 81–88

Bleyl R: Fibrinolyse durch Leukozyten. Therapeutische und experimentelle Fibrinolyse. Internationales Symposium (29.IX.–1.X.) Ulm (Donau), 1967, pp 59–62

Blicharski J: Lipids in blood cells (in Polish). Folia Biol, 1953, 1, 209–221

Block M, Jacobson LO, Bethard WI: Preleukemic acute human leukemia. JAMA, 1953, 152, 1018–1019

Blume RS, Bennett JM, Yankee RA, Wolff SM: Defective granulocyte regulation in the Chediak-Higashi syndrome. N Engl J Med, 1968, 279, 1009–1010

Bogdanowicz J (ed): Pertussis (in Polish). Polish Medical Publisher, Warsaw, 1954

Boggs DR: The cellular composition of inflammatory exudates in human leukemia. Blood, 1960, 15, 466–470

Boggs DR, Athens JW, Haab OP, Raab SO, Cartwright GE, Wintrobe MM: Induced inflammatory exudates in normal man. A method designed to study the qualitative and quantitative cellular response to a pyogenic stimulus. Am J Pathol, 1964, 44, 61–66

Boggs DR, Hyde F, Srodes C: An unusual pattern of neutrophil kinetics in sickle cell anemia. Blood, 1973, 41, 59–65

Bogusz J, Lisiewicz J: Blood and blood forming organs in hyperthyroidism. A review. Hematologia (Budap), 1968, 2, 293–400

Bogusz J, Mirecka J, Kahl J, Lisiewicz J: Alterations in the granulocyte alkaline phosphatase activity after surgical treatment of hyperthyreosis with reference to other changes in white blood cell system (in Polish). Przegl Lek, 1967, 23, 611–614

Boivin P, Hakim J, Mandreau J, Galand C, Degos F, Schaison G: Déficit en 3-phosphoglycérate kinase érythrocytaire et leukocytaire. Etude des propriétes de l'enzyme, de la fonction phagocytaire des polynucléaires et revue de la littérature. Nouv Rev Fr Hematol, 1974, 14, 495–508

Boll ITM, Kuhn A: Granulocytopoiesis in human bone marrow cultures studied by means of kinematography. Blood, 1965, 26, 449–453

Boll ITM, Wujanz GI: Die alkalische Leukozytenphosphatase bei der Diagnose der akuten hepatitis. Dtsch Med Wschr, 1969, 94, 318–322

Bölling R, Kleeberg UR: Granulocyte metabolism and function in patients with leukemia. Second Meeting of the European and African Division of the International Society of Haematology, Prague, 1973, pp 451–458

Bolotina A Jr, Mikhailova IM: Remarks on phagocytosis in the non-active stage of rheumatic fever (in Russian). Vopr Revm, 1971, 11, 17–24

Borchardt L: Übergang von Agranulocytose in Myeloblastenleukämie? Med Klin, 1930, 10, 341–343

Borel JF, Keller HU, Sorkin E: Studies on chemotaxis. XI. Effect on neutrophils of lysosomal and other subcellular fractions from leukocytes. Int Arch Allergy, 1969, 35, 194–205

Bork K: The chemotactic effect of blister roof, blister fluid and blister floor on polymorphonuclear leukocytes in dermatitis herpetiformis Duhring. Arch Dermatol Forsch, 1975, 252, 47–51

Bork K, Denk B: Defective polymorphonuclear leukocyte function in chronic granulomatous muco-cutaneous candidiasis. Arch Dermatol Res, 1975, 254, 233–238

Bottomley RH: Comparison of alkaline phosphatase from human normal and leukemic leukocytes. Cancer Res, 1969, 29, 1866–1867

Bourne HR, Lehrer RJ, Cline MJ, Melmon KL: Cyclic 3,5-adenosinemonophosphate in the human leukocyte: synthesis, degradation and the effect on neutrophil candidacidal activity. J Clin Invest, 1971, 50, 920–929

Boxer LA, Greenberg MS, Boxer GJ, Stossel TP: Autoimmune neutropenia. N Engl J Med, 1975, 293, 748–753

Boxer LA, Hedley-Whyte T, Glader B: A primary defect in neutrophil mobility. Clin Res, 1974, 22, 384

Boxer LA, Hedley-Whyte T, Stossel TP: Neutrophil actin dysfunction and abnormal neutrophil behavior. N Engl J Med, 1974, 291, 1093–1099

Boxer LA, Rister M, Allen JM, Baehner RL: Improvement of Chediak-Higashi leukocyte function by cyclic guanosine monophosphate. Blood, 1977, 49, 9–17

Boxer LA, Stossel TP: Effects of anti-human neutrophil antibodies in vitro. J Clin Invest, 1974, 53, 1534–1545

Boxer LA, Watanabe AM, Rister M, Besch HR, Allen JM, Baehner RL: Correction of leukocyte function in Chediak-Higashi syndrome by ascorbate. N Engl J Med, 1976, 295, 1041–1045

Boyden S: The chemotactic effect of mixtures of antibody and antigen on polymorphonuclear leukocytes. J Exp Med, 1962 115, 453–466

Brachmachari PN, Maiti CR: Agranulocytosis following antimony therapy in kala-azar. J Indian Med Assoc, 1955, 25, 408–410

Brandt IK, De Luca VA Jr: Type III glycogenosis: A family with an unusual tissue distribution of the enzyme lesion. Am J Med, 1966, 40, 779–781

Brandt J: Reduced number of peripheral blood granulocytes in chronic myeloid leukaemia during administration of clofazimine (B 663). Scand J Haematol, 1972, 9, 159–166

Brandt L: Stimulating effect of clofazimine (B 663) on the phagocytic capacity of human granulocytes in vitro and in vivo. XIV International Congress of Hematology. Sao Paulo, Brazil, (July 16–21) 1972, Abstracts 130

Braun EH, Buchwold AE, Emson HE, Russel AV: Familial neonatal neutropenia with maternal leucocyte antibodies. Blood, 1960, 16, 1745–1747

Braunsteiner H, Dienstl F, Sailer S, Sauchhofer F: Über den Nachweis einer sauren Lipase in weissen Blutzellen. Acta Haematol (Basel), 1965, 33, 335–340

Brayton RG, Stokes P, Louria DB: Polymorphonuclear leukocyte mobilization in man. Clin Res, 1964, 12, 221

Breton-Gorius J: Structures périodiques dans les granulations éosinophiles et neutrophiles des leucocytes polynucleaires du sang de l'homme. Nouv Rev Fr Hematol, 1966, 6, 195–208

Breton-Gorius J, Houssay D, Vilde JL, Dreyfus B: Partial myeloperoxidase deficiency in a case of preleukaemia. II. Defects of degranulation and abnormal bactericidal activity of blood neutrophils. Br J Haematol, 1975, 30, 279–288

Bretz U, Dewald D, Baggiolini M, Vischer TL: In vitro stimulation of lymphocytes by neutral proteinases from human polymorphonuclear leukocyte granules. Schweiz Med Wschr, 1976, 106, 1373–1374

Bridges RB, Kraal JH, Huang LJT, Chancellor MB: Effects of tobacco smoke on chemotaxis and glucose metabolism of polymorphonuclear leukocytes. Infect Immun, 1977, 15, 115–123

Brière J, Castro-Malaspina H, Tanzer J, Bernard J: Les leucemies myeloides subaugues a chromosome de Philadelphia. Nouv Rev Fr Hematol, 1975, 15, 407–424

Brogan AB: Phagocytosis by polymorphonuclear leukocytes from patients with renal failure. Br Med J, 1967, 3, 596–599

Brubaker LH: Unsticky neutrophils. N Engl J Med, 1974, 291, 674–675

Brumpt L, Ho-Thi-Sang: Les granulocytes mélanifères du paludisme. Bull Soc Pathol Exot, 1953, 46, 506–510

Brun J, Perrin-Fayolle A, Sedallian A: Gentamicin in pneumology: a clinical and bacteriological study. Lyon Med, 1967, 218, 1263–1265

Brunelli MA, Bagnara GP, Astaldi G, Carnevali C, Topuz U, Rizzoli C: A preliminary study on humoral control of granulopoiesis in primary myelofibrosis and chronic granulocytic leukaemia. Boll Ist Sieroter Milan, 1976, 55, 431–435

Brunning RD, Parkin J, Dick F, Nesbit M: Unusual inclusions occurring in the blasts of four patients with acute leukemia and Down's syndrome. Blood, 1974, 44, 735–741

Bryan HG, Nixon RK: Dyskeratosis congenital and familial pancytopenia. JAMA, 1965, 192, 203–208

Bryniak C, Bunsch-Welkens K, Doleżal M, Janik J: The leukergy test in newborns. Part V. Sex-dependence of leukergy (in Polish). Ginekol Pol, 1974, 45, 571–574

Bryniak C, Lisiewicz J: Neutrophil alkaline phosphatase and lymphocyte acid phosphatase in the premature infant (in Polish). Ginekol Pol, 1975, 46, 865–868

Bull JM, DeVita VT, Carbone PP: In vitro granulocyte production in patients with Hodgkin's disease and lymphocytic, histiocytic, and mixed lymphomas. Blood, 1975, 45, 833–842

Burch GE, Walsh JJ, Magabagab WJ: Asian influenza—clinical picture. Arch Intern Med, 1959, 103, 696–707

Burdick CO: Lipidosis of the spleen with thrombocytopenic purpura, leukocytosis, and amyloidosis. Arch Pathol, 1965, 79, 583–587

Burgess AM: Notes on the diagnosis of pulmonary tuberculosis, with special reference to the leucocyte count. RI Med J, 1968, 51, 552–554

Burke V, Colebatch JH, Anderson CM, Somons MJ: Association of pancreatic insufficiency and chronic neutropenia in childhood. Arch Dis Child, 1967, 42, 147–150

Burkens JCJ: Agranulocytose gevolgd door leucaemia. Ned Tijdschr Geneeskd, 1931, 75, 2722–2724

Bussel A, Benbunan M, Tanzer J, Bernard P: Report of a simple method of collecting leucocytes from patients with chronic myeloid leukaemia. In Goldman JM, Lowenthal RM (eds): Leucocytes: Separation, Collection and Transfusion. Academic Press, London, New York, San Francisco, 1975, pp 112–119

Bussolati C, Sperzani G: Il nuovo quadro clinico della malattia brucellare trattata con antibiotici. Gaz Sanit, 1965, 35, 1–7

Bybee JD, Rogers DE: The phagocytic activity of polymorphonuclear leucocytes obtained from patients with diabetes mellitus. J Lab Clin Med, 1964, 64, 1–13

Caban J, Okulski J, Mirecka J, Lisiewicz J: Activity of alkaline phosphatase of blood neutrophils in patients with tetanus. Pol Med J, 1970, 9, 626–628

Canellos GP, Whang-Peng J, DeVita VT: Chronic granulocytic leukemia without the Philadelphia chromosome. Am J Clin Pathol, 1976, 467–470

Cantow EF, Kostinas JE: Studies on infectious mononucleosis. IV. Changes in the granulocytic series. Am J Clin Pathol, 1966, 46, 43–47

Cantow EF, Kostinas JE: Studies on infectious mononucleosis. V. The Arneth count (preliminary observations). Am J Med Sci, 1967, 253, 221–224

Capo C, Bongrand P, Benoliel AM, Depieds R: Phagocytosis. J Theor Biol, 1974, 47, 177–188

Cardinali G, Innamorati G, Temperini U: La fosfatasa alkalina leucocitaria in gravidanza e nel puerperio. Prog Med (Roma), 1970, 26, 193–196

Cartier P, Habibi B, Leroux JP, Marchand JC: Anémie hémolytique congénitale associée à un déficit en phospho-glycérate-kinase dans les globules rouges, les polynucléaires et les lymphocytes. Nouv Rev Fr Hematol, 1971, 11, 565–570

Cartwright GE, Athens JW, Wintrobe MM: The kinetics of granulopoiesis in normal man. Blood, 1964, 24, 780–785

Casey TP: Drug-induced blood dyscrasias. NZ Med J, 1968, 67, 599

Castro O, Andriole VT, Finch SC: Whole blood phagocytic and bactericidal activity for Staphylococcus aureus. J Lab Clin Med, 1972, 80, 857–870

Cattan A, Amiel J, Schlumberger JR, Schneider M, Schwarzenberg L, Mathe G: Rôle des cellules leucémique dans l'apparition des phénoménes hémorragic au cours des leucemies aiguës. Nouv Rev Fr Hematol, 1966, 6, 705–712

Cattan A, Bresson ML, Schwarzenberg L, Seman G: Nouvelles données sur les activités fibrinolitique et coagulante des leucocytes. Coagulation, 1968, 1, 37–42

Celin LE: Hämatorheologische Varänderungen bei Trauma. Bibl Haematol, 1963, 67, 16–20

Chandra RK: Reduced bactericidal capacity of polymorphs in iron deficiency. Arch Dis Child, 1973, 48, 864–866

Chandra RK: Disorders of neutrophil function. Lancet, 1974, 1, 1052–1053

Chang YH, Gralla EJ: Suppression of urate crystal-induced canine joint inflammation by heterologous anti-polymorphonuclear leukocyte serum. Arthritis Rheum, 1968, 11, 145–147

Chatterjee HN, Basu DK, Chakravarty PK: A study of cholera stools and associated clinical features. J Hyg Epidem (Praha), 1958, 2, 172–183

Chediak M: Nouvelle anomalie leucocytaire de caractère constitutionnel familial. Rev Hematol, 1952, 7, 362–366

Chen LT, Weiss L: The development of vertebral bone marrow of human fetuses. Blood, 1975, 46, 389–408

Chervenick PA, Boggs DR: In vitro growth of granulocytic and mononuclear cell colonies from blood of normal individuals. Blood, 1971, 37, 131–134

Chiaroni T, Nardi E, Valentivo P: Gas-chromatography of leukocyte lipids in myeloid and lymphoid leukemia. Ital J Biochem, 1966, 15, 443–445

Chikkappa G, Boecker WR, Borner G, Carsten AL, Conkling K, Cook L, Cronkite EP, Dunwoody S: Return of alkaline phosphatase in chronic myelocytic leukemia cells in diffusion chamber cultures (37288). Proc Soc Exp Biol Med, 1973, 143, 212–214

Chikkappa G, Borner G, Burlington H, Chanana AD, Cronkite EP, Öhls A, Pavelec M, Robertson JS: Periodic oscillation of blood leukocytes, platelets and reticulocytes in a patient with chronic myelocytic leukemia. Blood, 1976, 47, 1023–1030

Chiyoda S, Miura Y: Alkaline phosphatase activity in chronic myelogenous leukemia cells in cultures. Acta Haematol Jap, 1977, 40, 172–176

Chlebowski J: Remarks on moniliasis (in Polish). Przegl Lek, 1955, 7, 198–201

Christie KE, Solberg CO, Larsen B, Grov A, Tonder O: Influence of IgG, F(ab)$_2$ and IgM on the phagocytic and bactericidal activities of human neutrophil granulocytes. Acta Pathol Scand, Sec C, 1976, 84, 119–123

Cichocki T, Mirecka J, Bogusz J, Lisiewicz J, Kahl J: Activity of acid phosphatase and of beta-glucuronidase of granulocytes in some post-surgery states (in Polish). Pol Przegl Chir, 1968, 40, 579–584

Civeira OF, Navarro AM: Esplenitis brucelosisa. Medicina (Madrid), 1953, 21, 137–156

Clark RA, Kimball HR: Defective granulocyte chemotaxis in the Chediak-Higashi syndrome. J Clin Invest, 1971, 50, 2645–2652

Clark RA, Klebanoff SJ: Neutrophil-mediated tumor cell cytotoxicity: role of peroxidase system. J Exp Med, 1975, 141, 1442–1447

Clark RA, Klebanoff SJ, Einstein AB, Fever A: Peroxidase-H_2O_2-halide system: cytotoxic effect on mammalian tumor cells. Blood, 1975, 45, 161–170

Clark RA, Root RK, Kimball HR, Kirkpatrick CH: Defective neutrophil chemotaxis and cellular immunity in a child with recurrent infections. Ann Intern Med, 1973, 78, 515–519

Clarke AE: Hydrolytic enzymes of human polymorphonuclear leukocytes and rat monocytes. Aust J Exp Biol Med Sci, 1965, 43, 201–204

Clemmensen O, Andersen V, Hansen NE, Karle H, Koch C: Sequential studies of lymphocytes, neutrophils and serum proteins during prednisone treatment. Acta Med Scand, 1976, 199, 105–111

Cline MJ: Ribonucleic acid biosynthesis in human leukocytes. Effects of phagocytosis on RNA metabolism. Blood, 1966, 28, 188–200

Cline MJ: Isolation and characterisation of RNA from human leukocytes. J Lab Clin Med, 1966, 68, 33–34

Cline MJ: Phagocytosis and synthesis of ribonucleic acid from human granulocytes. Nature, 1966, 212, 1431–1432

Cline MJ: A new white cell test which measures individual phagocyte function in a mixed leukocyte population. I. A neutrophil defect in acute myelocytic leukemia. J Lab Clin Med, 1973, 81, 311–316

Cline MJ: The White Cells. Harvard University Press, Cambridge, Massachusetts, 1975, pp 5–221

Cocchi P, Marianelli L: Phagocytosis and intracellular killing of Pseudomonas aeruginosa in premature infants. Helv Paediatr Acta, 1967, 22, 110–114

Cochran AJ, Mackie RM, Ross CE, Ogg LJ, Jackson AM: Leukocyte migration inhibition by cancer patients sera. Int J Cancer, 1976, 18, 274–281

Cochrane CG, Revak SD, Aikin BS, Wuepper KD: The structural characteristics and activations of Hageman factor. In Lepow I, Ward P (eds): Inflammation: Mechanisms and Control. Academic Press, New York, 1972, pp 119–138

Coen R, Grush O, Kauder E: Studies of bactericidal activity and metabolism of the leukocyte in full-term neonates. J Pediatr, 1969, 75, 400–406

Coiffier B, Souillet G, Frobert Y, Revol L., German D: Mise en evidence d'une activité anti-polynucleaire neutrophile par inhibition de la phagocytose du staphylocoque doré dans le serum de malades ayant recu des concentres leucocytaires. Lyon Med, 1976, 235, 963–967

Coleman CN, Johns DG, Chabner BA: Studies on the mechanism of resistance to cytosine arabinoside: problems in the determination of related enzyme activities in leukemia cells. Ann NY Acad Sci, 1975, 255, 247–251

Coltman CA Jr, Uhl GS, Bearden JD, Ratkin GA: Marrow engraftment with extreme leucocytosis in a patient with non-Hodgkin's lymphoma. In Goldman JM, Lowenthal RM (eds): Leucocytes: Separation, Collection and Transfusion. Academic Press, London, New York, San Francisco, 1975, pp 385–394

Conod EJ, Conover JH, Hirschhorn K: Demonstration on human leukocyte degranulation induced by sera from homozygotes and heterozygotes for cystic fibrosis. Pediatr Res, 1975, 9, 724–729

Cooper MR, DeChatelet LR, LaVia MD: Complete deficiency of leukocyte glucose-6-phosphate dehydrogenase with defective bactericidal activity. J Clin Invest, 1970, 49, 21a

Cooper MR, DeChatelet LR, McCall CE, Spurr CL: The activated phagocyte of polycythemia vera. Blood, 1972, 40, 366–374

Cooper MR, Heise E, Richard F, Kaufman J, Spurr CL: A prospective study of histocompatible leucocyte and platelet transfusions during chemotherapeutic induction of acute myeloblastic leukaemia. In Goldman JM, Lowenthal RM (eds): Leucocytes: Separation, Collection and Transfusion. Academic Press, London, New York, San Francisco, 1975, pp 436–449

Copeland JL, Karrh LR, McCoy J, Guckian JC: Bactericidal activity of polymorphonuclear leukocytes from patients with severe bacterial infections. Tex Rep Biol Med, 1971, 29, 555–562

Corrigan JJ Jr, Sieber OF Jr, Ratajczak H, Bennett BB: Modification of human neutrophil response to endotoxin with polymyxin B sulfate. J Infect Dis, 1974, 130, 384–387

Costello Ch: Turner's syndrome: defective neutrophil handling of Candida albicans. IRCS Med Sci, 1975, 3, 389

Coutellier J: Valeur diagnostique de l'étude des leucocytes dans le paludisme aiguë. Bull Soc Pathol Exot, 1956, 49 265–269

Craddock CG, Perry S, Lawrence JS, Buxbaum L, Piepes G: The physiology of granulocitic cells in normal and leukemic states. Am J Med, 1960, 28, 711–714

Craddock MB, Yawata Y, Dansanten L: Acquired phagocyte dysfunction: a complication of hypophosphatemia of parenteral hyperalimentation. N Engl J Med, 1974, 290, 1403–1407

Cramer E, Auclair C, Hakim J: Metabolic activity of phagocytosing leukemia: ultrastructural observation of a degranulation defect. Blood, 1977, 50, 93–106

Cress CH, Clare FB, Gellhorn E: The effect of anoxic and anemic anoxia on the leukocyte count. Am J Physiol, 1943, 140, 299–302

Creveld van J, Mochtar JA: Fibrinolysis in acute leukemia. Ann Pediatr, 1960, 194, 65–75

Creveld van S, Huijing F: Differential diagnosis of the type of glycogen storage disease in two adult patients with long history of glycogenosis. Metabolism, 1964, 13, 191

Cronkite EP: Kinetics of granulocytopoiesis. Natl Cancer Inst Monogr 30: Human Tumor Cells Kinetics, 1969, 51–53

Cronkite EP, Fliedner TM: Granulopoiesis. N Engl J Med, 1964, 270, 1347–1403

Cruickshank JM, Morris R, Butt WR, Corker CS: Interrelationships between levels of plasma oestradiol, urinary total oestrogens and blood haemoglobin and neutrophil counts. J Obstet Gynaecol Br Commonw, 1972, 79, 450–454

Curnutte JT, Whitten DM, Babior BM: Defective superoxide production by granulocytes from patients with chronic granulomatous disease. N Engl J Med, 1974, 290, 593–597

Custo R, Domingo A, Rosel-Perez M: Studies on glycogen metabolism in human leukemic cells. I. Glycogen content, glycogen synthetase forms and their metabolic interconversion. Rev Esp Fisiol, 1975, 31, 309–316

Cutting HO, Lang JE: Familial benign chronic neutropenia. Ann Intern Med, 1964, 61, 876–887

Czarnetzki BM, König W, Lichtenstein LM: Release of eosinophil chemotactic factor from human polymorphonuclear neutrophils by calcium ionophore A23187 and phagocytosis. Nature, 1975, 258, 725–726

Czauderna A: Alkaline phosphatase activity of neutrophil granulocytes in peripheral blood of infants with diarrhea (in Polish). Pediatr Pol, 1973, 48, 1453–1459

Dąbski H: Two cases of agranulocytosis in influenza (in Polish). Pol Tyg Lek, 1959, 14, 1533–1535

Dacie J: Haemolytic Anaemias. Part I—The congenital anaemias. Grune-Stratton, New York, 1960

Dacie J: Haemolytic Anaemias. Part II—The autoimmune haemolytic anaemias. Grune-Stratton, New York, 1962

Dacremont G, Hildebrand J: Characterization of two gangliosides from human leukemic polymorphonuclear leukocytes. Biochim Biophys Acta, 1976, 424, 315–322

Dale DC, Fauci AS, DuPont Guerry, IV, Wolff SM: Comparison of agents producing a neutrophilic leukocytosis in man. Hydrocortisone, prednisone, endotoxin and etiocholanolone. J Clin Invest, 1975, 56, 808–813

Davidova EV: Mobile activity of neutrophils as an index of rheumatic process activity in children (in Russian). Vopr Ochr Mater Dets, 1970, 15, 19–21

Davidson WM: Inherited variations in leukocytes. Semin Hematol, 1968, 5, 255

Davidson WM, Milner RDG, Lawler SD: Giant neutrophil leukocytes: an inherited anomaly. Br J Haematol, 1960, 6, 339–340

Davidson WM, Smith DR: A morphological sex difference in the polymorphologic leukocytes. Br Med J, 1954, 2, 6–9

Davidson WM, Tanaka KR: Polymorphonuclear leukocyte (PMN) function and metabolism in uremia. Clin Res, 1976, 23, 442 A

Davies JE, Whittaker JA, Khurshid M: The effect of cytotoxic drugs on neutrophil phagocytosis in vitro and in patients with acute myelogenous leukaemia. Br J Haematol, 1976, 32, 21–27

Davies W, Thomas M, Linkson P, Penny R: Phagocytosis and the gamma globulin monolayer: analysis by particle electrophoresis. J Reticuloendothel Soc, 1975, 18, 136–148

Davis AT, Brunning RD, Quie PG: Polymorphonuclear myeloperoxidase deficiency in a patient with myelomonocytic leukemia. N Engl J Med, 1971, 285, 789–790

Davis RB, Chakrabarty GN: Jarisch-Herxheimer reaction with interesting blood count. J Indian Med Assoc, 1969, 53, 83–85

Davis WC, Douglas SD: Defective granule formation and function in the Chediak-Higashi syndrome in man and animals. Semin Hematol, 1972, 9, 431–450

Day NK, Geiger H, Stround R, DeBracco M, Moncada B, Windhorst D, Good RA: C_{1r} deficiency: an inborn error associated with cutaneous and renal disease. J Clin Invest, 1972, 51, 1102–1108

DeBuse PJ: The nitroblue tetrazolium test in malnourished children in Papua New Guinea. Aust Pediatr J, 1974, 10, 334–336

DeChatelet LR: Absence of measurable leukocyte alkaline phosphatase activity from leukocytes of patients with chronic granulocytic leukemia. Clin Chem, 1970, 16, 798–801

DeChatelet LR: Oxidative bactericidal mechanisms of polymorphonuclear leukocytes. J Infect Dis, 1975, 131, 295–303

DeChatelet LR, Cooper MR, McCall CE: Stimulation of the hexose monophosphate shunt in human neutrophils by ascorbic acid: mechanism of action. Antimicrob Agents Chemother, 1972, 1, 12–16

DeChatelet LR, McPhail LC, Mullikin D, McCall CE: An isotopic assay for NADPH oxidase activity and some characteristics of the enzyme from human polymorphonuclear leukocytes. J Clin Invest, 1975, 55, 714–721

DeChatelet LR, Volk JV, McCall CE, Cooper MR: Studies on leukocyte phosphatase. II. Inhibition of leukocyte alkaline phosphatase by amino acids and its reversal by zinc. Clin Chem, 1971, 17, 210–213

De la Vega G, Freyre-Horta R, Benitez-Bibriesca L: Plasma factor affecting the NBT reducing capacity of neutrophils. N Engl J Med, 1973, 289, 271–272

DeMeo AN, Anderson BR: Defective chemotaxis associated with serum inhibitor in cirrhotic patients. N Engl J Med, 1972, 286, 735–740

De Vaal OM, Seynhaeve V: Reticular dysgenesis. Lancet, 1959, 2, 1123–1125

Dewald B, Rindler-Ludwig R, Bretz U, Baggiolini M: Subcellular localization and heterogeneity of neutral proteases in neutrophilic polymorphonuclear leukocytes. J Exp Med, 1975, 141, 709–723

Dhillon KS, MacLean LD, Meakins JL: Neutrophil function in surgical patients: correlation of neutrophil bactericidal function, serum albumin, and sepsis. Surg Forum, 1975, 26, 27–28

Diamant YZ, Thilo E, Sadowsky E, Polishuk WZ: Leukocyte alkaline phosphatase in pregnancy. Comparison with placental phosphatase activity. Clin Chim Acta, 1970, 29, 395–397

Diamant YZ, Zuckerman H, Sadowsky E, Polishuk WZ: Leukocyte alkaline phosphatase in cases of bleeding in the first half of pregnancy. Am J Obstet Gynec, 1970, 106, 872–874

Didisheim P, Bowie EJ, Owen CA: Intravascular coagulation-fibrinolysis (ICF) syndrome and malignancy: historical review and report of two cases with metastatic carcinoid and with acute myelomonocytic leukemia. In Mammen EF, Anderson SF, Barnhart MJ (eds): Disseminated Intravascular Coagulation. FK Schattauer Verlag, Stuttgart-New York, 1969 pp 215–231

Didisheim P, Trombold JS, Vandervoort RLE, Mibashan R: Acute promyelocytic leukemia with fibrinogen and factor V deficiency. Blood, 1964, 23, 717–728

Dignan PSJ, Mauer AM, Frantz C: Phocomelia with congenital hypoplastic thrombocytopenia and myeloid leukemoid reactions. J Pediatr, 1967, 70, 561–562

Dilworth JA, Hendley JO, Mandell GL: Attachment and ingestion of gonococci by human neutrophils. Infect Immun, 1975, 11, 512–516

Dimitrov NV, Douwes FR, Bartolotta B, Nochumson S, Toth AA: Metabolic activity of polymorphonuclear leukocytes in sickle cell anemia. Acta Haematol, 1972, 47, 283–291

Djaldetti M, Bessler H, Fishman P, van der Lyn E, Joshua H: Ultrastructural features of the granulocytes in Down's syndrome. Scand J Haematol, 1974, 12, 104–111

Djaldetti M, Joshua H, Kalderon M: Familial leukopenia-neutropenia in Yemenite Jews. Observations on eleven families. Bull Res Counc Israel E Exp Med, 1961, 9, 24–27

Djerassi I, Kim JS, Suvansri U, Ciesielka W, Lohrke J: Filtration leucopheresis: principles and techniques for harvesting and transfusion of filtered granulocytes and monocytes. In Goldman JM, Lowenthal RM (eds): Leucocytes: Separation, Collection and Transfusion. Academic Press, London, New York, San Francisco, 1975, pp 123–136

Döhle H: Leukozyteneinschlüsse bei Scharlach. Zbl Bakt, 1911, 1, 61–63

Donohue DM, Reiff RH, Hanson ML, Betson Y, Finch CA: Quantitative measurements of the erythrocytic and granulocytic cells of the marrow and blood. J Clin Invest, 1958, 37, 1571–1576

Dorr AD, Moloney WC: Acquired pseudo-Pelger anomaly of granulocytic leukocytes. N Engl J Med, 1959, 261, 742

Doscherholmen A, Mahmud K, Ripley D: Hypersegmentation in iron deficiency anemia. JAMA, 1974, 229, 1721–1722

Dossett JH, Williams RD, Quie PG: Studies on interaction of bacteria, serum factors and polymorphonuclear leukocytes in mothers and newborn. Pediatrics, 1969, 44, 49–50

Douglas SD: Analytic review. Disorders of phagocyte functions. Blood, 1970, 35, 851–866

Douglas SD, Schpfer K: The phagocyte in protein-calorie malnutrition. In Suskind RM (ed): Malnutrition and the Immune Response. Kroc Foundation Series, Raven Press, New York, 1977, pp 231–243

Dresch C, Faille A, Poirier O, Kadouche J: The cellular composition of the granulocyte series in normal human bone marrow according to the volume of the sample. J Clin Pathol, 1974, 27, 106–108

Drew SI, Terasaki PI, Billing RJ: Group-specific human granulocyte antigens on a chronic myelogenous leukemia cell line with a Philadelphia chromosome marker. Blood, 1977, 49, 715–718

Dreyfus B: Granulocytopathies acquises au cours des leucémies et des anémies réfractaires. Nouv Rev Fr Hematol, 1973, 13, 243–248

Drutz DJ, Cline MJ: Intermittent neutrophil-monocyte bactericidal defects in a patient with sarcoidosis. Am Rev Resp Dis, 1975, 112, 387–392

Duane GW: Periodic neutropenia. Arch Intern Med, 1958, 102, 462–463

Ebadi M, McCoy E: Progesterone-mediated increases of leucocyte alkaline phosphatase in rabbits. Biochim Biophys Acta, 1966, 130, 502–508

Eberhardt A: Effect of some non-specific factors on the phagocytic ability of neutrophil granulocytes. Acta Physiol Pol, 1971, 22, 899–900

Edelman R, Kulapongs P, Suskind RM, Olson RE: Leukocyte mobilization in Thai children with kwashiorkor. In Suskind RM (ed): Malnutrition and the Immune Response. Kroc Foundation Series, Raven Press, New York, 1977, pp 265–269

Edelson PJ, Stites DP, Gold S, Fudenberg HH: Disorders of neutrophil function. Defects in the early states of the phagocytic process. Clin Exp Immunol, 1973, 13, 21–28

Egeberg JC, Bro-Rasmusen F, Andersen V: Ultrastructure of the specific granules of human neutrophil granulocytes. Studies in fetal granulomatous disease and toxic granulation. Scand J Haematol, 1969, 6, 303–311

Eiseman G, Stefanini M: Thromboplastic activity of leukemic white cells. Proc Soc Exp Biol Med, 1954, 86, 763–765

Ekert H: Disseminated intravascular coagulation. Aust Paediatr J, 1969, 5, 219–225

Elder MG, Bonello F, Ellul J: Neutrophil alkaline phosphatase levels in normal and abnormal pregnancy. Am J Obstet Gynecol, 1971, 111, 663–665

El-Haalem H, Fletcher J: Defective neutrophil function in chronic granulocytic leukaemia. Br J Haematol, 1976, 34, 95–103

Elkeles G: Vergleichende Untersuchungen am Blute von Fleckfieberkranken. Zbl Bakt (Natur-wiss), 1917, 79, 260–290

Elliott PW, Blackford F: Nuclear alteration of the cells in the peripheral blood associated with the virus of influenza A (Asian infection and inoculation). J Indian Med Assoc, 1958, 51, 1651–1655

Elsbach P, Zucker-Franklin D, Sansarinoo C: Increased lecithin synthesis during phagocytosis by normal leukocytes and by leukocytes in chronic granulomatous disease. N Engl J Med, 1969, 280, 1319–1320

Engel E: Blood and skin chromosomal alterations of a clonal type in a leukemic man previously irradiated for a lung carcinoma. Cytogenetics, 1964, 3, 228–230

Erdogan G: The thromboplastic activity of leukemic white blood cells. Blut, 1968, 17, 276–278

Ermakov VV, Kobalskii VV: Biological Role of Selenium (in Russian). Nauka, Moskva, 1974, pp 298

Eschenbach C, Seebach G: Anomalie der Lysosomenmembrane von neutrophilen Granulozyten als Ursache der progressiven septischen Granulomatose. Virchows Arch (Zellpathol), 1971, 7, 16–26

Esmann V: The metabolism of $(1-^{14}C)$-, $(2-^{14}C)$-, $(3,4-^{14}C)$-, and $(6-^{14}C)$-glucose in normal and diabetic polymorphonuclear leukocytes and during phagocytosis. Diabetologia, 1968, 4, 188–190

Esmann V: The diabetic leukocyte. Enzyme, 1972, 13, 32–55

Estensen RD, Reusch ME, Epstein ML, Hill HR: Role of Ca^{2+} and Mg^{2+} in some human neutrophil functions as indicated by ionophore A23187. Infect Immun, 1976, 13, 146–151

Evans DI, Holzel A: Cyclical neutropenia. Proc Roy Soc Med, 1968, 61, 302–304

Fekete LL, Lever WF, Klein E: Inhibition of lipemia clearing activity by human white blood cell and platelet components. J Lab Clin Med, 1958, 52, 680–686

Fenczyn J: Clinics of Lung Tuberculosis (in Polish). Edition of the Section of Medical Students of the Jagiellonian University, Cracow, 1948

Fernandez DJ, Roha H: Caracteristicas da reacao inflamatoria em pacientes com forma hepa-tosplênica de esquistossomose mansonica e calazar. Rev Inst Med Trop (S Paulo), 1967, 9, 129–134

Fialkow PJ, Jacobson RJ, Papayannopoulou T: Chronic myelocytic leukemia: clonal origin in a stem cell common to the granulocyte, erythrocyte, platelet and monocyte. Am J Med, 1977, 63, 125–129

Fichtelius KE, Gisslen H, Hassler O: On the mechanism of the lymphocytosis following pertus-sis vaccination. Acta Haematol (Basel), 1957, 17, 106–110

Filyushina ZG: Allergic alteration of the blood neutrophils in the dynamics in patients with antibiotic-induced occupational disease (in Russian). Gig Tr Prof Zabol, 1974, 5, 12–14

Fink ME, Calabresi P: The granulocyte response to an endotoxin (Pyrexal) as a measure of functional marrow reserve in cancer chemotherapy. Ann Intern Med, 1962, 57, 732–733

Firkin BG, Williams WJ: The incorporation of radioactive phosphorus into the phospholipids of human leukemic leukocytes and platelets. J Clin Invest, 1961, 40, 423–426

Fischer CD, Da Cista M, Rothenberg SP: The heterogeneity and properties of folate binding proteins from chronic myelogenous leukemia cells. Blood, 1975, 46, 855–867

Fischer TN, Gingsberg HS: The reaction of influenza viruses with guinea pig polymorphonu-clear leucocytes. II. The reduction of white blood cell glycolysis by influenza viruses and receptor-destroying enzyme (RDE). Virology, 1956, 2, 637–642

Fischer TN, Gingsberg HS: The reaction of influenza viruses with guinea pig polymorphonu-clear leucocytes. III. Studies on the mechanism by which influenza viruses inhibit phago-cytosis. Virology, 1956, 2, 656–664

Fleck L, Szyszkowicz-Lille I, Ruszczyk K: Leukergy and leukoagglutination (in Polish). Med Dosw Mikrobiol, 1957, 8, 433–436

Fleming A: On a remarkable bacteriolytic element found in tissue and secretions. Proc Roy Soc (Biol), 1922, 93, 306–317

Fliedner TM, Cronkite EP, Killmann SA, Bond UP: Granulocytopoiesis. II. Emergence and pattern of labelling of neutrophilic granulocytes in human. Blood, 1964, 24, 683–700

Fliedner U, Meuret G, Senn H: Normal granulocyte collection with a modified repetitive cycle filtration leukapheresis. Blut, 1974, 39, 265–276

Forman ML, Stiehm ER: Impaired opsonic activity but normal phagocytosis in low birth weight infants. N Engl J Med, 1969, 281, 926–931

Forman NE, Abilgaard CF, Bolger JF, Johnson A, Schulman I: Generalized Schwartzman reaction: role of the granulocyte in intravascular coagulation and renal cortical necrosis. Br J Haematol, 1969, 16, 507–515

Fortynova J, Pospisilova V: Untersuchung der Plasmatischen Atmosphäre der Leukozyten in Hinblick auf das Vorhandensein von Gerinnungsfaktoren. Folia Haematol (Leipzig), 1964, 82, 220–237

Fraumeni JF Jr: Bone marrow depression induced by chloramphenicol or phenylbutazone. Leukemia and other sequelae. JAMA, 1967, 201, 828

Freeman AI, Journey LJ: Ultrastructural studies on monocytic leukaemia. Br J Haematol, 1971, 20, 225–231

Freeman G: The anticoagulant effect of bacterial polysaccharides in normal and thrombocytopenic plasma of leukemia. Blood, 1952, 7, 235–242

Fretland A: Problemer omkring to malariatifelle—et tilfelle av agranulocytose after behandling med atebrin. Tijd Nor Laegeforen, 1958, 78, 14–16

Fricker-Alder H: Die Aldersche Granulationsanomalie. Nach Untersuchungen des erstbeschreibenen Falles und Überblick über den heutigen Stand der Kenntnisse. Schweiz Med Wschr, 1958, 88, 989–990

Frottier J, Moda J: Leukocytosis and polynucleosis in infectious disease. Sem Hop Paris, 1975, 51, 659–666

Fruhman GJ: Inhibition of neutrophil mobilization by colchicine. Proc Soc Exp Biol Med, 1960, 104, 284–285

Gaertner H, Lisiewicz J: Der Einfluss von Ribonukleinase auf die Thrombininaktivierung und auf die Antithrombinwirkung des Heparins in vitro. Folia Haematol, 1962, 79, 258–271

Gahrton G: Glycogen synthesis in normal, leukemic and polycythemic leukocytes. Acta Med Scand, 1966, 189, 497–498

Gahrton G, Zetterberg A: Cytochemical population analyses of glycogen in neutrophil leukocytes of chronic myelocytic leukaemia during busulfan treatment. Eur J Clin Invest, 1972, 2, 412–416

Gairdner D, Marks J, Roscoe JD: Blood formation in infancy: normal erythropoiesis. Arch Dis Child, 1952, 27, 214–216

Gajda A: White blood cells in diphtheria with special reference to eosinophils (in Polish). Patol Pol, 1962, 13, 467–478

Galbraith PR: Studies on control of granulopoiesis in man. II. Influence of circulating neutrophil count on release of labelled bone marrow cells. Can Med Assoc J, 1974, 111, 919–923

Galbraith PR, Abu Zahra HT: Granulocytopoiesis in chronic granulocytic leukemia. Br J Haematol, 1972, 22, 135–143

Galbraith PR, Advincula EG: Observations on the myelocyte to tissue transit time (MTT) in acute leukaemia and other proliferative disorders. Br J Haematol, 1972, 22, 453–467

Galbraith PR, Broxmeyer HE: Studies on control of granulopoiesis in man. I. Relationship of leukocyte colony-stimulating activity in vitro to neutrophil count in vitro. IMA J, 1974, 111, 141–144

Galbraith PR, Valberg LS, Brown M: Patterns of granulocyte kinetics in health, infection and carcinoma. Blood, 1965, 25, 683–684

Gale RP, Zighelboim J: Modulation of polymorphonuclear leukocyte-dependent antibody-dependent cellular cytotoxicity. J Immunol, 1974, 113, 1793–1800

Gale RP, Zighelboim J: Polymorphonuclear leukocytes in antibody-dependent cellular cytotoxicity. J Immunol, 1975, 114, 1047–1051

Gallin JI: Abnormal chemotaxis: cellular and humoral components. In Bellanti JA, Dayton D (eds): The Phagocytic Cell in Host Resistance. National Institute of Child Health, New York, Raven Press, 1975, pp 227–249

Gallin JI, Rosenthal AS: The regulatory role of divalent cations in human granulocyte chemotaxis. J Cell Biol, 1974, 62, 594–609

Gallo RC, Perry S: Enzyme abnormality in human leukaemia. Nature, 1968, 218, 465

Gans H: Fibrinolytic properties of protease derived from human, dog and rabbit leukocytes. Thromb Diath Haemorrh, 1964, 10, 379–389

Garcia-Tamayo F, Ayala L, Kumate J: La prueba del nitroazul de tetrazolio en la amibiasis hepatica de los ninos. Bol Med Hosp Infant, 1974, 31, 683–690

Garg SK, Silber R: Decreased leukocyte alkaline phosphatase in monocytic leukemia. Am J Clin Pathol, 1972, 58, 668–674

Geddes AD, Kirchen ME, Marshal GJ: Localization of leukocyte alkaline phosphatase activity in human neutrophils. Acta Haematol, 1975, 53, 145–151

Gerber AC, Carson JH, Hadorn B: Partial purification and characterization of a chymotrypsin-like enzyme from human neutrophil leucocytes. Biochim Biophys Acta, 1974, 364, 103–112

Gibb RP, Stowell RE: Glycogen in human blood cells. Blood, 1949, 4, 569–570

Gibiński K, Gonciarz Z: The leukocyte proteolysis of blood proteins. Pol Arch Med Wewn, 1970, 44, 377–382

Gibiński K, Lipiński B, Trusz-Gluza M: The leukocyte digestion of fibrinogen degradation products (FDP). Thromb Diath Haemorrh, 1971, 26, 523–525

Gibiński K, Zahorska-Markiewicz B, Markiewicz A: Plasma fibrinolytic and leukocyte proteolytic activities: differentiation by activating and inhibiting factors. Acta Med Pol, 1970, 11, 97–101

Gierek T, Lisiewicz J, Astaldi G, Pilch J: Lymphocytes, neutrophils and serum immunoglobulins in patients with precancerous states of the larynx. The Laryngoscope, 1979, 89, 1145–1150

Gierek T, Lisiewicz J, Pilch J: Intracellular enzymatic response of lymphocytes and neutrophils in patients with cancer of the larynx. Folia Haematol, 1977, 104, 208–215

Gierek T, Lisiewicz J, Pilch J: The intracellular enzymatic response of neutrophils and lymphocytes in patients with precancerous states and cancer of the larynx. J Maxillofac Surg, 1979, 7, 172–176

Gierek T, Lisiewicz J, Pilch J, Namysłowski G: Effect of radiotherapy on the neutrophil and the lymphocyte enzymatic equipment and serum immunoglobulins in patients with cancer of the larynx. Folia Haematol, 1979, 1, 22–31

Gierek T, Lisiewicz J, Pilch J, Sąsiadek U: The neutrophil cytochemical equipment in patients with precancerous states of the larynx. Rev Roum Med—Med Int, 1978, 16, 33–36

Gigante D, Magalini SI, Dell'Amore M, Mascioli G, Ghiucini F: Studies on components of normal and leukemic leukocytes. Haematologica, 1962, 47, 203–205

Gilman PA, Jackson DP, Guild HG: Congenital agranulocytosis: prolonged survival and terminal acute leukemia. Blood, 1969, 34, 827–830

Girolami A: Correlazione tra uricemia e fibrinolisi nelle leucemie. Haematologica, 1967, 52, 469–478

Gitlin D, Vawter G, Craig JM: Thymic alymphoplasia and congenital aleukocytosis. Pediatrics, 1964, 33, 184–185

Giudice CR: Alterationes hematicas en la brucelosis. Sem Med (B Aires), 1956, 108, 275–279

Gladstone GP, Walton E: Effect of iron on the bactericidal proteins from rabbit PMN. Nature, 1970, 227, 849–851

Glick AD, Horn RG: Identification of promonocytes and monocytoid precursors in acute leukaemia of adults: ultrastructural and cytochemical observations. Br J Haematol, 1974, 26, 395–403

Godes IE: Alkaline phosphatase activity of leukocytes in tuberculosis (in Russian). Klin Med (Mosk), 1969, 47, 88–91

Godwin HA, Ginsburg AD: May-Hegglin anomaly: a defect in megacariocyte fragmentation? Br J Haematol, 1974, 26, 117–128

Goetzl EJ: Plasma and cell-derived inhibitors of human neutrophil chemotaxis. Ann NY Acad Sci, 1975, 256, 210–221

Goetzl EJ, Austen KF: A method for assessing the in vitro chemotactic response of neutrophils utilizing ^{51}Cr-labeled human leukocytes. Immunol Commun, 1972, 1, 421–430

Goetzl EJ, Austen KF: A neutrophil-immobilizing factor derived from human leukocytes. I. Generation and partial characterization. J Exp Med, 1972, 136, 1564–1580

Goetzl EJ, Austen KF: Active site of chemotactic factors and the regulation of the human neutrophil chemotactic response. Antibiot Chemother, 1974, 19, 218–232

Goh KO: Chronic myelocytic leukemia in identical twins. Arch Intern Med, 1967, 120, 214–215

Goh KO, Swisher SN: Specificity of the Philadelphia chromosome: cytogenetic studies in cases of chronic myelocytic leukemia and myeloid metaplasia. Ann Intern Med, 1964, 61, 609–610

Goihman-Yahr M, Rodriguez-Ochoa G, Aranzazu N, Convit J: Polymorphonuclear activation in leprosy. I. Spontaneous and endotoxin-stimulated reduction of nitroblue tetrazolium: effects of serum and plasma on endotoxin-induced activation. Clin Exp Immunol, 1975, 20, 257–264

Gola A: Leucocyte and plasma lipids in chronic granulocytic leukaemia. Haematologia, 1976, 10, 243–247

Gold SB, Hanes DM, Stites DP, Fudenberg HH: Abnormal kinetics of degranulation in chronic granulomatous disease. N Engl J Med, 1974, 291, 332–337

Gold SB, Hanes DM, Stites DP, Ponce B, Fudenberg HH: Abnormal kinetics of polymorphonuclear leukocyte (PMN) degranulation in chronic granulomatous disease (CGD). Blood, 1973, 42, 981a

Golde DW, Rothman B, Cline MJ: Production of colony-stimulating factor by malignant leukocytes. Blood, 1974, 43, 749–756

Goldfinger SE, Howell RR, Seegmiller JE: Suppression of metabolic accompaniments of phagocytosis by colchicine. Arthritis Rheum, 1965, 8, 1112–1113

Goldman JM: Acute promyelocytic leukaemia. Br Med J, 1974, 1, 380–382

Goldman JM, Lowenthal RM (eds): Leucocytes: Separation, Collection and Transfusion. Academic Press, London, New York, San Francisco, 1975

Goldman JM, Th'ng KH: Phagocytic function of leucocytes from patients with acute myeloid and chronic granulocytic leukaemia. Br J Haematol, 1973, 25, 299–308

Goldstein IM: Polymorphonuclear leukocyte lysosomes and immune tissue injury. Prog Allergy, 1976, 20, 301–340

Goldstein IM, Eyre HJ, Terasaki P, Henderson ES, Graw RG: Leukocyte transfusions: role of leukocyte alloantibodies in determining transfusion response. Transfusion, 1971, 11, 19–24

Goldstein IM, Hoffstein ST, Weissmann G: Influence of divalent cations upon complement-mediated enzyme release from human polymorphonuclear leukocytes. J Immunol, 1975, 115, 665–670

Goldstein IM, Hoffstein ST, Weissmann G: Mechanism of lysosomal enzyme release from human polymorphonuclear leukocytes: effects of phorbol myristate acetate. J Cell Biol, 1975, 66, 647–652

Goldstein IM, Horn JK, Kaplan HB, Weissmann G: Calcium-induced lysozyme secretion from human polymorphonuclear leukocytes. Biochem Biophys Res Commun, 1974, 60, 807–812

Goldstein IM, Wünschmann B, Astrup T, Henderson ES: Effects of bacterial endotoxin on the fibrinolytic activity of normal human leukocytes. Blood, 1971, 37, 447–453

Gomez-Estrada H, Garcia-Gonzales JL, Aragon-Mendia M, Diaz-Gomez A, Arellano-Blanco J, Fernandez-Quintero P: Disfagocitosis neonatal por deficiencia de tetrapéptido. Arch Invest Med (Mex), 1975, 6, 403–412

Gomez-Estrada H, Terese-Antillon A, Fernandez-Quintere P: Induction of phagocytosis by immunotherapy against leukemic leukocytoblasts. Arch Invest Med, 1976, 7, 57–60

Gonciarz Z, Koźmiński R, Wilk M, Rybicka J: The leukocyte proteolytic properties as a diagnostic aide in differentiation of leukemias. Pol Arch Med Wewn, 1970, 4, 385–388

Good RA, Quie PG, Windhorst DB, Page AR, Rodey GE, White J, Wolfson JJ, Holmes BH: Fatal (chronic) granulomatous disease of childhood: a hereditary defect of leukocyte function. Semin Hematol, 1968, 5, 215–254

Gordon AS: Plasma factors influenzing leukocyte release in rats. Ann NY Acad Sci, 1964, 113, 766–789

Górski J, Kordecki R, Reutt H: Effect of physical exercise on phagocytic capacity of neutrophils (in Polish). Med Pracy, 1969, 20, 113–117

Gottfried EL: Lipids of human leukocytes; relation to cell type. J Lipid Res, 1967, 8, 321–322

Gowland E: Studies on the migration of polymorphonuclear leukocytes from skin lesion in man. J Pathol Bacteriol, 1964, 87, 347–349

Graf M, Tarlov A: Agranulocytosis with monohistiocytosis associated with ampicillin therapy. Ann Intern Med, 1968 69, 91–95

Graham RC Jr: Disorders of polymorphonuclear leukocytes relevant to infection. Cleveland Clin Quarterly, 1975, 42, 33–47

Graham RC, Karnovsky MJ, Shafer AW, Glass EA, Karnovsky ML: Metabolic and morphological observations on the effect of surface-active agents on leukocytes. J Cell Biol, 1967, 32, 629–647

Gralnick HR: Myelofibrosis in chronic granulocytic leukemia. Blood, 1971, 37, 152–155

Gralnick HR, Abrell E: Studies of the procoagulant activity of promyelocytes in acute promyelocytic leukaemia. Br J Haematol, 1973, 24, 89–99

Gray GR, Stamatoyannopoulos G, Naiman SC, Kliman MR, Klebanoff SJ, Austin T, Yoshida A, Robinson GCF: Neutrophil dysfunction, chronic granulomatous disease, and non-spherocytic haemolytic anaemia caused by complete deficiency of glucose-6-phosphate dehydrogenase. Lancet, 1973, 2, 530–534

Greenberg MS, Zanger B, Wong H: Studies in granulocytopenic subjects. Blood, 1967, 30, 891–893

Greenberg PL, Schrier SL: Granulopoiesis in neutropenic disorders. Blood, 1973, 41, 753–769

Gregory EM, Fridovich I: Oxygen toxicity and the superoxide dismutase. J Bacteriol, 1973, 114, 1193–1197

Grignaschi VJ, Sperperato AM, Etcheverry MJ, Macario AJL: Un nuevo cuadro citoquimico: negatividad espontanea de las reacciones de peroxidasas, oxidasas y lipidos en la progenie neutrofila y en los monocitos de dos hermanos. Rev Asoc Med Argent, 1963, 77, 218–221

Grogan JB, Smith GV: Neutrophil function in clinical kidney allograft recipients. Surgery, 1975, 78, 316–321

Grozdea J, Colombies P, Kessous A. Correlations between the Ph[1] clone and leukocyte alkaline phosphatase levels during chronic myeloid leukemia in pregnancy. Soc Biol, Compte Rendus, 1975, 169, 1376–1379

Grybowska J: Leukergy in rheumatic fever (in Polish). Pediatr Pol, 1958, 23, 563–570

Guichard A, Alex R, Paliard P, Moulin G: A propos d'un cas de distomatose hépatique dépistée par une éosinophilie médullaire. Lyon Med, 1959, 201, 519–525

Gullberg R, Riezenstein P: Granulocyte release of vitamin B_{12}-binders in vivo and in vitro in leukaemia and non-neoplastic leucocytosis. Scand J Haematol, 1975, 15, 377–383

Gunawardena DA, Gunawardena KA, Ratnayaka RM, Vasanthanathan NS: The clinical spectrum of Sweet's syndrome (acute febrile neutrophilic dermatosis)—a report of eighteen cases. Br J Dermatol, 1975, 92, 363–373

Gupta KS, Kohli SS, Sharma BN: Acute promyelocytic leukaemia. Indian J Cancer, 1969, 6, 53–57

Gupta RC, Robinson WA: Efficacy of lithium in rheumatoid arthritis with granulocytopenia (Felty's syndrome). A preliminary report. Arthritis Rheum, 1975, 18, 179–184

Hahneman BM, Alt HL: Cyclic neutropenia in a father and daughter. JAMA, 1958, 168, 270

Hakim J, Boivin P, Troube H, Boucherot J: Activités fonctionnelles et enzymatiques des granulocytes du sang de malades ayant une anémie réfractaire acquise. Nouv Rev Fr Hematol, 1974, 14 397–408

Halikowski B, Kowalczykowa J: Pneumonia in Children (in Polish). Polish Medical Publishers, Warsaw, 1968

Halvorsen K: Neonatal leukopenia due to fetomaternal leucocyte incompatibility. Acta Paediatr Scand, 1965, 54, 86–89

Handin RI, Stossel TP: Phagocytosis of antibody-coated platelets by human granulocytes. N Engl J Med, 1974, 290, 989–993

Hankiewicz J, Świerczek E: Lysozyme—biochemical and clinical problems (in Polish). Post Hig Med Dosw, 1976, 5, 609–623

Hansen NE: Plasma lysozyme—a measure of neutrophil turnover. An analytical review. Ser Haematol, 1974, 7, 1–87

Hansen NE, Grube G: Eine weitere Besonderheit des Keuchhustenblides. Kinderaerztl Prax, 1954, 22, 49–53

Hański W: A case of generalized moniliasis (in Polish). Pol Tyg Lek, 1956, 11, 1382–1385

Hargraves MM: Discovery of the LE cell and its morphology. Mayo Clin Proc, 1969, 44, 579–582

Harker GW, Rothstein G, Clarkson DW, Athens JW: Stimulation of neutrophil production by lithium. Clin Res, 1975, 23, 103 A

Harker GW, Rothstein G, Clarkson D, Athens JW, MacFarlane JL: Enhancement of colony-stimulating activity production by lithium. Blood, 1977, 49, 263–267

Hartl W, Genth E: In vitro binding of complement globulin on leucocytes by sera of patients with agranulocytosis. XIV International Congress of Hematology, Sao Paulo, 1972, Abstracts, 213

Haschen RJ, Krug K: Distribution patterns of proteolytic enzymes in normal and leukemic human leukocytes. Nature, 1966, 209, 511–512

Haschen RJ, Krug K: Proteolitische Enzyme in normale und leukämischen Leukozyten. Folia Haematol, 1966, 85, 284–287

Hattersley PG, Engels JL: Neutrophilic hypersegmentation without macrocytic anemia. West J Med, 1974, 121, 179–184

Hayhoe FGJ: Clinical and cytological recognition and differentiation of the leukemias. In Zaraforetis CJD (ed): Proc Int Conf Leukemia-Lymphoma, Lea and Febiger, Philadelphia. 1968, p 307

Hegglin R: Gleichzeitige Konstitutionelle Veränderungen an Neutrophilen und Thrombozyte. Helv Med Acta, 1945, 12, 439–440

Hegglin R, Gross R, Löhr GW: Anomalie Hegglin-May—polyphyle Reifungstörung. Schweiz Med Wschr, 1964, 94, 1357–1364

Heimpel H, Bauke J: Präleukämien. Med Klin, 1972, 67, 1004–1011

Helldén L, Ericson T, Lindhe J: Neutrophil chemotactic substances in different fractions of soluble dental plaque material. Scand J Dent Res, 1973, 81, 276–284

Heller A, Gross R: Histochemical findings on preleukemic states. Blut, 1974, 28, 452–456

Henderson LW, Miller ME, Hamilton RW, Norman ME: Hemodialysis leukopenia and polymorph random mobility—a possible correlation. J Lab Clin, 1975, 85, 191–197

Hennekeuser HH, Möbius W: Untersuchungen zur Bedeutung des peroxidase-Nachweises bei akuter myeloischer Leukämie. Blut, 1974, 29, 317–322

Henry RL: Leukocytes and thrombosis. Thromb Diath Haemorrh, 1965, 13, 35–46

Henson PM, Johnson HB, Spiegelberg HI: The release of granule enzymes from human neutrophils stimulated by aggregated immunoglobulins of different classes and subclasses. J Immunol, 1972, 109, 1182–1192

Henson PM, Oades ZG: Stimulation of human neutrophils by soluble and insoluble immunoglobulin aggregates. Secretion of granule constituents and increased oxidation of glucose. J Clin Invest, 1975, 56, 1053–1061

Herrlich A, Mayer A: Die Pocken—Erreger, Epidemiologie und linisches Bild. Georg Thieme Verlag, Stuttgart, 1960

Hester JP, McCredie KB, Freireich EJ, Rossen RD: Relationship of the HL-A system to leuco-agglutinins in recipients of granulocyte transfusion. In Goldman JM, Lowenthal RM (eds): Leukocytes: Separation, Collection and Transfusion. Academic Press, London, New York, San Francisco, 1975, pp 456–463

Heyne K, Kemmer C, Rudolph S: Ultrastructure of phagocytizing granulocytes in chronic granulomatous disease of childhood. Pathol Microbiol (Basel), 1972, 38, 133–143

Higashi O: Congenital gigantism of peroxidase granules. First case ever reported of qualitative abnormality of peroxidase. Tohoku J Exp Med, 1954, 39, 315–316

Higby DJ, Henderson ES, Holland JF: Granulocyte transfusion therapy: a randomised clinical trial. In Goldman JM, Lowenthal RM (eds): Leucocytes: Separation, Collection and Transfusion. Academic Press, London, New York, San Francisco, 1975, pp 307–315

Higgins GR, Swanson Y, Yamazaki J: Granulocytasthenia. A unique leukocyte dysfunction associated with decreased resistance to infection. Clin Res, 1970, 18, 209–210

Higushi T: A comparative study of 6-merkaptopurine metabolism in human leukemic lekocytes and L1210 cells. Acta Haematol Jap, 1975, 38, 259–266

Hill HR, Quie PG: Defective neutrophil chemotaxis associated with hyperimmunoglobulinemia E. In The Phagocytic Cell in Host Resistance. National Institute of Child Health, New York, Raven Press, 1975, pp 249–267

Hill HR, Sauls HA, Dettloff JL, Quie PG: Impaired leukotactic responsiveness in patients with juvenile diabetes mellitus. Clin Immunol Immunopathol, 1974, 2, 395–403

Hill NO, Khan A, Hill JM, Loeb E, MacLellan A, Dandona S: Granulocyte preparation by continuous flow filtration leucapheresis. In Goldman JM, Lowenthal RM (eds): Leucocytes: Separation, Collection and Transfusion. Academic Press, London, New York, San Francisco, 1975, pp 168–173

Hillestad LK: Acute promyelocytic leukemia. Acta Med Scand, 1957, 159, 189–194

Hirsch JG: Studies of the bactericidal action of phagocytin. J Exp Med, 1956, 103, 589–611

Hirsch JG, Cohn ZA: Degranulation of polymorphonuclear leukocytes following phagocytosis of microorganisms. J Exp Med, 1960, 112, 1005–1006

Hirschhorn R, Weissmann G: Isolation and properties of human leukocyte lysosomes in vitro. Proc Soc Exp Biol Med, 1965, 119, 36–38

Hitzig WH: Familiäre Neutropenie mit dominanten Erbgang und Hypergammaglobulinämie. Helv Med Acta, 1959, 26, 779–780

Hoffman TA, Bullock WE: A statistical approach to the polymorphonuclear leukocyte bactericidal assay. J Lab Clin Med, 1973, 81, 148–156

Hoffstein S, Soberman R, Goldstein I, Weissmann G: Concanavalin A induced microtubule assembly and specific granule discharge in human polymorphonuclear leukocytes. J Cell Biol, 1976, 68, 781–787

Hohn DC, Lehrer RI: NADPH oxidase deficiency in X-linked chronic granulomatous disease. J Clin Invest, 1975, 55, 707–713

Holemans R, Młynarczyk EJ, Mann LS, Smalley RV: Hypofibrinogenaemia in leukemia. Lancet, 1967, 2, 97

Holland JF, Senn HJ, Banerjee T: Quantitative studies of localized leukocyte mobilization in acute leukemia. Blood, 1971, 37, 499–502

Holley TR, Van Epps DE, Harvey RL, Anderson RE, Williams RC Jr: Effect of high doses of radiation on human neutrophil chemotaxis, phagocytosis and morphology. Am J Pathol, 1974, 75, 61–72

Holmes B, Gray GR, Good RA: Chronic granulomatous disease of childhood. In Good RA, Fisher DW (eds): Immunobiology. Sinauer, Stamford, Conn, 1971

Holmes B, Page AR, Good RA: Studies of the metabolic activity of leukocytes from patients with a genetic abnormality of phagocytic function. J Clin Invest, 1967, 46, 1422–1432

Holmes B, Park BH, Malawista SE, Quie PG, Nelson DL, Good RA: Chronic granulomatous disease in females: a deficiency of leukocyte glutathione peroxidase. N Engl J Med, 1970, 283, 217–221

Holmes B, Quie PG, Windhorst DB, Good RA: Fatal granulomatous disease of childhood: an inborn abnormality of phagocytic function. Lancet, 1966, 1, 1225

Homan-Müller JWT, Weening RS, Roos D: Production of hydrogen peroxide by phagocytizing human granulocytes. J Lab Clin Med, 1975, 85, 198–207

Hong R, Schubert WK, Perrin EV, West SD: Antibody deficiency syndrome associated with beta-2-macroglobulinemia. J Pediatr, 1962, 61, 831–832

Horland AA, Wolman SR, Distenfeld A: Another variant translocation in chronic myelogenous leukemia. N Engl J Med, 1976, 294, 164–165

Horn RG, Collins RD: Studies on the pathogenesis of the generalized Schwartzman reaction. The role of granulocytes. Lab Invest, 1968, 18, 101–107

Horn RG, Spicer SS, Wetzel BK: Phagocytosis of bacteria by heterophil leukocytes, acid and alkaline phosphatase cytochemistry. Am J Pathol, 1964, 45, 327–330

Howell RR, Seegmiller JE: A mechanism of action of colchicine. Arthritis Rheum, 1962, 5, 303–304

Hsia DYY: Study of hereditary metabolic disease using in vitro techniques. Metabolism, 1970, 19, 309–310

Huestis DW, Goodsite LM, Price MJ, White RF: Granulocyte collection with the Haemonetics Blood Cell Separator. In Goldman JM, Lowenthal RM (eds): Leucocytes: Separation, Collection and Transfusion. Academic Press, London, New York, San Francisco, 1975, pp 208–219

Huët GJ: Über eine blisher unbekannte Familiare Anomalie der Leukozyten. Klin Wschr, 1932, 11, 1264

Huguley CM Jr: Hematological reactions. JAMA, 1966, 196, 404–405

Huijing F: Phosphorylase kinase in leucocytes of normal subjects and of patients with glycogen-storage disease. Biochim Biophys Acta, 1967, 147, 601–603

Huijing F, Obbink HJK, van Creveld S: The activity of the debranching-enzyme system in leukocytes. A genetic study of glycogen storage disease type III. Acta Genet (Basel), 1968, 18, 128–136

Huijing F, Sandberg DH: Phosphorylase kinase defect: a generalized disorder. South Med J, 1970, 63, 1482–1483

Hulewicz-Grabowska L: Generalized moniliasis in a 5-year-old boy (in Polish). Pediatr Pol, 1957, 12, 1379–1384

Humbert JR, Gross GP, Vatter AE, Hathaway WE: Nitroblue tetrazolium reduction by neutrophils: biochemical and ultrastructural effects of methylene blue. J Lab Clin Med, 1973, 82, 20–30

Humbert JR, Hutter JJ Jr, Thoren CH: Decreased neutrophil bactericidal activity in acute leukemia of childhood. Cancer, 1976, 37, 2194–2200

Humbert JR, Lurtz ML, Hathaway WE: Increased reduction of nitroblue tetrazolium by neutrophils of newborn infants. Pediatrics, 1970, 45, 125–126

Hume PD, Fleming KA, Tavadia HB, Simpson HW: Arneth-Cooke count: timing cancer therapy (circadian rhythm). Lancet, 1975, 1, 802

Hurley IV: Substances promoting leukocyte migration. Ann NY Acad Sci, 1964, 116, 2918

Huth K, Löffler H, Lechlemayer U: Verbrauchskoagulopathie bei Unreifzelligen Leukosen. Verh Dtsch Ges Inn Med, 1968, 74, 147–149

Ignarro LJ, Lint TF, George WJ: Hormonal control of lysosomal enzyme release from human neutrophils. Effects of autonomic agents on enzyme release, phagocytosis, and cyclic nucleotide levels. J Exp Med, 1974, 139, 1395–1414

Inoue S, Ravindranath Y, Thompson RI: Cytogenetics of juvenile type chronic granulocytic leukemia. Cancer, 1977, 39, 2017–2024

Ishiwara T, Kumatori T: Chromosome studies on Japanese exposed to radiation resulting from the nuclear bomb explosions. In Human Radiation Cytogenetics. North Holland, Amsterdam, 1967, pp 144–148

Issidorides MR, Stefanis CN, Varsou E, Katsorchis T: Altered chromatin ultrastructure in neutrophils of schizophrenics. Nature, 1975, 258, 612–614

Itoga T, Laszlo J: Döhle bodies and other granulocyte alterations with cyclophosphamide. Blood, 1962, 20, 668–670

Ivady G, Dux E, Illyes M: Untersuchungen über die Phagocytosebereitschaft der Leukozyten von an interstitieller Phneumonie erkrankten Säuglingen. Z Kinderheilkd, 1961, 85, 378–386

Ivanova LA, Udovichenko NA: Significance of alkaline and acid phosphatases of blood neutrophils in diagnosing chronic dust-induced bronchitis. Gig Tr Prof Zabol, 1975, 4, 18–21

Iwaszko-Krawczuk W: Phagocytic activity of leukocytes in newborns (in Polish). Pediatr Pol, 1974, 49, 543–548

Iyer GNY, Islam MF, Quastel JH: Biochemical aspects of phagocytosis. Nature, 1961, 1, 535–541

Jacobs AA, Low IE, Paul BB, Strauss RR, Sbarra AJ: Mycoplasmacidal activity of peroxidase-H_2O_2-halide systems. Infect Immun, 1972, 5, 127–131

Jacques PJ: Endocytosis. In Dingle JT, Fell BH (eds): Lysosomes in Biology and Pathology. North Holland, Amsterdam, 1969, 2, pp 395–420

Janicki K, Ronikier A, Śliwczyńska B, Lisiewicz J, Moszczyński P, Kwiatkowski A: Effect of testosterone on the activity of granulocyte alkaline phosphatase in patients with chronic granulocytic leukemia. Endokrynol Pol, 1977, 28, 139–143

Janis MG, Brauer MJ: Leukocyte alkaline phosphatase activity in sickle cell disease. Clin Res, 1976, 24, 480A

Jankowski A, Rudkowski Z, Płotnicki B: Serum immunoglobulin level and NBT test results depending on cupremia in children (in Polish). Pol Tyg Lek, 1975, 30, 2179–2180

Janoff A: Purification of human granulocyte elastase by affinity chromatography. Lab Invest, 1973, 29, 458–464

Janoff A, Basch RS: Further studies on elastase-like esterases in human leukocyte granules. Proc Soc Exp Biol Med, 1971, 136, 1045

Jansa P: Skin window in clinical routine. Folia Haematol, 1973, 99, 121–122

Japa J: A study of the mitotic activity of normal human bone marrow. Br J Exp Pathol, 1942, 23, 272

Jeannet M: Aspects immunologiques des transfusions de granulocytes. Schweiz Med Wschr, 1976, 106, 1336–1340

Jemelin M, Fornerod M, Frei J: Impaired phagocytosis in leukocytes from newborn infants. A study of glycolysis and activities of phosphoglycerate kinase and pyruvate kinase. Enzyme, 1971, 12, 642–646

Jensen DP, Brubaker LH, Nolph KD, Johnson CA, Nothum RJ: Hemodialysis coil-induced transient neutropenia and overshoot neutrophilia in normal man. Blood, 1973, 41, 399–408

Jensen KG: Transplacental passage of leucocyte agglutinins occurring on account of pregnancy. Danish Med Bull, 1960, 7, 55

Jensen MS, Bainton DF: Temporal changes in pH within the phagocyting vacuole of the polymorphonuclear neutrophilic leukocyte. J Cell Biol, 1973, 56, 379–388

Jeremin B: Clinical picture of the zinc fever (observation of 43 cases) (in Polish). Biul Inst Med Morskiej, 1973, 24, 233–235

Jirillo E, Pasquetto N, Monno RA, De Rinaldis P, Fumarola D, Pantaleo R: Leukocyte inhibiting factor (LIF) production from human lymphocytes stimulated by bacterial lipopolysaccharides. Boll Ist Sieroter Milan, 1976, 55, 560–567

John TJ, Sieber OF Jr: Chemotactic migration of neutrophils under agarose. Life Sci, 1976, 18, 177–182

Johnson U, Ohlsson K, Olsson I: Effects of granulocyte neutral proteases on complement components. Scand J Immunol, 1976, 5, 421–426

Johnston RB, Baehner RL: Chronic granulomatous disease: correlation between pathogenesis and clinical findings. Pediatrics, 1971, 48, 730–734

Jordan SW, Larsen WE: Ultrastructure studies of the May-Hegglin anomaly. Blood, 1965, 25, 921–925

Jordans GHW: The familial occurrence of fat containing vacuoles in the leucocytes diagnosed in two brothers suffering from dystrophia musculorum progressiva (Erb). Acta Med Scand, 1953, 145, 419–423

Jungi WF, Meuret G, Senn HJ: Granulozytenclearance und Granulozytenkinetik bei myeloproliferativen Syndromen. Schweiz Med Wschr, 1974, 104, 133–134

Kamada N, Okada K, Oguma N, Tanaka R, Mikami M, Uchino H: C-G translocation in acute myelocytic leukemia with low neutrophil alkaline phosphatase activity. Cancer, 1976, 37, 2380–2387

Kampine JP, Kanfer NJ, Gal AE, Bradley RM, Brady RO: Response of hydrolipid hydrolases in spleen and liver to increased erythrocytorrhexis. Biochim Biophys Acta, 1967, 137, 135–137

Kane SP, Hoffbrand AV, Neale G: Indices of granulocyte activity in inflammatory bowel disease. Gut, 1974, 15, 953–959

Kanfer JN, Blume RS, Yankee RA, Wolff SM: Alteration of sphingolipid metabolism in leucocytes from patients with Chediak-Higashi syndrome. N Engl J Med, 1968, 279, 410–412

Kaplan AP, Goetzl EJ, Austen KF: The fibrinolytic pathway of human plasma. II. The generation of chemotactic activity by activation of plasminogen proactivator. J Clin Invest, 1973, 52, 2591–2595

Kaplan AP, Kay AB, Austen KF: A prealbumin activator of prekallikrein. III. Appearance of chemotactic activity for human neutrophils by the conversion of human prekallikrein to kallikrein. J Exp Med, 1972, 135, 81–97

Kaplan EL, Laxdal T, Quie PG: Studies of polymorphonuclear leukocytes from patients with chronic granulomatous disease of childhood: bactericidal capacity for streptococci. Pediatrics, 1968, 41, 591–592

Kaplan SS, Finch SC, Basford RE: Polymorphonuclear leukocyte activation: effects of phospholipase C. Proc Soc Exp Biol Med, 1972, 140, 540–543

Kaplow LS: A histochemical procedure for localizing and evaluating leukocyte alkaline phosphatase activity in smears of blood and marrow. Blood, 1955, 10, 1023–1029

Kaplow LS: Cytochemistry of leukocyte alkaline phoshpatase. Am J Clin Pathol, 1963, 39, 459–460

Kapustin AV: Frequency of drumsticks in neutrophil nuclei of adult women. Sud Med Ekspert, 1974, 17, 25–27

Karle H, Hansen NE, Killman SA: Intracellular lysozyme in mature neutrophils and blast cells in acute leukemia. Blood, 1974, 44, 247–255

Karle H, Hansen NE, Plesner T: Neutrophil defect in multiple myeloma. Studies on intraneutrophilic lysozyme in multiple myeloma and malignant lymphoma. Scand J Haematol, 1976, 17, 62–70

Karnovsky ML: The metabolism of leukocytes. Semin Hematol, 1968, 5, 156–165

Karnovsky ML, Wallach DF: The metabolic basis of phagocytosis. III. Incorporation of inorganic phosphate into various classes of phosphatides during phagocytosis. J Biol Chem, 1961, 236, 1895–1901

Karpas A: A human haemic cell line capable of cellular and humoral killing of normal and malignant cells. Br J Cancer, 1977, 35, 152–160

Kasha M, Khan AU: The physics, chemistry and biology of singlet molecular oxygen. Ann NY Acad Si, 1970, 171, 2–23

Kass L: Histone abnormalities in adult acute leukaemias. Blood, 1975, 45, 477–484

Kattlove HE, Williams JC, Gaynor E, Spivack M, Bradley RM, Brady RO: Gaucher's cells in chronic myelocytic leukemia: an acquired abnormality. Blood, 1969, 33, 379–380

Kauer GL Jr, Engle RL Jr: Eosinophilic leukemia with Ph[1]-positive cells. Lancet, 1964, 2, 1340

Kay AB, Austen KF: The IgE-mediated release of an eosinophil leukocyte chemotactic factor from human lung. J Immunol, 1971, 107, 899–902

Kędrowa S: Pancytopenia complicating viral hepatitis (in Polish). Pol Tyg Lek, 1966, 21, 2018–2019

Keller HU, Hess MW, Cottier H: Inhibiting effect of human plasma and serum on neutrophil random migration and chemotaxis. Blood, 1974, 44, 843–848

Kelley WN: Hypoxanthine-guanine phosphoribosyltransferase deficiency in the Lesch-Nyhan syndrome and gout. Fed Proc, 1968, 27, 1047

Kennedy CC: The leukocyte count in Weil's disease. Ulster Med J, 1958, 27, 43–46

Kerby GP: The occurrence of acid mucopolysaccharides in human leukocytes. J Clin Invest, 1955, 34, 944–946

Kernbaum S: Pouvoir candidacide des polynucléaires neutrophiles humains et chimiothérapie antibactérienne. Pathol Biol, 1974, 22, 789–794

Keusch GT, Urrutia JJ, Fernandez R, Guerrero O, Casteneda G: Humoral and cellular aspects of intracellular bacterial killing in Guatemalan children with protein-calorie malnutrition. In Suskind RM (ed): Malnutrition and the Immune Response. Kroc Foundation Series, Raven Press, New York, 1977, pp 245–251

Khodyaeva MI: Cytochromoxidase activity of neutrophil leukocytes in pulmonary tuberculosis (in Russian). Vrach Delo, 1975, 11, 56–58

Kidson C: Lipid synthesis in human leukocytes in acute leukemia. Aust Ann Med, 1961, 10, 282–283

Kidson C: Leukocyte metabolism in myeloproliferative states. Aust Ann Med, 1962, 11, 50–51

Killmann SA, Cronkite EP, Fliedner TM, Bond VP: Mitotic indices of human bone marrow cells. I. Number and cytologic distribution of mitoses. Blood, 1962, 19, 743

Kirchmayer St, Stalowa I, Biernacka B, Ślizowska H: Measurement of proteolytic activity of leukoblasts—a new diagnostic method. Pol Arch Med Wewn, 1970, 44, 365–368

Kitaev MI, Zasukhina IB: The mechanism of damage to neutrophils in allergic reactions in tuberculosis. J Hyg Epidemiol Microbiol Immunol (Praha), 1975, 19, 85–92

Klebanoff SJ: Myeloperoxidase–halide–hydrogen peroxide antibacterial system. J Bacteriol, 1968, 95, 2131–2138

Klebanoff SJ: Antimicrobial systems of the polymorphonuclear leukocyte. In Bellanti JA, Dayton DH (eds): The Phagocytic Cell in Host Resistance. National Institute of Child Health, New York, Raven Press, 1975, pp 45–61

Klebanoff SJ, Hamon CB: Role of myeloperoxidase-mediated antimicrobial systems in intact leukocytes. RES J Reticuloendothel Soc, 1972, 12, 170–196

Klebanoff SJ, White LR: Iodination defect in the leukocytes of a patient with chronic granulomatous disease of childhood. N Engl J Med, 1969, 280, 460–466

Knudtzon S: In vitro growth of granulocytic colonies from circulating cells in human cord blood. Blood, 1974, 43, 357–361

Kobielowa Z, Kolanowska H, Szumera B, Jaworek Z: NBT reduction test in evaluation of peripheral blood neutrophil function (in Polish). Przegl Metod AM Cracow, 1973, 8, 89–96

Koch C: Neutrophil granulocyte function in vitro. Acta Pathol Microbiol Scand, Sec B, 1974, 82, 127–135

Koch C: Acquired defect in the bactericidal function of neutrophil granulocytes during bacterial infections. Acta Pathol Microbiol Scand, Sec B, 1974, 82, 439–447

Koch C, Hiby N: NBT staining of human neutrophil granulocytes. Acta Pathol Microbiol Scand, Sec B, 1973, 81, 787–794

Koch C, Sögaard H, Christensen MF: Inheritance of chronic granulomatous disease in females. Acta Paediatr Scand, 1973, 62, 659–665

Kohler WC, Karacan I, Rennert OM: Discovery of circadian rhythm for low molecular weight RNA in human leucocytes. Nature (London), 1972, 239, 94–96

Kolanowska H, Mazurek A, Grządzielska E: NBT test in acute pneumonia in newborns and children (in Polish). Pediatr Pol, 1976, 8, 917–923

Komp DM, Donaldson MH, Charlottenville V: Sepsis and the Shwartzman reaction. Am J Dis Child, 1970, 119, 114–116

Konrad APN, Carthy DJ, Mauer AM, Valentine WN, Paglia DE: Erythrocyte and leukocyte phosphoglycerate kinase deficiency with neurologic disease. J Pediatr, 1973, 82, 456

Kontras SB, Bodenbender JG: Studies of the inflammatory cycle in juvenile diabetes. Am J Dis Child, 1968, 116, 130–131

Kostman R: Infantile genetic granulocytosis. Acta Pediatr, Suppl, 1956, 105, 454

Kostrzewski J: Typhus exanthématique sporadique en Pologne. Ann Inst Pasteur, 1956, 91, 15–24

Kostrzewski J: Typhoid Fever in Cracow and in Some Other Localities (in Polish). Scientific Medical Institute, Warsaw, 1947

Koszewsky BJ, Vahabzadeh H, Wilrodt BS: Hemosiderin content of leucocytes in animals and man and its significance in the physiology of granulocytes. Am J Clin Pathol, 1967, 48, 474–483

Kotlarek-Haus S: L'activité enzymatique de certaines peptidases des leucocytes du sang humain chez la sujets sains et au cours des affections pathologiques. Pol Arch Med Wewn, 1970, 44, 369–375

Kotlarek-Haus S, Gabryś K: Leukocytosis, granulocytosis and activity of some white blood cells enzymes in patients treated with Proresid (SPP-SPG) (in Polish). Pol Tyg Lek, 1971, 26, 1815–1817

Kowalczyk Z: The glycogen content in white blood cells in women during delivery and in neonatals (in Polish). Pediatr Pol, 1969, 35, 621

Kowalewski J, Szymanek D: Leukergy in diseases of the liver parenchyma (in Polish). Pol Arch Med Wewn, 1953, 23, 610

Krasik ID, Kuznik BI: Relationship between fibrinolytic activity and leukocyte content in the blood of patients with leukemias (in Russian). Probl Gematol, 1972, 17, 41–44

Krauser RE, Schumacher HR: The arthritis of Sweet's syndrome. Arthritis Rheum, 1975, 18, 35–41

Kretschmer RR, Osuna ML, Valenzuela RH: Reversible neutrophil defect in ataxia telangiectasia. Pediatrics, 1972, 50, 147–150

Kruse H: Zytochemie der Leukozyten in Kindersalter. II. Veränderungen zytochemischer Reaktionen der nuetrophilen Granulozyten im Verlaufe von Leukosen. Folia Haematol (Leipzig), 1975, 102, 1–12

Kruse H: Zytochemie der Leukozyten im Kindersalter. IV. Die Adwendung zytochemischer Untersuchungen bei der Differenzierung und prognostischen Beurteilung von akuten Leukosen. Folia Haematol (Leipzig), 1975, 102, 389–402

Kryshen PF, Shamshonkova GP: Clinical significance of the neutrophilic vulnerability in chronic enterocolitis (in Russian). Vrach Delo, 1975, 5, 98–101

Kuang-Li C: Acute agranulocytosis in kala-azar. Analysis of 56 cases. Chin J Intern Med, 1959, 7, 268–273

Kulapongs P, Suskind R, Vithayashai V, Olson RE: Cell-mediated immunity and phagocytosis and killing function in children with severe iron-deficiency anaemia. Lancet, 1974, 1, 689–694

Kustova NI: Reaction of leukocytolysis in rheumatism and similar infectious-allergic diseases. Kardiologiya, 1974, 14, 120–121

Kuvin SF, Brecher G: Differential neutrophil counts in pregnancy. N Engl J Med, 1962, 266, 877

Kuznik BI: Leukocytes and their role in hemostasis (in Russian). Probl Gematol, 1966, 11, 49–55

Kuznik BI, Kuzmenko EL, Alnokov GP: On the role of leukocytes in the process of blood coagulation in chronic lymphocytic leukemia (in Russian). Probl Gematol, 1969, 14, 3–7

Lachman PJ, Kay AB, Thompson RA: The chemotactic activity for neutrophil and eosinophil leukocytes of the trimolecular complex of the fifth, sixth, and seventh components of human complement (C567) prepared in free solution by the "reactive lysis" procedure. Immunology, 1970, 19, 895–899

Laforce PM, Mills DM, Iverson K, Cousins R, Everett ED: Inhibition of leukocyte candidacidal activity by serum from patients with disseminated candidiasis. J Lab Clin Med, 1975, 86, 657–666

Lalezari P, Bernard GE: An isologue antigen-antibody reaction with human neutrophils, related to neonatal neutropenia. J Clin Invest, 1966, 45, 1741–1750

Lalezari P, Jiang AF, Yegen L, Santorineou M: Chronic autoimmune neutropenia due to anti-Na_2-antibody. N Engl J Med, 1975, 293, 744–747

Lalezari P, Murphy CB, Allen FH: NB 1, a new neutrophil specific antigen involved in the pathogenesis of neonatal neutropenia. J Clin Invest, 1971, 50, 1108–1115

Lalezari P, Nussbaum M, Gelman S, Spaet TH: Neonatal neutropenia due to maternal isoimmunization. Blood, 1960, 15, 236–243

Lalezari P, Radel E: Neutrophil-specific antigens: immunology and clinical significance. Semin Hematol, 1974, 11, 281–290

Lapin J, Hornick A: Ameboid mobility of human leukocytes. Blood, 1956, 11, 225

Larsen JW Jr, Weis KR, Lenihan JP Jr, Crumrine M, Heggers JP: Significance of neutrophils and bacteria in the amniotic fluid of patients in labor. Obstet Gynecol, 1976, 47, 142–147

Ławkowicz W, Krzemińska-Ławkowiczowa J: Hematology of children's age (in Polish). Polish Medical Publishers, Warsaw, 1969

Lawler SD: The cytogenetics of chronic granulocytic leukemia. Clin Haematol, 1977, 6, 55–75

Lawrence DA, Weigle WO, Spiegelberg HL: Immunoglobulins cytophilic for human lymphocytes, monocytes, and neutrophils. J Clin Invest, 1975, 55, 368–387

Laws WC, Bohannon RA, Robinson AJ, Aggeler PM: Acute promyelocytic leukemia with hypofibrinogenemia. Calif Med, 1968, 109, 219–223

Lazarus GS, Brown RS, Daniels JR, Fullmer HM: Human granulocyte collagenase. Science, 1968, 159, 1483–1485

Lazarus GS, Daniels JR, Brown RS, Bladen HA, Fullmer HM: Degradation of collagen by a human granulocyte collagenolytic system. J Clin Invest, 1968, 47, 2622

Lazarus GS, Neu HC: Agents responsible for infection in chronic granulomatous disease of childhood. J Pediatr, 1975, 86, 415–417

Lazarus GS, Vethamanay VG, Schneck L, Volk BV: Fine structure and histochemistry of peripheral blood cells in Niemann-Pick disease. Lab Invest, 1967, 17, 155–170

Leale M: Recurrent furunculosis in an infant showing an unusual blood picture. JAMA, 1910, 54, 1854

Lechat ME, Bias WB, Guinto RS, Cohen BH, Tolentino JG, Abalos RM: A study of various blood group system in leprosy patients and controls in Cebu, Philippines. Int J Lepr, 1968, 36, 17–31

Leder H: Der Blutmonozyt. Springer-Verlag, Berlin, 1967

Leffell MS, Spitznagel JK: Fate of human lactoferrin and myeloperoxidase in phagocytizing human neutrophils: effects of immunoglobulin G subclasses and immune complexes coated on latex beads. Infect Immun, 1975, 12, 813–820

Lehrer RI: Antifungal effects of peroxidase systems. J Bacteriol 1969, 99, 361–365

Lehrer RI: The role of phagocyte function in resistance to infection. Calif Med (West J Med), 1971, 114, 17–25

Lehrer RI, Cline MJ: Interaction of Candida albicans with human leukocytes and serum. J Bacteriol 1969, 98, 996–1004

Lehrer RI, Cline MJ: Leukocyte myeloperoxidase deficiency and disseminated candidiasis: the role of myeloperoxidase in resistance to Candida infection. J Clin Invest, 1969, 48, 1479–1488

Lehrer RI, Cline MJ: Leukocyte candidacidal activity and resistance to systemic candidiasis in patients with cancer. Cancer, 1971, 27, 1211–1217

Lehrer RI, Goldberg LS, Apple MA, Rosenthal NP: Refractory megaloblastic anemia with myeloperoxidase-deficient neutrophils. Ann Intern Med, 1972, 76, 447–453

Lehrer RI, Hanifin J, Cline MJ: Defective bactericidal activity in myeloperoxidase-deficient human neutrophils. Nature, 1969, 233, 78–79

Leitzmann C, Vithayasai V, Windecker P, Suskind RM, Olson PE: Phagocytosis and killing function of polymorphonuclear leukocytes in Thai children with protein-calorie malnutrition. In Suskind RM (ed): Malnutrition and the Immune Response. Kroc Foundation Series, Raven Press, New York, 1972, Vol. 7, pp 253–257

Lejman K: Cellular defense of the body in untreated primary syphilis and in cases treated with penicillin and arsenic compounds. Morphology of treponemas. Hematology of syphilitic infiltration and of lymph nodes in primary syphilis (in Polish). Pol Dermatol Wenerol, 1952, 1, pp 7–64

Lennard ES, Petering HG, Alexander JW: A metabolic and nutritional evaluation of burn neutrophil function. Tex Med, 1974, 70, 81–91

L'Esperance P, Brunning R, Good RA: Congenital neutropenia: in vitro growth of colonies mimicking the disease. Proc Natl Acad Sci USA, 1973, 70, 669–672

Levin AI, Marmolevskaya GS, Kudryavtseva VM, Lipovetskaya LI: Autoallergic reaction of neutrophils in tonsillogenic lesion of the heart of rheumatic and nonrheumatic etiology. Klin Med (Mosk), 1971, 49, 126–130

Levine S: Chronic familial neutropenia with marked periodontal lesions: report of a case. Oral Surg, 1959, 12, 310

Lewis GP: Pharmacological mediators of immediate hypersensitivity. I. Polymorph and platelet factors. Prog Immunol, 1974, 4, 295–297

Lewis JH, Szeto JLF, Bayer WL, Curiel DC: Leukofibrinolysis. Blood, 1972, 50, 844–855

Lewis SM, Dacie JV: The aplastic anemia—paroxysmal nocturnal hemoglobinuria syndrome. Br J Haematol, 1967, 14, 236–240

Lichtman MA: Cellular deformability during maturation of the myeloblast. Possible role in marrow egress. N Engl J Med, 1970, 281, 943–948

Lim SD, Kim WS, Kim CS, Good RA, Park BH: NBT responses of neutrophils and monocytes in leprosy. Int J Lepr, 1974, 42, 150–153

Lindenbau J, Lieber CS: Hematologic effects of alcohol in man in absence of nutritional deficiency. N Engl J Med, 1969, 280, 333–335

Lisiewicz J: White blood cell system reactions in lung tuberculosis (in Polish). Wiad Gruz Chor Pluc, 1963, 4, 5–13

Lisiewicz J: The use of normal leukocyte extracts in the thromboplastin generation test (in Polish). Pol Arch Med Wewn, 1965, 9, 1349–1354

Lisiewicz J: Thromboplastic, antiheparin and antithrombin activity in leukaemic leukocytes. Haematologia (Budap), 1968, 2, 43–50

Lisiewicz J: Studies on the influence of normal and leukaemic leukocytes on blood coagulation. Ann Med Sec Pol Acad Sci, 1969, 13, 233–278

Lisiewicz J: Hemorrhage in Leukemias. Polish Medical Publishers, Warsaw, 1976

Lisiewicz J: The lysosomal enzymes of lymphocytes in human fetuses. Boll Ist Sieroter Milan, 1976, 55, 264–265

Lisiewicz J: Clinical defects of neutrophil chemotaxis. Wiad Lek, 1978, 31, 395–398

Lisiewicz J: Immunologic properties and transfusion of neutrophils. Wiad Lek, 1978, 31, 335–340

Lisiewicz J: Mechanisms of hemorrhage in leukemias. Sem Thromb Hemost, 1978, 4, 241–267

Lisiewicz J: Intracellular enzymatic deficiencies as a basis of phagocytic defects of neutrophils (in Polish). Przegl Lek, 1979, 36, 617–621

Lisiewicz J, Aleksandrowicz J, Sąsiadek U, Bodzoń A, Płonka I, Ważewska-Czyżewska M: Effect of thymus gland extract on activity of acid phosphatase of neutrophils (in Polish). Przegl Lek, 1976, 33, 848–853

Lisiewicz J, Aleksandrowicz J, Ważewska-Czyżewska M, Sąsiadek U, Bodzoń, A, Kulig D, Kowalczyk K: The effect of diet poor in magnesium and zinc on lysosomal acid phosphatase activity in neutrophil granulocytes of mouse blood (in Polish). Med Dosw Microbiol, 1977, 29, 73–77

Lisiewicz J, Borkowski W, Moszczyński P, Mermon S: Neutrophil alkaline phosphatase activity in the early puerperium. Ind Med Gaz, 1974, 14, 183–185

Lisiewicz J, Gierek T, Piastucka B, Namysłowski G, Pilch J: Effect of radiotherapy on lysosomal enzyme of neutrophils in patients with cancer of the larynx. Rev Esp Oncologia, 1978, 25, 429–436

Lisiewicz J, Gierek T, Pilch J: N-acetyl-beta-glucosaminidase, beta-glucuronidase and acid phosphatase of peripheral blood neutrophils in patients with cancer of the larynx. Rev Esp Oncologia, 1976, 23, 233–239 and Nowotwory, 1977, 27, 141–146

Lisiewicz J, Gierek T, Pilch J: Deficiency of beta-glucuronidase in neutrophils from patients with precancerous state of the larynx. Folia Haematol, 1978, 105, 194–199

Lisiewicz J, Gierek T, Pilch J, Piastucka B, Namysłowski G: Enzymes of neutrophils from patients with precancerous states of the larynx. Rev Esp Oncologia, 1978, 25, 7–11

Lisiewicz J, Malkiewicz-Wąsowicz B, Biernacka B: Thromboplastic activity of chronic myelogenous leukaemia granulocytes. Folia Haematol, 1973, 99, 57–64

Lisiewicz J, Moszczyński P: Leukocytosis and fibrinolytic activity of the blood in leukemic patients. Rev Roum Med Int, 1975, 13, 37–44

Lisiewicz J, Moszczyński P: Neutrophil alkaline phosphatase in patients with internal diseases treated with testosterone (in Polish). Endokrynol Pol, 1975, 26, 253–258

Lisiewicz J, Moszczyński P, Mirecka J, Nowicka E: Neutrophil alkaline phosphatase in patients with untreated pulmonary tuberculosis (in Polish). Pol Tyg Lek, 1972, 27, 1594–1595

Lisiewicz J, Naskalski J, Sznajd J: Antiheparin activity of chronic granulocytic leukemia granulocytes in the light of chromatographic studies (in Polish). Pol Arch Med Wewn, 1966, 433–439

Lisiewicz J, Piotrowski J, Sąsiadek U, Wąs K, Piastucka B, Fijałkowska M, Tacik M, Klimczyk K: The lysosomal acid phosphatase of neutrophilic granulocytes in pregnant women. Gin Pol, 1977, 48, 685–689

Lisiewicz J, Pituch A, Litwin JA: Sanarelli-Shwartzman phenomenon in rats induced by human leukaemic cells. Thromb Diath Haemorrh, 1973, 127, 314–323

Liso V, Traccoli G, Grande M: Cytochemical study of acute promyelocytic leukaemia. Blut, 1975, 30, 261–268

Litwin J, Stacher A: Therapiebedingte Veränderungen zytochemischer Befunde akuter Leukämien. Blut, 1974, 28, 161–165

Liyamaswas S, Nobthai A, Piankijagum A: Neutrophil lobe count in normals and thalassemia patients. J Med Assoc Thai, 1975, 58, 474–477

Lockwood WR, Allison F: Electron micrographic studies of phagocytic cells. I. Morphological changes of the cytoplasm and granules of rabbit granulocytes associated with ingestion of rough pneumococcus. Br J Exp Pathol, 1963, 44, 593–594

Loginskii BE, Mazurok AA, Chuma VB: Role of alkaline phosphatase of neutrophils in the differential diagnosis of different types of malignant lymphomas (in Russian). Vrach Delo, 1975, 3, 43–46

Logoida DM: Disseminated intravascular coagulation and its role in the pathogenesis of hemorrhagic syndrome in some types of acute leukemia (in Russian). Probl Gematol, 1970, 15, 15–19

Lonsdale D, Deodhar SD, Mercer RD: Familial granulocytopenia and associated immunoglobulin abnormality. Report of three cases in young brothers. J Pediatr, 1967, 71, 790–791

Lorenz E, Messner H, Mutz I: Leucocytokinetic studies during viral hepatitis. Z Kinderheilkd, 1972, 113, 171–174

Lou FT: Infectious mononucleosis. A review of 572 cases. Chinese Med J, 1959, 79, 175–177

Lowenthal RM, Grossman L, Goldman JM, Storring RA, Buskard NA, Park DS, Murphy BC, Galton AG: Granulocyte transfusion therapy: a comparison of the use of cells obtained from normal donors with those from patients with chronic granulocytic leukaemia. In Goldman JM, Lowenthal RM (eds): Leucocytes: Separation, Collection and Transfusion. Academic Press, London, New York, San Francisco, 1975, pp 363–379

Lozzio BB, Lozzio CB, Machado E: Brief communication: human myelogenous (Ph1+) leukemia cell line: transplantation into athymic mice. J Natl Cancer Inst, 1976, 56, 627–629

Lozzio CB, Lozzio BB: Human chronic myelogenous leukemia cell-line with positive Philadelphia chromosome. Blood, 1975, 45, 321–334

Lutas EM, Zucker-Franklin D: Formation of lipid inclusions in normal human leukocytes. Blood, 1977, 49, 309–320

Lutyński R, Nowicki J, Stanecka B, Zadura S, Ziemichód T: A fever epidemic in Cracow (in Polish). Przegl Lek, 1957, 13, 33–38

Lyulka AN, Kovalchuk LA, Dyachuk IA: Functional activity of neutrophils in patients with thyretoxicosis before and after surgical treatment (in Russian). Probl Endokrinol, 1974, 20, 31–35

MacDougall LG, Anderson R, McNab GM, Katz J: The immune response in iron-deficient children: impaired cellular defense mechanism with altered humoral components. J Pediatr, 1975, 86, 833–843

Mackey MC, Glass L: Oscillation and chaos in physiological control systems. Science, 1977, 197, 287–289

MacLennan ICM, Howard A, Gotch FM, Quie PG: Effector activating determinants on IgG. I. The distribution and factors influencing the display of complement, neutrophil and cytotoxic B-cell determinants on human IgG subclasses. Immunology, 1973, 25, 459–469

Mahmoud AAF, Kellermeyer RW, Warren KS: Monospecific antigranulocyte sera against human neutrophils, eosinophils, basophils, and myeloblasts. Lancet, 1974, 2, 1163–1166

Mahuren JD, Coburn SP: Pyridoxal phosphate in lymphocytes, polymorphonuclear leukocytes and platelets in Down's syndrome. Am J Clin Nutr, 1974, 27, 521–527

Maiolo AT, Cazzaniga E, Cortelezzi A, De Pangher V, Foa P, Lombardi L, Mozzana R, Polli EE: In vitro production of lymphocyte and granulocyte proliferation inhibitors (chalones?) from living cells. Boll Ist Sieroter Milan, 1975, 54, 235–243

Maj S, Zdebska E: Effect of hydroxyurea treatment on free nucleotides in leukemic leukocytes (in Polish). Acta Haematol Pol, 1975, 6, 211–216

Majda A, Beer Z: Differential leukocyte count in healthy blood donors (in Polish). Problemy Krwiodawstwa i Leczenia Krwią. Polish Medical Publishers, Warsaw, 1965, pp 60-65

Majerus PW, Lastra RR: Fatty acid biosynthesis in human leukocytes. Biochim Biophys Acta, 1967, 84, 8–10

Majeski JA, McClellan MA, Alexander JW: Evaluation of leukocyte chemotactic response in the presence of antibiotics. Surg Forum, Burns, Wounds, Sepsis, 1975, 26, 83–85

Malaskova V: The positive PAS reaction to glycogen in blast cells in acute leukemia of adults. Vnitr Lek 1975, 21, 667–680

Malawista SE: Sols, gels, and colchicine: a common formulation for the effects of colchicine in gouty inflammation and on cell division. Arthritis Rheum, 1964, 7, 325–326

Malawista SE, Bodel PT: The dissociation by colchicine of phagocytosis from increased oxygen consumption in human leukocytes. J Clin Invest, 1967, 46, 786–787

Malemud ChJ, Janoff A: Human polymorphonuclear leukocyte elastase and cathepsin G mediate the degradation of lapin articular cartilage proteoglycan. Ann NY Acad Sci, 1975, 256, 254–262

Malfatti S, Cantoni PE: Anomalie qualitative del granulocita neutrofilo. Clin Terap, 1975, 73, 305–326

Malkiewicz B, Pajdak W, Okulski J, Lisiewicz J: Recherches sur l'activité thromboplastique des éosinophiles d'un malade atteint de leucémie éosinophilique. Haematologia (Budap), 1971, 5, 439–446

Manai G, Mandelli F, Magalini S, Bordoni C: Effects of fractions from leukemic white cells on blood coagulation. Haematol Lat, 1961, 4, 115–121

Mandell GL: Intraphagosomal pH of human polymorphonuclear neutrophils. Proc Soc Exp Biol Med 1970, 134, 447–449

Mandell GL: Influence of type of ingested particle on human leukocyte metabolism. Proc Soc Exp Biol Med, 1971, 137, 1228–1230

Mandell GL: Functional and metabolic derangements in human neutrophils induced by a glutathione antagonist. J Reticuloendothel Soc, 1972, 11, 129–137

Mandell GL: Bactericidal activity of aerobic and anaerobic polymorphonuclear neutrophils. Infect Immun, 1974, 9, 337–341

Mandell GL: Effect of temperature on phagocytosis by human polymorphonuclear neutrophils. Infect Immun, 1975, 12 221–223

Mandell GL, Fullen LF: Nitroblue tetrazolium dye test, a diagnostic aid in tuberculosis. Am Rev Resp Dis, 1972, 105, 123–124

Mandell GL, Hook E: Leukocyte function in chronic granulomatous disease of childhood. Am J Med, 1969, 47, 473–474

Mandell GL, Rubin W, Hook EW: The effect of an NADH oxidase inhibitor (hydrocortisone) on polymorphonuclear leukocyte bactericidal activity. J Clin Invest, 1970, 49, 1381–1382

Mangalik A, Robinson WA: Cyclic neutropenia: the relationship between urine granulocyte colony stimulating activity and neutrophil count. Blood, 1973, 41, 79–84

Marchal G, Deprez V, Blanc G: Syndrome agranulocytaire par chimiothérapie, transformé en crypto-leucémie aiguë à évolution lente. Sang, 1944, 16, 133

Marks PA, Gellhorn A, Kidson C: Lipid synthesis in human leukocytes, platelets, and erythrocytes. J Biol Chem, 1960, 235, 2579–2580

Marmont AM, Raffo MR: Erythrocyte-granulocyte rosette. Schweiz Med Wschr, 1976, 106, 1375

Marmont AM, Raffo MR: The erythrocyte-granulocyte rosette, an immune cellular interaction found in some cases of autoimmune hemolytic anemias. Nouv Rev Fr Hematol, 1976, 16, 221–228

Marsh JC, Levitt M: Neutrophilia inducing activity in plasma of neutropenic human beings. Blood, 1971, 37, 647–656

Marsh JC, Perry S: The granulocyte response to endotoxin in patients with hematologic disorders. Blood, 1964, 23, 581–584

Martin NH, Roka L: Beeinflüssung der Blutgerinnung durch Leukozyten. Klin Wschr, 1951, 29, 510–512

Mason DY: Intracellular lysozyme and lactoferrin in myeloproliferative disorders. J Clin Path, 1977, 30, 541–546

Masson PL, Heremans JF, Schonne E: Lactoferrin, an iron-binding protein in neutrophilic leukocytes. J Exp Med, 1969, 130, 643–658

Mathur TN: The total and differential leukocyte count in brucellosis. Indian Med Gaz, 1955, 90, 51–54

Matsaniotis N, Kiossoglou KA, Karpouzas J, Anastasea-Vlachou K: Chromosomes in Kostmann's disease. Lancet, 1966, 2, 104

Matsuda J: Studies on NBT-test methodological and clinical significance. Jap J Clin Hematol, 1975, 16, 599–613

Matsuoka M, Mattori A, Mizushina T, Jinbo Ch: The ultrastructure of the cryofibrinogen in acute promyelocytic leukemia displaying the defibrination syndrome and fibrillar inclusions in promyelocytes. Acta Med Biol, 1969, 17, 49–64

Matula G, Paterson PhY: NBT test in a patient on steroides. Lancet, 1971, 1, 803–804

Matula G, Paterson PhY: Spontaneous in vitro reduction of nitroblue tetrazolium by neutrophils of adult patients with bacterial infection. N Engl J Med, 1971, 285, 311–317

Mauer AM: Diurnal variation of proliferative activity in human bone marrow. Blood, 1965, 26, 1–7

Mauer AM, Krill CE: A study of the mechanisms for granulocytopenia. Ann NY Acad Sci, 1964, 113, 1003

Maughan WZ, Bishop CR, Pryor TA, Athens JW: The question of cycling of the blood neutrophil concentrations and pitfalls in the statistical analysis of sampled data. Blood, 1973, 41, 85–91

May R: Leukozyten Einschlüsse. Dtsch Arch Klin Med, 1909, 96, 1

McAdam KP, Anders RF, Smith SR, Russel DA, Price MA: Association of amyloidosis with erythema nodosum leprosum reactions and recurrent neutrophil leucocytosis in leprosy. Lancet, 1975, 2, 572–573

McCall CE, Caves J, Cooper R, De Chatelet L: Functional characteristics of human toxic neutrophils. J Infect Dis, 1971, 124, 68–75

McCall CE, Katayama I, Cotran RS, Finland M: Lysosomal and ultrastructural changes in human "toxic" neutrophils during bacterial infection. J Exp Med, 1969, 129, 267–279

McCall MS, Sutherland DA, Eisentrant AM, Lanz H: The tagging of leukemic leukocytes with radioactive chromium and measurement of the in vivo cell survival. J Lab Clin Med, 1955, 45, 717

McCarty DJ: Pathophysiologie de la goutte. Congres International de la Goutte et de la Lithiasis urique. Evian, 1964, (Sep 4–6), p 161

McCullough NB: Microbial and host factors in the pathogenesis of brucellosis. In Mudd S (ed): Infectious Agents and Host Reactions. WB Saunders, Philadelphia, London, Toronto, 1970, pp 324–345

McCullough J, Weiblen BJ, Deinard AR, Boen J, Fortuny IE, Quie PG: In vitro function and post-transfusion survival of granulocytes collected by continuous-flow centrifugation and by filtration leukapheresis. Blood, 1976, 48, 315–326

McFarland W, Libre EP: Abnormal leukocyte response in alcoholism. Ann Intern Med, 1963, 59, 865

McMillan R, Scott JL, Marino JV: The in vivo survival of leukocytes labeled in vitro with radioactive chromate. Blood, 1966, 28, 1009

McRipley RJ, Sbarra A: Role of the phagocyte in host-parasite interactions. XI. Relationship between stimulated oxidative metabolism and hydrogen peroxidase formation and intracellular killing. J Bacteriol, 1967, 94, 1417–1424

McRipley RJ, Sbarra A: Role of the phagocyte in host-parasite interactions. XII. Hydrogen peroxidase-myeloperoxidase bactericidal system on the phagocyte. J Bacteriol, 1967, 94, 1425–1430

McRipley RJ, Selvaraj RJ, Glovsky MM, Sbarra AJ: The role of the phagocyte in host-parasite interactions. V. Phagocytic and bactericidal activities of leukocytes from patients with different neoplastic disorders. Cancer Res, 1971, 27, 674–685

McRipley RJ, Selvaraj RJ, Glovsky MM, Sbarra AJ: The role of the phagocyte in host-parasite interaction. VI. The phagocytic and bactericidal capabilities of leukocytes from patients undergoing X-irradiation. Radiat Res, 1967, 31, 706–720

Mdzewski B: Neutrophil alkaline phosphatase in hematological syndromes (in Polish). Pol Arch Med Wewn, 1963, 33, 511–518

Mdzewski B, Łakowicz W, Kolakowska-Polubiec K: Lysosomes of blast cells in various cytochemical types of acute leukemia. Acta Haematol Pol, 1977, 8, 7–13

Mechank M: Untersuchungen über das Gewicht des Knochenmarkes des Menschen. Z Ges Anat, 1926, 79, 58

Mecheva IC, Gurian IE: Cytochemical studies of glycogen in leukocytes from the blood of patients with various form of pulmonary tuberculosis (in Russian). Probl Tuberk, 1968, 46, 68–73

Medenica R, Maurice P, Cruchaud A, Wyss M: Transfusions granulocytaires. Schweiz Med Wschr, 1976, 106, 1369–1370

Mehta H, Shetty U, Parekh JG: Leucocyte alkaline phosphatase activity—its utility in diagnosis. Indian J Med Sci, 1974, 28, 12–18

Melamed MR, Adams LR, Traganos F, Kamentsky LA: Blood granulocyte staining with acridine orange changes with infections. J Histochem Cytochem, 1974, 22, 526–530

Melmon KL, Cline MJ: The interaction of leukocytes and the kinin system. Biochem Pharmacol, 1968, 17, 271–272

Merker H, Castoldi GL, Linde AH: Cholindehydrogenase in den Phagocytes des Blutes und des entzündlichen Exudats. Schweiz Med Wschr, 1965, 95, 1446–1450

Merkiel K, Kemona H, Iwaszko-Krawczuk W, Prokopowicz J: NBT-reduction in granulocytes of newborns. Pediatr Pol, 1977, 52, 406–408

Merkiel K, Prokopowicz J: The immune processes in malignant diseases. Przegl Lek, 1977, 34, 585–588

Merkiel K, Prokopowicz J, Krawczuk J: The lysozyme activity in the serum after surgical treatment of digestive tract tumors. Proceedings of 2nd Conference of Polish Immunological Society, Warsaw, 1977, p 127

Messner RP, Jelinek J: Receptors for human gamma-globulin on human neutrophils. J Clin Invest, 1970, 49, 2165

Messner RP, Reed WP, Palmer DL: Transient defect in leukocytic intracellular bactericidal capacity. Clin Immunol Immunopathol, 1973, 1, 523–525

Meuret G, Fliedner TM: Neutrophil and monocyte kinetics in a case of cyclic neutropenia. Blood, 1974, 43, 565–571

Meuret G, Hoffman G, Fliedner TM, Rau M, Oehl S, Walz R, Klein-Wisenberg A: Neutrophil kinetics in man. Studies using autotransfusion of ^{3}H-DFP labeled blood cells and autoradiography. Blut, 1973, 26, 97–109

Miale JB: Laboratory medicine: Hematology. The CV Mosby Company, Saint Louis, 1972

Michałowicz R: Development of research on leukergy (in Polish). Post Hig Med Dosw, 1967, 21, 453–462

Michaux JL, Van den Berghe H, Rodhain J, Sokal G, David G, Hulhoven R: Etude simultanée du caryotype et de l'histologie médullaire dans la léucémie myrloide chronique a chromosome Ph_1. Nouv Rev Fr Hematol, 1975, 15, 575–588

Mickenberg ID, Root RK, Wolff SM: Leukocytic function in hypogammaglobulinemia. J Clin Invest, 1970, 49, 1528–1538

Mikułowski W, Rogalska-Chrzanowska E: Leukemoid reaction in the bone marrow of 5-year-old child (in Polish). Pol Tyg Lek, 1956, 11, 1919–1921

Milhorat AT, Small SM, Diethelm O: Leukocytosis during various emotional states. Arch Neurol Psychiat, 1942, 47, 779

Miller ME: Phagocytosis in the newborn infant: humoral and cellular factors. J Pediatr, 1969, 74, 255–256

Miller ME: Chemotactic function in the human neonate. Humoral and cellular aspects. Pediatr Res, 1971, 5, 487–492

Miller ME: Developmental maturation of human neutrophil motility and its relationship to membrane deformability. In Bellanti JA, Dayton D (eds): The Phagocytic Cell in Host Resistance. National Institute of Child Health, New York, Raven Press, 1975, pp 295–309

Miller ME: Pathology of chemotaxis and random mobility. Semin Hematol, 1975, 12, 59–82

Miller ME, Norman ME, Koblenzer PJ: A new familial defect of neutrophil movement. J Lab Clin Med, 1973, 82, 1–8

Miller ME, Oski FA, Harris MB: Lazy leukocyte syndrome. Lancet, 1971, 1, 665–669

Miller ME, Seals J, Kaye R, Levitsky LC: A familial plasma-associated defect of phagocytosis. A new cause of recurrent bacterial infections. Lancet, 1968, 2, 60–63

Mirecka J, Lisiewicz J, Okulski J: Activity of neutrophil alkaline phosphatase in patients with streptococcal pneumonia (in Polish). Pol Tyg Lek, 1970, 25, 922–924

Mishler JM, Higby DJ, Cohen E, Rhomberg W, Nicora RW, Holland JF: Evaluation of donor-recipient serological discordance and effectiveness of granulocyte replacement therapy. In Goldman JM, Lowenthal RM (eds): Leucocytes: Separation, Collection and Transfusion. Academic Press, London, New York, San Francisco, 1975, pp 427–435

Mishler JM, Higby DJ, Rhomberg W, Nicora RW, Holland JF: Leucapheresis: increased efficiency of collection by the use of hydroxyethyl starch and dexamethasone. In Goldman JM, Lowenthal RM (eds): Leucocytes: Separation, Collection and Transfusion. Academic Press, London, New York, San Francisco, 1975, pp 61–74

Miyamoto K: Phagocytic activity of leucocytes in premature infants. II. Correlation of the plasma components and phagocytic activities of leucocytes in premature and full-term infants. J Med Sci (Hiroshima), 1965, 14, 19

Moeschlin S, Wagner K: Agranulocytosis due to the occurrence of leukocyte-agglutinins (Pyramidon and cold agglutinins). Acta Haematol, 1952, 8, 29

Morenz J: Leukotaxisdefekte der neutrophilen Granulozyten und Monozyten. Folia Haematol, 1977, 104, 153–192

Mori W, Asakawa H, Taguchi T: Antiserum against leukemic cell ferritin as a diagnostic tool for malignant neoplasms. Natl Cancer Inst J, 1975, 55, 513–518

Morimoto M: Cytochemical studies on non-specific esterase in leukemic cells, especially in monocytic leukemia. Nogoya Med J, 1975, 20, 69–93

Morita T, Wenzl JE, Kimmelstiel P: The relationship of neutrophilic and eosinophilic leukocytes to the glomerular capillary basement membrane in acute proliferative glomerulonephritis. Lab Invest, 1971, 25, 445–450

Morley AA, Carew JP, Baikie AG: Familial cyclical neutropenia. Br J Haematol, 1967, 13, 719–720

Moroni M, Copsoni F, Caredda F, Lazzarin A, Besana C: Dimostrazione di un difetto granulocitario in soggetti anziani e correlazione con la presenza di auto-anticorpi. Boll Ist Sieroter Milan, 1976, 55, 317–322

Morris RB, Nichols BA, Bainton DF: Ultrastructure and peroxidase cytochemistry of normal human leukocytes at birth. Dev Biol, 1975, 44, 223–237

Morris TCM, Butler M, Muldrew JG: Changes in granulopoiesis detected by in vitro colony formation in acute lymphatic leukaemia. Br J Cancer, 1977, 35, 868–874

Moszczyński P: Effect of cyclophosphamide on neutrophil alkaline phosphatase activity (in Polish). Wiad Lek, 1976, 29, 1249–1251

Moszczyński, P: Effect of stilbestrol on neutrophil alkaline phosphatase activity (in Polish). Endokrynol, Pol, 1976, 27, 259–264

Moszczyński, P, Wiernikowski A: Alkaline phosphatase activity of neutrophils in acute poisoning with carbon monoxide. Pol Tyg Lek, 1977, 32, 53–56

Movat HZ, Steinberg SG, Habal FM, Ranadive NS: Demonstration of a kinin-generating enzyme in the lysosomes of human polymorphonuclear leukocytes. J Lab Invest, 1973, 29, 669–684

Mowat AG, Baum J: Chemotaxis of polymorphonuclear leukocytes from patients with rheumatoid arthritis. J Clin Invest, 1971, 50, 2541–2549

Mowat AG, Baum J: Chemotaxis of polymorphonuclear leukocytes from patients with diabetes mellitus. N Engl J Med, 1971, 284, 621–624

Mowat AG, Baum J: Polymorphonuclear leukocyte chemotaxis in patients with bacterial infections. Br Med J, 1971, 3, 617–619

Mrševič D, Stefanowić S, Djerdjević V: Contribution to the study of the appearance and presence of megakaryocytes in the circulation of human embryos during the early phases of intrauterine development. Acta Anat, 1972, 76, 47–55

Nadler SH, Hansen HJ, Sprague CC, Sherman H: The effect of 6-mercaptopurine on the incorporation of labelled amino acids into cellular protein of chronic granulocytic leukemia leukocytes. Blood, 1961, 18, 336

Najjar VA: The physiological role of gamma-globulin. Adv Enzymol, 1974, 41, 129–178

Najjar VA, Constantopoulos A: A new phagocytosis-stimulating tetrapeptide hormone, "tuftsin," and its role in disease. J Reticuloendothel Soc, 1972, 12, 197–215

Najjar VA, Nishioka K: "Tuftsin": A physiological phagocytosis stimulating peptide. Nature, 1970, 228, 672

Nanoishvilli BR, Zurabashvili ZA: The ultrastructure of formed white blood elements (neutrophils) in schizophrenia. Folia Haematol (Leipz), 1976, 2, 160–165

Nathan DG, Baehner RL, Weaver DK: Failure of nitroblue tetrazolium reduction in the phagocytic vacuoles of leukocytes in chronic granulomatous disease. J Clin Invest, 1969, 48, 1895–1896

Nathan DG, Oski FA (eds): Hematology of Infancy and Childhood. WB Saunders Philadelphia, London, Toronto, 1974

Nazarenko VG: The neutrophil damage factor and the tuberculin hemolysis reaction in the diagnosis of tuberculous meningitis in adults (in Russian). Probl Tuberk, 1975, 6, 59–62

Neuwirtová R, Setková O, Housková J, Poch T, Dorazilová V, Donner L: Phagocytic activity of leukaemic blasts. Acta Haematol, 1975, 53, 17–24

Newton RM, Ward VG: Leukopenia associated with eristocetin (Spontin) administration. JAMA, 1958, 166, 1956–1957

Ng RP, Chan TK, Todd D: NBT (nitroblue-tetrazolium dye) test—false-negative and false-positive results. Lancet, 1972, 1, 1341–1342

Nilzen A: Phagocytic activity of leukocytes in rhinitis allergica. Allerg Immunol, 1975, 21, 29–32

Nishimura ET, Whest GM, Yang HY: Ultrastructural localization of peroxidatic catalase in human peripheral blood leukocytes. Lab Invest, 1976, 34, 60

Nishioka K, Constantopoulos A, Satoh PS, Najjar VA: The characteristics, isolation and synthesis of the phagocytosis stimulating peptide Tuftsin. Biochem Biophys Res Commun, 1972, 47, 172–179

Nowell PC, Hungerford DA: A minute chromosome in human chronic granulocytic leukemia. Science, 1960, 132, 1497

Nunziante CA, Granata A: Cytoanalyse chimique quantitative des leucocytes dans le sang péripherique au cours de l'ankylostomiase. Sang, 1956, 27, 593–597

Nydegger UE, Miescher A, Anner RM, Greighton DW, Lambert PH, Miescher PA: Serum and cellular factor involvement in nitroblue tetrazolium (NBT) reduction by human neutrophils. Klin Wschr, 1973, 51, 377–382

Ockerman PA, Jelke H, Kaijser K: Glycogenosis type VI (liver phosphorylase deficiency). Acta Paediatr Scand, 1966, 55, 10

Ohlsson K: Properties of leukocyte protease. Clin Chim Acta, 1971, 32, 399–405

Ohlsson K, Olsson I: The neutral proteases of human granulocytes. Isolation and partial characterization of two granulocyte collagenases. Eur J Biochem, 1973, 36, 473–481

Okuda K: Effects of cytochalasin B on the intracellular bactericidal activity of human neutrophils. Antimicrob Agents Chemother, 1975, 7, 736–741

Okulski J, Caban J, Lisiewicz J: Serum alkaline phosphatase in patients with tetanus (in Polish). Pol Tyg Lek, 1969, 24 1484–1485

Olds JW, Reed WP, Eberle B, Kisch AI: Corticosteroids, serum, and phagocytosis: in vitro and in vivo studies. Infect Immun, 1974, 9, 524–529

Oleś A, Kurzeja K, Suliński S: First cases of Q fever in Poland (in Polish). Pol Tyg Lek, 1956, 11, 1950–1955

Oliver JM: Impaired microtubule function correctable by cyclic GMP and cholinergic agonists in the Chediak-Higashi syndrome. Am J Pathol, 1976, 85, 395–418

Oliver JM, Spielberg SP, Pearson CB, Schulman JD: Microtubule assembly and function in normal and glutathione synthetase-deficient polymorphonuclear leukocytes. J Immunol, 1978, 120, 1181–1186

Olofsson T, Olsson I, Kostman R, Malmstroem S, Thilen A: Granulopoiesis in infantile genetic agranulocytosis. In vitro cloning of marrow cells in agar culture. Scand J Haematol, 1976, 16, 18–24

O'Riordan ML: Distinguishing between the chromosomes involved in Down's syndrome (trisomy 21) and chronic myeloid leukemia (Ph^1) by fluorescence. Nature, 1971, 230, 167

Oss CJ, Gillman CF, Bronson PM, Border JR: Phagocytosis-inhibiting properties of human serum alpha-1 acid glycoprotein. Immunol Commun, 1974, 3, 321–328

Oss CJ, Woeppel MS, Marquart SE: Immunoglobulins as aspecific opsonins. III. The opsonizing power of fragments of polyclonal and monoclonal immunoglobulin G. J Reticuloendothel Soc, 1973, 13, 221–230

Ostojska J: Enzymatic and phagocytic activity of neutrophils in children with Down's syndrome (in Polish). Pediatr Pol, 1972, 47, 1221–1229

Ottesen J: On the age of human white cells in peripheral blood. Acta Physiol Scand, 1954, 32, 75

Ove P, Kremer WB, Laszlo J: Increased DNA polymerase activity in human leukaemic cells. Nature, 1968, 220, 713

Owusu SK: Complete deficiency of glucose-6-phosphate dehydrogenase and neutrophil dysfunction. Lancet, 1973, 2, 796

Oye E: Recherches sur la composition de la moelle osseuse chez les enfants. V. Le myélogramme dans la diphtérie. Rev Belg Path, 1952, 21, 385–388

Pabst HF, Holmes B, Quie PG: Immunologic abnormalities in Job's syndrome. Pediatr Res, 1971, 5, 380

Padgett GA, Reiquam CW, Gorham JR, Henson JB, O'Mary CC: Comparative studies of the Chediak-Higashi syndrome. Am J Pathol, 1967, 51, 553–556

Page AR, Berendes H, Warner J, Good RA: The Chediak-Higashi syndrome. Blood, 1962, 20, 330–331

Page AR, Good RA: Studies on cyclic neutropenia. A clinical and experimental investigation. Am J Dis Child, 1957, 94, 623

Pajdak W, Sznajd J: Phosphatases of leukocytes. II. Isolation and characteristics of acid phosphatase in leukocytes from healthy subjects and from patients with chronic granulocytic leukemia (in Polish). Przegl Lek, 1972, 29, 301–312

Palmblad J: Fasting (acute energy deprivation) in man: effect on polymorphonuclear granulocyte function, plasma iron and serum transferrin. Scand J Haematol, 1976, 17, 217–226

Parameshwaran N: The sex chromatin body and neutrophil "drumstick" appendage. Ceylon Med J, 1971, 16, 39–46

Park BH, Firkin SM, Smithwick EM: Infection and nitroblue-tetrazolium reduction by neutrophils. Lancet, 1968, 2, 532–534

Park BH, Holmes B, Good RA: Metabolic activities in leukocytes of newborn infants. J Pediatr, 1970, 76, 237–241

Parkinson CF, Carter PB: Phagocytosis of mycoplasma salivarium by human polymorphonuclear leukocytes and monocytes. Infect Immun, 1975, 11, 405–414

Paukovits WR, Paukovits JB: Separation, identification and mechanism of action of the granulocytic chalone. Boll Ist Sieroter Milan, 1975, 54, 177–186

Payne R: Neonatal neutropenia and leukoagglutinins. Pediatrics, 1964, 33, 194

Pelger K: Demonstratie van een paar zeldzaam voorkomende typen van bloedlichaampjes en bespreking der patienten. Discuss Med Tijdschr Geneesk, 1928, 72, 1178

Pellegrini MSF: Le varie fasi maturative dei granulociti neutrofili umani studiati al microscopio elettronico. Boll Soc Ital Biol Sper, 1974, 50, 17–20

Perillie PE, Finch SC: Quantitative studies on the local exudative cellular reaction in acute leukemia. J Clin Invest, 1964, 43, 425

Perillie PE, Kaplan SS, Lefkowitz E, Rogaway W, Finch SC: Studies of muramidase (lysozyme) in leukemia. JAMA, 1968, 203, 317–322

Perillie PE, Nolan JP, Finch SC: Studies of the resistance to infection in diabetes mellitus: local exudative cellular responses. J Lab Clin Med, 1962, 59, 1108–1115

Perry S, Godwin HA, Zimmerman TS: Physiology of granulocyte. I. JAMA, 1968, 203, 437–444

Perry S, Godwin HA, Zimmerman TS: Physiology of granulocyte. II. JAMA, 1968, 203, 1125–1137

Phelps P: Polymorphonuclear leukocyte mobility in vitro. IV. Colchicine inhibition of chemotactic activity formation after phagocytosis of urate crystals. Arthritis Rheum, 1970, 13, 1

Phelps P, McCarty DJ Jr: Crystal induced inflammation in canine joints. II. Importance of polymorphonuclear leukocytes. J Exp Med, 1966, 124, 115–116

Phillips CW Jr, Kimbrough GR, Weaver JA, Tucker AL: Rocky Mountain spotted fever with thrombocytopenia. STN Med P, 1960, 53, 867–869

Pietrzyk J: Cytochemistry of neutrophils in diabetic children (in Polish). Doct Diss, Medical Academy, Cracow, 1979

Pietrzyk JA, Palimąka W: Immune system in patients with diabetes mellitus (in Polish). Wiad Lek, 1979, 32, 323–326

Pilgrim U, Gingrat JJ, Ruckli B, Hitzig WH: Nitroblue tetrazolium (NBT) reduction in granulocytes in children with acute leukemia. Preliminary report. Schweiz Med Wschr, 1974, 104, 147

Piotrowski J, Lisiewicz J, Sąsiadek U, Wąs K: Lysosomal acid phosphatase of lymphocytes from pregnant women with Rh-incompatibility (in Polish). Pol Tyg Lek, 1977, 5, 108–113

Piquet H, Greze A, Hayet U: Hypofibrinogenopenie par coagulation intravasculaire disséminée au cours d'une leucemie aiguë a promyelocytes. Coagulation (Lyon), 1969, 2, 71–73

Pituch A: Peripheral blood neutrophils in children in remission of acute lymphoblastic leukaemia. Acta Med Pol, 1977, 18, 69–84

Plum CM, Warburg M, Danielsen J: Defective maturation of granulocytes, retinal cysts and multiple skeletal malformations in a mentally retarded girl. Acta Haemat, 1978, 59, 53–63

Polishuk WZ, Diamant YZ: Leukocyte alkaline phosphatase monitoring of ovarian function in normal and clomiphene-treated cycles. Fertil Steril, 1973, 24, 245–251

Polishuk WZ, Diamant YZ, Zuckerman H: Leukocyte alkaline phosphatase in pregnancy and the puerperium. Am J Obstet Gynecol, 1970, 107, 604–609

Polliack A: Acute promyelocytic leukemia with disseminated intravascular coagulation. Am J Clin Pathol, 1971, 56, 155–161

Polliack A, McKenzie S, Gee T, Lampen N, de Harven E, Clarkson BD: A scanning electron microscopic study of 34 cases of acute granulocytic, myelomonocytic, monoblastic, and histiocytic leukemia. Am J Med, 1975, 59, 308–315

Popławski A, Prokopowicz J, Niewiarowski S: Antiheparin activity in subcellular fractions of human granulocytes. Thromb Diath Haemorrh, 1969, 21, 170–171

Powell HC, Wolf PL: Neutrophilic leukocyte inclusion in colchicine intoxication. Arch Pathol Lab Med, 1976, 100, 136–138

Power DL, Mandell GL: Intra-leukocytic bacteria in endocarditis. JAMA, 1974, 227, 312

Pringle EM, Young, WF, Haworth EM: Syndrome of pancreatic insufficiency, blood dyscrasia and metaphyseal dysplasia. Proc Roy Soc Med, 1968, 61, 776

Pritchard JA: Leukocyte alkaline phosphatase activity in pregnancy. J Lab Clin Med, 1957, 50, 432

Prokopowicz J: Distribution of fibrinolytic and proteolytic enzymes in subcellular fraction of human granulocytes. Thromb Diath Haemorrh, 1968, 19, 84–89

Prokopowicz J: Purification of plasminogen from human granulocytes using DEAE-sephadex column chromatography. Biochim Biophys Acta, 1968, 154, 91–95

Prokopowicz J, Merkiel K, Krawczuk J: Bactericidal activity of plasma and leukocytes after surgical treatment of digestive tract tumors. Proceedings of VII Conference of Commission of Tumor Biology of Polish Academy of Science. Onkologia Doświadczalna, 1977

Prokopowicz J, Stormorken H: Fibrinolytic activity of leukocytes in smears of bone marrow and peripheral blood. Scand J Haematol, 1968, 15, 1–9

Propp RP, Alper LA: C_3' synthesis in the human fetus and lack of transplacental passage. Science, 1968, 162, 672

Pružanski W, Leers WD, Wardlaw AC: Bactericidal and bacteriolytic activity of leukemic sera. Cancer Res, 1973, 33, 2048–2053

Pryadkina MD, Fradkin VA, Kuznetsova LS, Raetskaia EK: The response of blood neutrophils (the PPN test) to pertussis allergen in children with pertussis and children immunized with ADPT vaccine. Zh Mikrobiol Epidemiol Immnobiol, 1975, 1, 78–80

Qualliotine D, DeChatelet LR, McCall CE, Cooper MR: Stimulation of oxidative metabolism in polymorphonuclear leukocytes by catecholamines. J Reticuloendothel Soc, 1972, 11, 263–276

Quie PG: Pathology of bactericidal power of neutrophils. Semin Hematol, 1975, 12, 143–160

Quie PG, White JG, Holmes B, Good RA: In vitro bactericidal capacity of human polymorphonuclear leukocytes: diminished activity in chronic granulomatous disease of childhood. J Clin Invest, 1967, 46, 668

Quigley HJ: Peripheral leukocyte thromboplastin in promyelocytic leukemia (abstr 2199). Fed Proc, 1967, 26, 648

Quigley HJ, Dawson AE, Hyun BH, Custer RP: The activity of alkaline phosphatase in granular leukocytes during pregnancy and the puerperium: a preliminary report. Am J Clin Pathol, 1960, 33, 109

Rabinovitch M: Phagocytosis: the engulfment stage. Semin Hematol, 1968, 5, 134–155

Rachmilewitz D, Rachmilewitz EA, Polliack A, Hershko Ch: Acute promyelocytic leukemia: a report of five cases with comment on the diagnostic significance of serum vitamin B_{12} determination. Br J Haematol, 1972, 22, 87–92

Radwańska U, Michalewska D, Sotnik D, Fojudzki E, Strzykała K: Neutrophil alkaline phosphatase in girls during menstrual cycle (in Polish). Pediatr Pol, 1971, 11, 1373–1378

Raichs A, Girald M, Gil JL, Uguet JA, Novarro DM, Aztarain E, Torres A: Granulocytic function in the hemopathies: qualitative and quantitative aspects. XIV International Congress of Hematology, Sao Paulo, Brazil, 1972, Abstracts, 123

Rainer H, Höcker P, Deutsch E, Stacher A, Moser K: Biochemische Unterschiede der DNA-Polymerasen leukämischer Zellen. Blut, 1974, 28, 256–263

Rajan KT: Lysosomes and gout. Nature (London), 1966, 210, 959

Rastuntsev LP: Functional changes in neutrophils according to cytochemical findings in suppurative and serous viral meningitis. Zh Nevropatol Psikhiatr, 1973, 73, 177–180

Ratzan KR, Giraudo C, Amado C, Lauredo I, Horowitz G: Effect of sodium cyanate upon the function of normal human polymorphonuclear leukocytes. J Infect Dis, 131 Suppl, 1975, 73–80

Rebuck JW, Crowley JH: A method of studying leukocytic functions in vivo. Ann NY Acad Sci, 1955, 59, 757

Reed WP, Palmer DL, Williams RC, Kish AL: Bubonic plague in the Southwestern United States. Medicine, 1970, 272, 1263–1268

Reilly WA: The granules in the leukocytes in gargyolism. Am J Dis Child, 1941, 62, 489

Repine JE, Clowson CC, Brunnung RD: Primary leukocyte alkaline phosphatase deficiency in an adult with repeated infections. Br J Haematol, 1976, 34, 87–94

Rey JJ, Wolf PL: Extreme leukocytosis in accidental electric shock. Lancet, 1968, 1, 18

Reyero C, Dorner F: Purification of arginases from human leukemic lymphocytes and granulocytes: study of their physicochemical and kinetic properties. Eur J Biochem, 1975, 56, 137–147

Ricci P, Bagnara GP, Brunelli MA: Granulopoiesis in "smoldering" leukemia in vitro. Boll Soc Ital Biol Sper, 1975, 51, 1001–1006

Rich KC, Neumann CG, Stiehm ER: Neutrophil chemotaxis in malnourished Ghanaian children. In Suskind RM (ed): Malnutrition and the Immune Response. Kroc Foundation Series, Raven Press, New York, 1977, pp 271–275

Riddle JM, Barnhard MI: Ultrastructural study of fibrin dissolution via emigrated polymorphonuclear neutrophils. Am J Pathol, 1964, 45, 805–823

Riddle JM, Barnhard MI: The eosinophils as a source for profibrinolysin in acute inflammation. Blood, 1965, 25, 776–794

Riddle JM, Bluhm GB, Barnhart MI: Ultrastructural study of leucocytes and urates in gouty arthritis. Ann Rheum Dis, 1967, 25, 389–401

Rindler R, Braunsteiner H: Soluble proteins from human leukocyte granules. I. Esterase activity of cationic proteins. Blut, 1973, 27, 26

Rindler R, Braunsteiner H: Cationic proteins from human neutrophil granulocytes. Evidence for their chymotrypsin-like properties. Biochim Biophys Acta, 1975, 379, 606–617

Rindler R, Hörtnagl H, Schmalzl F, Braunsteiner H: Hydrolysis of a chymotrypsin substrate and of naphthol AS-D chloracetate by human leukocyte granules. Blut, 1973, 26, 239

Rindler R, Schmalzl F, Braunsteiner H: Esterases in human neutrophil granulocytes: evidence for their protease nature. Br J Haematol, 1974, 27, 57–64

Rindler R, Schmalzl F, Braunsteiner H: Isolierung und Charakterisierung der chymotrypsinnählichen Protease aus neutrophilen Granulozyten des Menschen. Schweiz Med Wschr, 1974, 104, 132–133

Rindler R, Schmalzl F, Hörtnagl H, Braunsteiner H: Naphthol AS-D chloracetate esterases in granule extracts from human neutrophil leukocytes. Blut, 1971, 23, 223

Robineaux R, Kourilsky R, Buffe D: Recherches sur la formation de la cellule de Hargraves. Am Inst Pasteur, 1956, 91, 109–112

Robinson WA, Pike BL: Leukopoietic activity of human bone marrow cells in vitro. In Stohlman F Jr (ed): Hemopoietic Cellular Proliferation. Grune-Stratton, New York, 1970, p 249

Rocklin RE: Partial characterization of leukocyte inhibitory factor by concanavalin A stimulated human lymphocytes (LIF con A). J Immunol, 1975

Rodey GE, Jacob HS, Holmes B, McArthur JR, Good RA: Leukocyte G-6-PD levels and bactericidal activity. Lancet, 1970, 1, 355

Rodin AE, Haggard ME, Nichols MM, Gustavson LP: Infantile genetic agranulocytosis. Am J Child, 1973, 126, 818–821

Rodriguez V, Burgess M, Bodey GP: Management of fever of unkown origin in patients with neoplasms and neutropenia. Cancer, 1973, 32, 1007–1012

Rohde L, Grottum KA: Virushepatitt og pancytopeni. T Nor Laegeforen, 1967, 87, 1906–1908

Rohmann H: Über die Phagocytoze der Leukozyten bei Diabetikern. Folia Haematol (Leipz), 1966, 85, 267–269

Rohrer GF, Wartburg JP, Aebi H: Myeloperoxidase aus menschlichen Leukozyten. I. Isolierung und Charakterisierung des Enzyms. Biochem Z, 1966, 344, 478

Roos D, Weening WS, Voetman AA, van Schaik LJ, Bot AAM, Meerhof LJ, Loos JA: Protection of phagocytic leukocytes by endogenous glutathione: studies in a family with glutathione reductase deficiency. Blood, 1979, 53, 851–866

Rosenbaum MJ, Muehl P, Sullivan EJ, Edwards EA, Krumpe P, Miller CH: NBT reduction by human neutrophils stimulated by adenoviruses in vitro. Proc Soc Exp Biol Med, 1974, 146, 868–875

Rosenbloom FM, Kelley WN, Miller J, Henderson JF, Seegmiller JE: Inherited disorder of purine metabolism: correlation between central nervous dysfunction and biochemical defects. JAMA, 1967, 202, 275

Rosenblum AL, Carbone PP: Androgenic hormones and human granulopoiesis in vitro. Blood, 1974, 43, 351–356

Rosenblum D, Petzold SJ: Neutrophil alkaline phosphatase: comparison of enzymes from normal subjects and patients with polycythemia vera and chronic myelogenous leukemia. Blood, 1975, 45, 335–343

Resenszajn L, Klajman A, Yaffe D, Efrati P: Jordan's anomaly in white blood cells. Blood, 1966, 28, 258–265

Rosnay C: L'hématologie du typhus exanthématique. Doin, 1947

Rosner F, Valmont I, Kozzin PP, Caroline L: Leukocyte function in patients with leukemia. Cancer, 1970, 25, 835–842

Rosner F, Weisfogel G, Feinerman A: Infantile amaurotic familial idiocy. Leukocyte granulation and leukocyte alkaline phosphatase. JAMA, 1968, 205, 873

Ross JD, Rosenbaum E: Paroxysmal nocturnal hemoglobinuria presenting in aplastic anemia in a child. Am J Med, 1964, 37, 130–132

Roth L, Turcanu P, Zosiñ I, Serban M, Harry J: Die Tuschephagozytose der Mono- und Granulozyten während der akuten und chronischen Verbrauchskoagulopathie. Folia Haematol (Leipz), 1975, 102, 431–437

Rothstein G, Bishop CR, Athens JW, Ashenbrucker HE: A method for leukokinetic study in the nonsteady state. Blood, 1971, 38, 302–311

Rowley JD: A new consistent chromosomal abnormality in chronic myelogenous leukaemia identified by quinacrine fluorescence and Giemsa staining. Nature, 1973, 243, 290–292

Rubio T, Riley HD, Nida JR, Brooksaler F, Nelson JD: Thrombocytopenia in Rocky Mountain spotted fever. Am J Dis Child, 1968, 116, 88–96

Ruddy S, Gigli I, Austen KF: The complement system of man. N Engl J Med, 1972, 287, 489–495, 545–549, 592–596, 662–664

Rudyk BJ: Toxic granulations in neutrophils and colored precipitation reaction of urine in patients with diseases of the hematopoietic system (in Polish). Przegl Lek, 1966, 7, 506–508

Ruutu F, Ruutu T, Vuopio P: Functions of neutrophils in preleukemia. Scand J Haematol, 1977, 18, 317–325

Ruutu T, Kosunen TU: Phagocytic activity of neutrophilic leukocytes of A_2 influenza patients. Acta Pathol Microbiol Scand, B, 1971, 79, 67–72

Ruzicka F, Pawlowsky J, Erber A: Three cases of eosinophilic leukemia with atypical granulation in the eosinophils and neutrophils. Blut, 1976, 32, 337–346

Ryan GB, Borysenko JZ, Karnovsky MJ: Factors affecting the redistribution of surface-bound concanavalin A on human polymorphonuclear leukocytes. J Cell Biol, 1974, 62, 351–356

Ryden SE, Silverman EM: The nitroblue tetrazolium test in tuberculosis. Am J Clin Pathol, 1974, 63, 431–432

Ryder RJW: Promyelocytic leukaemia and hypofibrinogenaemia. Acta Haematol (Basel), 1966, 35, 181–191

Rytömaa T: Granulocytic chalone. In Dutcher RM, Chieco-Bianchi L (eds): Unifying Concepts of Leukaemia. Bibl Haematol, 1973, 39, 885–889

Rytömaa T: Biology of the granulocyte chalone. Boll Ist Sieroter Milan, 1975, 54, 195–202

Rytömaa T, Vilpo JA, Levanto A: Effect of granulocytic chalone on acute myeloid leukaemia in man. Lancet, 1977, 8015, 771–774

Rytömaa T, Vilpo JA, Levanto A, Jones WA: Effect of granulocyte chalone on acute and chronic leukaemia in man. Scand J Haematol, 1976, Suppl, 27, 1–28

Saba HI, Roberts HR, Herion JC: Anti-heparin activity of lysosomal cationic proteins from polymorphonuclear leukocytes. Blood, 1968, 31, 369–380

Sabin FR, Cunningham RS, Doan CA, Kindwall JA: The normal rhythm of white blood cells. Johns Hopkins Med J, 1925, 37, 14

Salmon SE, Cline MJ, Schultz J, Lehrer RJ: Myeloperoxidase deficiency: a genetic leukocyte defect. N Engl J Med, 1970, 282, 252

Samuels AJ: Primary and secondary changes following the intramuscular injection of epinephrine hydrochloride. J Clin Invest, 1951, 30, 941

Sanchez Yllades L: Tuberculosis y sindromes mieloproliferativos en busca de los medios que perminan hacer un diagnostico differencial. Gaz Med Mex, 1964, 54, 43–76

Sandberg AA: Chromosomes and causation of human cancer and leukemia. VI. Blastic phase, cellular origin, and Ph^1 in CML. Cancer, 1971, 27, 176

Sandberg AA, Hossfield DK: Chromosomal abnormalities in human neoplasia. Am Rev Med, 1970, 21, 379–380

Sander GE, Allen RC, Mansell PA, Reed MA, Carter KJ, Steele RH, Carter RD, Krementz ET: Polymorphonuclear leukocyte chemiluminescence: decreased activity in terminal stages of malignant melanoma. IRCS Med Sci Pathol 1976, 4, 116

Sarin PS, Anderson PN, Gallo RG: Terminal deoxynucleotidyl transferase activities in human blood leukocytes and lymphoblast cell lines: high levels in lymphoblast cell lines and in blast cells of some patients with chronic myelogenous leukemia in acute phase. Blood, 1976, 47, 11–20

Sarnitski IP, Temnik IV: Some cytochemical indices of the functional activity of neutrophils in patients with lymphogranulomatosis (in Russian). Vrach Delo, 1975, 7, 77–80

Sbarra AJ, Karnovsky ML: The biochemical basis of phagocytosis. I. Metabolic changes during the ingestion of particles by polymorphonuclear leukocytes. J Biol Chem, 1959, 234, 1335–1362

Sbarra AJ, Selvaraj RJ, Paul BP, Poskitt PKF, Zgliczyński JM, Mitchell GW Jr, Louis F: Biochemical, functional and structural aspects of phagocytosis. Int Rev Exp Pathol, 1976, 16, 249–271

Sbarra AJ, Shirley W, Selyara J, McRipley RJ, Rosenbaum E: The role of phagocytic cells in host-parasite interactions. III. The phagocytic capabilities of leucocytes from myeloproliferative and other neoplastic disorders. Cancer Res, 1965, 25, 1199–1206

Schaefer R: Zur Differentialdiagnose der Agranulocytose. Dtsch Arch Klin Med, 1926, 151, 191

Schiffer CA, Sanel FT, Techmiller BK, Wiernik PH: Functional and morphologic characteristics of the leukemic cells of a patient with acute monocytic leukemia: correlation with clinical features. Blood, 1975, 46, 17–26

Schlesinger JJ, Ernst C, Weinstein J: Inhibition of human neutrophil chemotaxis by influenza virus. Lancet, 1976, 1, 650–651

Schmalzl F, Braunsteiner H: The application of cytochemical methods to the study of acute leukemia. Acta Haematol, 1971, 45, 209–217

Schreiner A, Solberg CO: Neutrophil dysfunction and granulomatosis in the preleukemic state. Scand J Infect Dis, 1976, 8, 53–55

Schultz J, Kaminker K: Myeloperoxidase of the leukocyte of normal human blood. I. Content and localization. Arch Biochem, 1962, 96, 465

Schultz J, Shmukler HR: Myeloperoxidase of the leukocyte of normal human blood. II. Isolation, spectrophotometry, and amino acid analysis. Biochemistry, 1964, 3, 1234

Schwarzenberg L, Schneider M, Mathé G: Factors influencing the clinical response to white blood cell transfusions in aplastic infected patients. In Goldman JM, Lowenthal RM (eds): Leucocytes: Separation, Collection and Transfusion. Academic Press, London, New York, San Francisco, 1975, pp 380–384

Seelich F: Sind lysosomale Enzyme an der Regulation der Zellvermehrung beteiligt? Osterr Z Oncol, 1975, 2, 31–37

Seip M: Systemic lupus erythematosus in pregnancy with haemolytic anaemia, leukopenia and thrombocytopenia in the mother and her newborn infant. Arch Dis Child, 1960, 35, 364

Seitz IF: Biochemistry of Normal and Leukemic Leucocytes, Thrombocytes and Bone Marrow Cells (in Russian). Meditsina, Leningrad, 1965

Selvaraj RJ, McRipley RJ, Sbarra AJ: The effect of phagocytosis and X-irradiation on human leukocyte metabolism. Cancer Res, 1967, 25, 2280–2286

Selvaraj RJ, McRipley RJ, Sbarra AJ: The metabolic activities of leukocytes from lymphoproliferative and myeloproliferative disorders during phagocytosis. Cancer Res, 1967, 25, 2287–2294

Selye H: Thrombohemorrhagic Phenomena. Charles C Thomas, Springfield, Ill, 1966

Senn HJ: Infektabwehr bei Hämoblastosen: Funktionelle Studien Über Leukozytenmobilization beim gesunden and kranken Menschen. Exp Med Pathol Klin, 36, Springer, Berlin, 1972

Senn HJ, Chu B, O'Malley J, Holland JF: Experimental and clinical studies on muramidase (lysozyme). VII. Muramidase activity of normal human blood cells and inflammatory exudates. Acta Haematol, 1970, 44, 65–77

Senn HJ, Holland JF: Leukocyte mobilization in health and acute leukemia. Blood, 1967, 30, 888

Senn HJ, Holland JF, Banerjee T: Kinetic and comparative studies of localized leucocyte mobilization in normal man. J Lab Clin Med, 1969, 74, 742

Senn HJ, Jungi WF: Neutrophil migration in health and disease. Semin Hematol, 1975, 12, 27–45

Senn HJ, Rhomberg WU, Jungi WF: Störung der leukozytären Abwehrfunktion als paraonco-plastisches Syndrom bei Hämoblastosen. Schweiz Med Wschr, 1971, 101, 466

Serafińska D: Antibacterial immunity in proliferative diseases of the hemopoietic system. I. Phagocytic capacity of leukocytes (in Polish). Acta Haematol Pol, 1970, 1, 95–101

Serafińska D, Lewicka T, Jasser S: Antibacterial immunity in proliferative diseases of the hematopoietic system. Acta Haematol Pol, 1973, 4, 55–64

Shakhabazian AA: Reaction of neutrophil damage in non-specific ulcerative colitis (in Russian). Sov Med, 1975, 4, 149–150

Shapera RM, Matsen JM: Nitroblue tetrazolium dye reduction by neutrophils from patients with streptococcal pharyngitis. Pediatrics, 1973, 51, 284–288

Shapiro AM, Guseva NG, Komissarova IA: Some data on the cytochemistry of peripheral blood neutrophils in scleroderma. Sov Med, 1971, 34, 36–39

Sharp GW: Reversal of diurnal leucocyte variations in man. J Endocrinol, 1960, 21, 107–114

Sharp GW: The effect of light on diurnal leucocyte variations. J Endocrinol, 1960, 21, 213–218

Shohet SB: Morphologic evidence for the in vivo activity of transfused chronic myelogenous leukemia cells in a case of massive staphylococcal septicemia. Blood, 1968, 32, 111–118

Shopsin B, Friedmann R, Gershon S: Lithium and leukocytosis. Clin Pharmacol Ther, 1971, 12, 923–928

Silber R, Unger KW, Ellman L: RNA metabolism in normal and leukaemic leukocytes: further studies on RNA synthesis. Br J Haematol, 1968, 14, 261

Silver RT, Beal GA, Schneiderman MA, McCullough NB: The role of mature neutrophil in bacterial infections in acute leukaemia. Blood, 1957, 12, 814–821

Simons K, Weber T: The vitamin B_{12}-binding protein in human leukocytes. Biochim Biophys Acta, 1966, 117, 201

Sinakos Z, Larrieu MJ: Leukocytes et fibrinolyse. Nouv Rev Fr Hematol, 1965, 5, 601–608

Skarnes RC, Watson DW: Characterization of leukin: an antibacterial factor from leukocytes active against Gram-positive pathogens. J Exp Med, 1956, 104, 829–845

Skotnicki AB: Pulmonary tuberculosis in the course of leukemias (in Polish). Patol Pol, 1975, 26, 397–407

Smetana K, Vlastiborová A, Iscenko I: Studies on micronucleoli of immature human leukemic neutrophils. Neoplasma, 1973, 20, 491–498

Smith CW, Hellers JC, Dupree E: A serum inhibitor of leukotaxis in a child with recurrent infections. J Lab Clin Med, 1972, 79, 878–885

Smith HL Jr, Baker FA: Pyrimidine metabolism in man. I. The biosynthesis of orotic acid. J Clin Invest, 1959, 38, 798

Smith LH, Baker FA, Sullivan M: Pyrimidine metabolism in man. II. Studies of leukemic cells. Blood, 1960, 15, 360

Smith SB, Revel JP: Mapping of concanavalin A binding sites on the surfaces of several cell types. Dev Biol, 1972, 28, 434–442

Smith WC, Kaneshiro MM, Goldstein BD, Parker JW, Lukes RJ: Gaucher cells in chronic gran-ulocytic leukemia. Lancet, 1968, 2, 780

Sneiderman CA, Wilson JW: Effects of corticosteroids on complement and the neutrophilic polymorphonuclear leukocytes. Transplant Proc, 1975, 7, 41–48

Söder PO, Nord CE, Lundblad G, Kjellman O: Investigation on lysozyme, protease and hyalu-ronidase activity in extracts from human leukocytes. Acta Chem Scand, 1970, 24, 129–136

288

Söderlund I, Engstedt L, Paléus S, Unger P: Induction of leucocytosis by means of hydrocortisone and/or muscular exercise. In Goldman JM, Lowenthal RM (eds): Leucocytes: Separation, Collection and Transfusion. Academic Press, London, New York, San Francisco, 1975, pp 97–103

Solberg CO: Protection of phagocytized bacteria against antibiotics. A new method for the evaluation of neutrophil granulocyte functions. Acta Med Scand, 1972, 191, 383–387

Solberg CO, Hellum KB: Neutrophil function in bacterial infections. Lancet, 1972, 2, 727–730

Solberg CO, Schreiner K, Hellum KB, Hamre E: Neutrophil granulocyte function in the early diagnosis of acute myelocytic and myeloblastic leukaemia. Acta Med Scand, 1975, 197, 147–151

Soonattrakul W, Andersen BR: NBT test in lymphomas. N Engl J Med, 1973, 288, 218

Sopata I, Dancewicz A: Neutral protease of human leukocytes degrading collagen (in Polish). Przegl Lek, 1974, 31, 435–439

Soriano RB, South MA, Goldman AA, Smith CW: Defect of neutrophil motility in a child with recurrent bacterial infections and disseminated cytomegalovirus infection. J Pediatr, 1973, 83, 951–958

Souillet G, Germain D, Carraz M, Veysseyre C, Frobert Y: Phagocytose et bactéricidie normales du polynucléaire neutrophile. Sem Hop Paris, 1975, 51, 1689–1700

Spatz N, Borches HG, Zobl H: Knochenmarkschädigung bei Virus-Hepatitis. Med Klin, 1968, 63, 1761–1765

Spector GI, Kevorkov NN: Autoallergic reaction of neutrophils in the diagnosis of pyelonephritis. Klin Med (Mosk), 1975, 53, 52–55

Spector GI, Kevorkov NN, Chumakov II: Allergic affection of neutrophils as a test for differential diagnosis of pyelonephritis and nephrotuberculosis. Urol Nefrol, 1975, 2, 26–29

Spiegelberg HL, Lawrence DA, Henson P: Cytophilic properties of IgA to human neutrophils. Adv Exp Med Biol, 1974, 45, 67–74

Spiers ASD, Baikie AG, Dartnall JA, Cox JI: Cytogenetic studies of the spleen in chronic granulocytic leukemia. Aust NZ Med, 1975, 5, 295–305

Spitznagel JK: Bactericidal mechanism of the granulocytes. Prog Clin Biol Res, 1977, 13, 103–113

Spitznagel JK, Chi HY: Cationic proteins and antibacterial properties of infected tissue and leukocytes. Am J Pathol, 1963, 43, 697–711

Stanbury JB, Wyngaarden JB, Fredrickson DS: The Metabolic Basis of Inherited Disease. McGraw-Hill, New York, 1972

Stavem P, Ly B, Egeberg O: Flaming promyelocytes in acute hypergranuiar promyelocytic leukaemia. Scand J Haematol, 1977, 19, 99–105

Steerman RL, Synderman R, Leikin SL, Colten HR: Intrinsic defect of the polymorphonuclear leukocyte resulting in impaired chemotaxis and phagocytosis. Clin Exp Immunol, 1971, 9, 939–946

Stefanini M, Mele RH, Skinner D: Transitory congenital neutropenia: a new syndrome. Report of two cases. Am J Med, 1958, 25, 749

Steinbrinck W: Über eine neue Granulationsanomalie der Leukozyten. Dtsch Arch Klin Med, 1948, 193, 577–580

Steinitz K, Bodur H, Arman T: Amylo-1,6-glucosidase activity in leukocytes from patients with glycogen storage disease. Clin Chim Acta, 1963, 8, 807

Stendahl O, Lindgren S: Function of granulocytes with deficient myeloperoxidase-mediated iodination in a patient with generalized pustular psoriasis. Scand J Haematol, 1976, 16, 144–153

Stepanova ZhV: Study of the neutrophil damage test in patients with mycoses (in Russian). Vestn Dermatol Venerol, 1975, 8, 41–45

Sternberger LA, Osserman EF, Seligman AM: Lysozyme and fibrinogen in normal and leukemic blood cells: a quantitative electron immunocytochemical study. Johns Hopkins Med J, 1970, 126, 188–209

Stevenson RD: Polymorph migration stimulator. A new factor produced by hydrocortisone-treated monocytes. Clin Exp Immunol, 1974, 17, 601–606

Stieglitz R, Kranz D: Panmyelophthisen nach Virushepatitis. Ber Dtsch Gesungh Wes, 1968, 23, 241–248

Stjernholm RL: The metabolism of human leukocytes. XII Congress of International Society of Hematology. Plenary Session Papers. New York, 1968, pp 175–186

Stjernholm RL, Allen RC, Steele RH, Waring WW, Harris JA: Impaired chemiluminescence during phagocytosis of opsonized bacteria. Infect Immun, 1973, 7, 313–314

Stolc V: Effect of pituitary factor on iodine uptake and cyclic adenosine 3',5'-monophosphate formation in human polymorphonuclear leukocytes. Biochem Med, 1975, 12, 226–233

Stollerman GH, Rytel M, Ortiz J: Accessory plasma factors involved in the bactericidal test for type-specific antibody to group A streptococci. II. Human plasma cofactor(s) enhancing opsonization of encapsulated organisms. J Exp Med, 1963, 117, 1–17

Stossel TP: Phagocytosis. N Engl J Med, 1974, 290, 717–723, 774–780, 833–839

Stossel TP, Alper CA, Rosen FS: Opsonic activity in the newborn. Role of properdin. Pediatrics, 1974, 52, 134

Stossel TP, Pollard TD, Mason RJ, Vaughan M: Isolation and properties of phagocytic vesicles from polymorphonuclear leukocytes. J Clin Invest, 1971, 50, 1745–1757

Stossel TP, Root RK, Vaughan M: Phagocytosis in chronic granulomatous disease and the Chediak-Higashi syndrome. N Engl J Med, 1972, 286, 120–123

Strauss RS, Bove KE, Jones JF, Mauer AM, Fulginiti VA: An anomaly of neutrophil morphology with impaired function. N Engl J Med, 1974, 290, 478–484

Strauss RG, Burrows SE: Activity of 5'-nucleotidase in polymorphonuclear leukocytes. Blood, 1975, 46, 655–656

Strausz I, Barcsák J, Kékes E, Szebeni A: Prednisolone-induced acute changes in circulating neutrophil granulocytes. I. In cases of normal granulocyte reserves. Haematologia (Budap), 1967, 1, 319–326

Strausz I, Barcsák J, Kékes E, Szebeni A: Prednisolone-induced acute changes in circulating neutrophil granulocytes. III. In cases of pernicious anaemia. Haematologia (Budap), 1968, 2, 109–115

Strouth JC, Zeman W, Merritt AD: Leukocyte abnormalities in familial amaurotic idiocy. N Engl J Med, 1966, 274, 36–38

Strumia MM: Agranulocytosis and acute leukemia. Am J Med, Sci, 1934, 187, 826

Stryckmans P, DeBusscher L: Neutrophil collection and transfusion for the treatment of infection in neutropenic patients. Eur J Cancer, 1975, 11 Suppl, 67–77

Sullivan JF, Dolan T, Meyers A, Treat K: Use of NBT dye test. Am J Dis Child, 1973, 125, 702–704

Sułowicz W, Dawidiuk W, Szczepaniec M, Jakóbiec M: Spontaneous nitroblue tetrazolium reduction test in women in the perinatal period. Gin Pol, 1977, 48, 967–971

Sultan Y, Delobel J, Caen J: Anomalies de l'hemostase primaire au cours des leucémies myeloides chroniques et des autres syndromes myeloproliferatifs. Actual Hematol, 1969, 3, 95–101

Sultan C, Gounault M, Varet B: Relationship between the cell morphology of acute myeloblastic leukaemia and the occurrence of a syndrome of disseminated intravascular coagulation. XIV International Congress of Hematology, Sao Paulo, 1972, Abstract, 603

Suzuki JB, Booth RR, Grecz N: Evaluation of phagocytic activity by ingestion of labelled bacteria. J Infect Dis, 1971, 123, 93–96

Suzuki Y, Suzuki K: Krabbe's globoid cell leukodystrophy: deficiency of galactocerebrosidase in serum, leukocytes, and fibroblasts. Science, 1971, 171, 73–75

Szathári E, Lehoczky D, Fehér T: Studies on the alkaline granulocyte phosphatase (GAP) in endocrine diseases. Folia Haematol (Leipz), 1971, 96, 197–204

Szczeklik A, Musiał J, Piętoń R: Eosinophil: structure, function and significance in clinic (in Polish). Post Hig Med Dosw, 1976, 5, 579–608

Szczepaniec M, Sułowicz W: The NBT test in selected respiratory diseases (in Polish). Pol Arch Med Wewn, 1976, 4, 335–344

Szczepańska H: Pertussis (in Polish). Polish Medical Publishers, Warsaw, 1961

Szczepkowska W, Urasiński I: Alkaline phosphatase activity in neutrophils in polycythemia vera and in secondary erythrocytaemias (in Polish). Pol Arch Med Wewn, 1973, 50, 269–277

Szmigiel Z: Immunology of leukemias. In Aleksandrowicz J, Sznajd J, Urbańczyk J (eds.): The Leukemias (in Polish). Polish Medical Publishers, Warsaw, 1967, pp 74–88

Szmigiel Z, Doleżal M, Kaczorowska A: Phagocytic activity of neutrophils in leukemias, inflammation and health (in Polish). Pol Tyg Lek, 1957, 12, 434–437

Szmigielski S: Peroxisomal enzymes in human granulocytes. I. Catalase and peroxidase. Folia Histochem Cytochem, 1972, 10, 47–49

Szmigielski S, Kołakowska-Polubiec K, Litwin J, Słomkowski M, Żupańska B: Histochemical studies on 5'-nucleotidase activity in blood and bone marrow cells. Pol Med J, 1967, 6, 631–635

Szmigielski S, Litwin J, Żupańska B, Królikowska J: Histochemical studies of the blood and blood forming organ cells (in Polish). Post Hig Med Dosw, 1965, 19, 1

Szmigielski S, Michalewska D: Improvement in the cytochemical localization of aryl sulphatase in bone marrow and blood cells by use of naphthyl-sulphate and naphthol-AS-BI-sulphate. Folia Haematol (Leipz), 1974, 101, 536–542

Szmitkowski M: Isolation, purification, and physicochemical properties of antihemophilic globulin from human granulocytes (in Polish). Doct Diss, Medical Academy, Białystok, Poland, 1973

Sznajd J: Isolation and characteristics of ribonucleases in healthy subjects and patients with chronic granulocytic leukemia (in Polish). Folia Med Cracov, 1972, 14, 297–333

Sznajd J, Lisiewicz J, Pajdak W, Naskalski J: The biochemistry of normal and leukemic leukocytes (in Polish). Przegl Lek, 1971, 7, 496–501

Sznajd J, Naskalski J, Lisiewicz J: Antiheparin activity of myeloperoxidase and ribonucleinase of chronic granulocytic leukemia leukocytes (in Polish). Pol Arch Med Wewn, 1969, 42, 207–214

Szpilman H, Prokopowicz J, Niewiarowski S: Distribution of procoagulant activity in the subcellular fractions of human granulocytes. Experientia, 1969, 25, 77–78

Takahashi I, Nakanishi T, Sakato J: Preleukemia: hematological disorders prior to onset of leukemia. Acta Med Okayama, 1975, 29, 437–444

Tan JS, Akabutu JJ, Mauer AM: Isolated neutrophil dysfunction in adults. A new entity. Proc Am Soc Clin Invest, 1971, 50, 90a

Tan JS, Anderson JL, Watanakunakorn C, Phair JP: Neutrophil dysfunction in diabetes mellitus. J Lab Clin Med, 1975, 85, 26–33

Tatarsky J, Sinakos Z, Larrieu MJ, Barnard J: Leucocytes et fibrinolyse. II. L'étude des leucocytes pathologiques. Nouv Rev Fr Hematol, 1967, 7, 95–108

Tempka T, Braun B: Das morphologische Varhalten des Sternpunktates in verschiedenen Stadien der perniziösen Anämie und seine Wandlungen unter den Einflusse der Therapie. Folia Haematol, 1932, 48, 355–365

Territo MC, Dawidson WD, Tanaka KR: Simultaneous measurement of bactericidal activity and glucose oxidation in the human granulocyte. Br J Haematol, 1974, 28, 217–220

Tijo JH, Carbone PP, Whang J, Frei E: The Philadelphia chromosome and chronic myelogenous leukemia. J Natl Cancer Inst, 1966, 36, 567

Timina VP: Role of autoimmune processes in pathogenesis of leukopenias and thrombocytopenias in patients with typhoid fever (in Russian). Z Mikrobiol Epid Immunol, 1967, 44, 99–102

Tindall JP, Beeker SK, Rosse WF: Familial cold urticaria. A generalized reaction involving leukocytosis. Arch Intern Med, 1969, 124, 129

Tisman G, Safire G, Wu G: Lithium carbonate test in blood disorders. Clin Res, 1976, 24, 103 A

Tokodi I, Pozsar BI: Protein synthesis in leukocytes of diabetic and normal subjects. Nature (London), 1967, 215, 300

Tomonaga M: Leukocyte drumsticks in chronic granulocytic leukemia and related disorders. Blood, 1961, 18, 581

Tough IM: Cytogenetic studies in cases of chronic myeloid leukemia with a previous history of radiation. In Hayhoe FGJ (ed): Current Research in Leukemia. Cambridge University Press, London, 1965, p 47

Toyota S: Studies of characteristics of leukocytes from a pediatric perspective. I. Studies on the morphology of leukocytes and bufty coat smears of umbilical cord blood. Hiroshima J Med Sci, 1968, 17, 313

Trever WR, Leighton EC, Peller RN, Bennett IL: Brucellosis. Arch Intern Med, 1959, 103, 381–396

Tropeano L, Cacciola E: On the thromboplastic activity of normal and leukemic leukocytes. Boll Soc Biol Sperim, 1957, 33, 977–980

Tryfiates GP, Laszlo J: Human leukemic polyribosomes. Proc Soc Exp Biol Med, 1967, 124, 1125

Tsan M, Douglass KH, McIntyre PA: Hydrogen peroxide production and killing of Staphylococcus aureus by human polymorphonuclear leukocytes. Blood, 1977, 49, 437–444

Tsan MP, McIntyre PA: Stimulation by propylthiouracil of the hexose monophosphate shunt in human polymorphonuclear leukocytes during phagocytosis. Br J Haematol, 1975, 31, 193–208

Ts'ao C, Ruder EA: Ultrastructural damage of leukocytes procured by the leukopak: vulnerability of leukocytes to mechanical injury. Transfusion, 1976, 16, 336–345

Tullis JL: Prevalence, nature and identification of leukocyte antibodies. N Engl J Med, 1958, 258, 569

Ullyot JL, Bainton DF: Azurophil and specific granules of blood neutrophils in chronic myelogenous leukemia: an ultrastructural and cytochemical analysis. Blood, 1974, 44, 469–482

Ullyot JL, Bainton DF, Farquhar MG: Cytochemical studies of human neutrophilic leukocyte granules. J Histochem Cytochem, 1970, 18, 681–682

Undritz E: Die Alius-Grignaschi-Anomalie der erblich-konstitutionelle Peroxydasedefekt der Neutrophilen und Monozyte. Blut, 1966, 14, 129–136

Undritz E: Die erblich-konstitutionellen morphologischen Anomalien der Leukozyten. In Mohr L, Staehelin R (eds): Handbuch der innere Medizing. H. Schwieck-München, Springer-Verlag, Berlin, Heidelberg, New York, 1974, 2, pp 355–466

Undritz E, Schali H: Eine neue Sippe mit erblichkonstitutioneller Hochsegmentierung der Neutrophilenkerne und das Knochenmarkbild beim homozytogen Trager dieser Anomalie. Schweiz Med Wschr, 1964, 94, 1365–1370

Urasiński I, Pochopień A: Enlargement of lymph nodes as rare initial symptom of exacerbation of chronic granulocytic leukemia (in Polish). Wiad Lek, 1972, 25, 801–807

Urrego SA, Epstein JA: Leukocyte alkaline phosphatase activity in symptomatic users of intrauterine contraceptive devices. Am J Obstet Gynecol, 1971, 110, 461–466

Valentine WN, Follette JH, Lawrence JS: The glycogen content of human leukocytes and various disease states. J Clin Invest, 1953, 32, 251

Valentine WN, Hsieh HS, Paglia DE, Anderson HM, Baughan MA, Jaffe ER, Garson OM: Hereditary hemolytic anemia associated with phosphoglycerate kinase deficiency in erythrocytes and leukocytes. A probable X-chromosome-linked syndrome. N Engl J Med, 1969, 280, 528

Valkov I, Topov I, Glukhchev G, Marinov M: Morphometric study on the nucleoli of mesothelial and tumour cells being in pleural cavity effusions. Arch Geschwulstforsch, 1977, 47, 220–225

Vietzke WM, Finch SC: Serum muraminidase in neutropenic states. Clin Res, 1968, 16, 543

Vildé JL: Etude de l'activite bactéricide des leucocytes dans diverses affections. Nouv Rev Fr Hematol, 1974, 14, 301–308

Vlastiborova A, Smetana K: Studies on nucleoli of human immature neutrophils. Folia Haematol (Leipz), 1972, 98, 253–262

Vogel JM, Kimball HR, Wolff SM, Perry S: Etiocholanolone in the evaluation of marrow reserves in patients receiving cytotoxic agents. Ann Intern Med, 1967, 67, 1226

Vogel JM, Yankee RA, Kimball HR: The effect of etiocholanolone on granulocyte kinetics. Blood, 1967, 30, 474

Wachstein M: The distribution of histochemically demonstrable glycogen in human blood and bone marrow cells. Blood, 1949, 4, 54

Wagner R: Studies on the physiology of the white blood cell: the glycogen content of leukocytes in leukemia and polycythemia. Blood, 1947, 2, 235

Walford RL: Leukocyte Antigens and Antibodies. Grune-Stratton, New York, 1960

Wantzin GL, Wantzin J: The NBT test: erratic behaviour in acute leukaemia. Blut, 1975, 31, 133–142

Ward PA: The chemosuppression of chemotaxis. J Exp Med, 1966, 124, 209–226

Ward PA: Natural and synthetic inhibitors of leukotaxis. In Lepow JH, Ward PA (eds): Inflammation Mechanisms of Control. Academic Press, New York, 1972, pp 301–308

Ward PA: Leukocytic muscular dystrophy. N Engl J Med, 1974, 292, 1134–1135

Ward PA, Berenberg JL: Defective regulation of inflammatory mediators in Hodgkin's disease. Supernormal levels of chemotactic-factor inactivator. N Engl J Med, 1974, 290, 76–80

Ward PA, Newman LJ: A neutrophil chemotactic factor from human C5. J Immunol, 1969, 102, 93–99

Ward PA, Remold HG, David JR: Leukotactic factor produced by sensitized lymphocytes. Science, 1969, 163, 1079

Warner HR, Athens JW: An analysis of granulocyte kinetics in blood and bone marrow, in leukopoiesis in health and disease. Ann NY Acad Sci, 1964, 113, 523

Warrell DA, Perine PL, Bryceson ADM, Parry EHO, Pope HM: Physiologic changes during the Jarish-Herxheimer reaction in early syphilis. Am J Med, 1971, 51, 176–185

Watanabe I, Donhaue S, Hoggatt N: Method for electron microscopic studies of circulating human leucocytes and observations on their fine structure. J Ultrastruct Res, 1967, 20, 366–382

Wawryk R, Kasperczak W, Śliwa J: Serum alkaline phosphatase activity and neutrophil alkaline phosphatase activity in physiologic term pregnancy (in Polish). Ginekol Pol, 1971, 42, 1115–1118

Ważewska-Czyżewska M: Skin window method of Rebuck in diagnosis of acute monocytic and eosinocytic leukaemia (in Polish). Przegl Lek, 1972, 29, 972–974

Ważewska-Czyżewska M, Mossor-Ostrowska J, Węsierska-Gądek J: Observations on the clinical course of leukaemia complicated with virus hepatitis. Pol Tyg Lek, 1977, 32, 1597–1600

Wechsler R, Wallace SL, Gerber D, Scherrer J: Colchicine and trimethylcolchicinic acid: a comparison of their effects on human white blood cells in vitro. Arthritis Rheum, 1965, 8, 1104

Weening RS, Roos D, Loos JA: Oxygen consumption of phagocytizing cells in human leukocyte and granulocyte preparations: a comparative study. J Lab Clin Med, 1974, 83, 570–576

Weisberger AS, Suhrland LG, Griggs RC: Incorporation of radioactive L-cystine and L-methionine by leukemic leukocytes in vitro. Blood, 1954, 9, 1095

Weissmann G, Zurier RB, Spieler PJ, Goldstein IM: Mechanisms of lysosomal enzyme release from leukocytes exposed to immune complexes and other particles. J Exp Med, 1971, 134, 149–165

Welsh IRH, Zeya HI, Spitznagel JK: Heterogeneity of lysosomes from human peripheral blood polymorphonuclear leukocytes. Fed Proc, 1971, 30, 599

West BC, Gelb NA, Kimball HR: Human blood granulocyte granules. Fed Proc, 1972, 31, 253 abstr

Westwick WJ, Allsop J, Gumpel JM, Watts RWE: Studies on pyrimidine biosynthesis in the granulocytes of patients receiving gold therapy for rheumatoid arthritis. Q J Med, 1974, 43, 231–243

Whang J, Frei E, Tijo JH, Carbone PP, Brecker G: The distribution of the Philadelphia chromosome in patients with chronic myelogenous leukemia. Blood, 1963, 22, 664

Whang-Peng J, Gralnick HR, Johnson RE, Lee EC, Lear A: Chronic granulocytic leukemia (CGL) during the course of chronic lymphocytic leukemia (CLL): correlation of blood, marrow and spleen morphology and cytogenetics. Blood, 1974, 43, 333–339

Wheldon TE, Kirk J, Finlay HM: Cyclical granulopoiesis in chronic granulocytic leukemia: a stimulation study. Blood, 1974, 43, 379–387

White JG: The Chediak-Higashi syndrome. Fine structure of giant inclusions in freeze-fractured neutrophils. Am J Pathol, 1973, 72, 503–520

Whittaker JA, Hughes HR, Khurshid M: The effect of cytotoxic and anti-inflammatory drugs on the phagocytosis of neutrophil leukocytes. Br J Haematol, 1975, 29, 273–278

Whittaker JA, Khurshid M, Hughes HR: Neutrophil function in chronic granulocytic leukaemia before and after busulfan treatment. Br J Haematol, 1974, 28, 541–549

Whittaker JA Sartain P, Shaheedy M: Hematological aspects of congenital syphilis. J Pediatr, 1965, 66, 629–636

Wickramasinghe SN, Bush V: An investigation into the development and fate of neutrophil giant metamyelocytes using the techniques of electron microscopy and high resolution autoradiography. Br J Haematol, 1977, 35, 659–664

Wiener L: A family with a high incidence of leukemia and unique Ph¹ chromosome findings. Blood, 1965, 26, 871

Wiik A, Munthe E: Complement-fixing granulocyte-specific antinuclear factors in neutropenic cases of rheumatoid arthritis. Immunology, 1974, 26, 1127–1134

Wilbur DW: The Neutrophil System. Publications of University of California, Livermore, 1966

Wilkinson PM, Summer C, Delamore IW: Granulocyte function in myeloblastic leukaemia. Br J Cancer, 1975, 32, 574–577

Williams HE, Field JB: Further studies on leukocyte phosphorylase in glycogen storage disease. Metabolism, 1963, 12, 464–466

Williams HE, Field JB: Studies on glycogen storage disease. III. Limit dextrinosis: a genetic study. J Pediatr, 1968, 72, 214–221

Williams HE, Kending EM, Field JB: Leukocyte debranching enzyme in glycogen storage disease. Pediatrics, 1963, 27, 103

Williams HE, Kending EM, Field JB: Leukocyte debranching enzyme in glycogen storage disease. III. Limit dextrinosis: a genetic study. J Clin Invest, 1963, 72, 656–658

Williams HE, Lundholm UI: UDPG-glycogen synthetase activity in human leukocytes. Biochim Biophys Acta, 1968, 158, 465

Williams WJ, Beutler E, Erslev AJ, Rundles WR: Hematology. McGraw-Hill, New York, Toronto, 1977

Windhorst DB, Holmes B, Good RA: A newly diagnosed X-linked trait in man with demonstration of the Lyon effect in carrier females. Lancet, 1967, 1, 737

Winkelstein A, Goldberg LS, Tishkoff GH, Sparkes RS: Leukocyte alkaline phosphatase and the Philadelphia chromosome. Arch Intern Med, 1967, 119, 291

Winkelstein JA, Drachman RH: Deficiency of pneumococcal serum opsonizing activity in sickle cell disease. N Engl J Med, 1968, 279, 459

Wintrobe MM, Lee GR, Boggs DR, Bithell TC, Athens JW, Foester J: Clinical Hematology. Lea and Febiger, Philadelphia, 1975

Wintroub BU, Goetzl EJ, Austen KF: A neutrophil-dependent pathway for the generation of a neutral peptide mediator: partial characterization of components and control by alpha-1-antitripsin. J Exp Med, 1974, 140, 812–824

Wojtecka-Łukasik E, Dancewicz AM: Human leukocyte collagenase: isolation, purification, properties (in Polish). Przegl Lek, 1974, 31, 431–435

Wolff SM, Dale DC, Clark RA Roct RK, Kimball HR: The Chediak-Higashi syndrome: studies of host defenses. Ann Intern Med, 1972, 76, 293–306

Wolfish NM, Wassef N, Gonzales H, Acharya C: Immunologic parameters of children with urinary tract infection: effects of trimethoprim-sulfamethoxasole. Can Med Assoc J, 1975, 112, 76–79

Wołosowicz N: Antifibrinolytic system of human granulocytes (in Polish). Pol Tyg Lek, 1978, 33, 651–652

Wołosowicz N, Prokopowicz J: Isolation and Purification of Antiplasmins from Human Granulocytes. Thromb Diath Haemorrh, 1970, 34, 343–347

Wong L, Wilson JD: The identification of Fc and C3 receptors on human neutrophils. J Immunol Meth, 1975, 7, 69–76

Wriedt K, Kaeder E, Mauer AM: Failure of myeloid differentiation as a cause of congenital neutropenia. J Pediatr, 1966, 68, 839

Wright DG, Kauffmann JC, Chusid MJ, Herzig GP, Gallin JI: Functional abnormalities of human neutrophil collected by continuous flow filtration leukopheresis. Blood, 1975, 46, 901–911

Wünschmann B, Goldstein I, Astrup T, Henderson E: Fibrinolytic activity of normal human leukocytes increased by bacterial endotoxin. XIII International Congress of Hematology (Aug 2–8), München, Abstract Volume, 1970, p 328

Xanthou M: Leucocyte blood picture in healthy full-term and premature babies during neonatal period. Arch Dis Child, 1970, 45, 242–249

Yoshinaga M, Yamamoto S, Kiyota S, Hayashi H: The natural mediator for PMN migration in inflammation. IV. In vitro production of a chemotactic factor by papain from immunoglobulin G. Immunology, 1972, 22, 393–399

Yunis AA, Harrington WJ: Patterns of inhibition by chloramphenicol of nucleic acid synthesis in human bone marrow and leukemic cells. J Lab Clin Med, 1960, 56, 831–832

Żaboklicki S, Zeman K: Reduction of NBT in neutrophils after physical exercise and in various periods of a day (in Polish). Pol Tyg Lek, 1976, 31, 1321–1324

Zacharski LR, Bowie EJW, Titus JL, Owen CA: Cell-culture synthesis of a factor VII-like activity. Mayo Clinic Proc, 1969, 44, 784–792

Zaharia L, Hill HM, Khan A, Loeb E, MacLellan A, Hill NO: Filtration leukapheresis for granulocyte transfusion. J Clin Hematol Oncol (Wadley Med Bull), 1976, 6, 1–9

Zajączkowski J: Problems of immunologic reactivity in patients with malignancies (in Polish). Wiad Lek, 1976, 29, 2009–2012

Zajączkowski J: Humoral and cellular immunity in children with acute lymphoblastic leukemia (in Polish). Pediatr Pol, 1977, 52, 225–228

Zajączkowski J, Kolanowska H, Pituch A: Nitroblue tetrazolium (NBT) test in children with acute lymphoblastic leukemia or malignant lymphomas. Rev Roum Med—Med Int, 1976, 14, 121–123

Zajączkowski J, Pituch A, Legutko L: Immunoglobulin and granulocyte cytochemical reactions in L-asparaginase treated children with acute lymphoblastic leukemia. Rev Roum Med—Med Int, 1976, 14, 191–195

Zajączkowski J, Pituch A, Legutko L: Immunoglobulin levels and cytochemical reactions in children with acute lymphoblastic leukemia (in Polish). Przegl Pediatr, 1976, 4, 349–353

Zajączkowski J, Pituch A, Legutko L, Pajdak E: Immunological aspects of L-asparaginase treatment in children with lymphoproliferative disease. Helv Paediatr Acta, 1975, 30, 441–446

Zatti M, Rossi F, Patriarca P: The H_2O_2 production by polymorphonuclear leucocytes during phagocytosis. Experientia, 1968, 24, 669–670

Zeigler Z: In vitro granulocyte-platelet rosette formation mediated by an IgG immunoglobulin. Haemostasis 1974, 3, 282–287

Zeya HJ, Keku E, Richards F, Spurr CL: Monocyte and granulocyte defect in chronic lymphocytic leucaemia. Am J Path, 1979, 95, 45–53

Zeya HJ, Keku E, Richards F, Spurr CL: Absence of neutral protease and alkaline phosphatase in neutrophils of a case of hairy cell leukemia. Am J Path, 1979, 95, 55–66

Zeya HJ, Spitznagel JK: Cationic proteins of polymorphonuclear leukocyte lysosomes. II. Composition, properties and mechanism of antibacterial action. J Bacteriol, 1966, 91, 755–762

Zgliczyński JM: The model of chlorinating action of myeloperoxidase of human neutrophils (in Polish). Przegl Lek, 1979, 3, 136–142

Zgliczyński JM, Stelmaszyńska T: Chlorinating ability of human phagocytising leucocytes. Eur J Biochem, 1975, 56, 157–162

Zgliczyński JM, Stelmaszyńska T, Ostrowski W, Naskalski J, Sznajd J: Myeloperoxidase of human leukemic leukocytes. Oxidation of amino acids in the presence of hydrogen peroxide. European J Biochem, 1968, 4, 540–547

Zhuklis Y: Serum of patients with pulmonary tuberculosis in potentiating the reaction of blood neutrophils to tuberculin (in Russian). Probl Tuberk, 1975, 76, 42–43

Zigmond SH, Hirsch JG: Leucocyte locomotion and chemotaxis. New methods for evaluation, and demonstration of a cell-derived chemotactic factor. J Exp Med, 1973, 137, 387–410

Zikovic M, Baum J: Chemotaxis of polymorphonuclear leukocytes from patients with systemic lupus erythematosus and Felty's syndrome. Immunol Commun, 1972, 1, 39–49

Zipursky A, Brown EJ: The ingestion of IgG-sensitized erythrocytes by abnormal neutrophils. Blood, 1974, 43, 737–742

Zittoun R, Berche PA: L'adhésivité au verre et le pouvoir phagocytaire des polynucléaires neutrophiles dans les syndromes myélo-prolifératifs et les anémies refractaires. Pathol Biol, 1973, 21, 271–277

Zucker-Franklin D, Hirsch JG: Electron miscroscope studies on the degranulation of rabbit peritoneal leukocytes during phagocytosis. J Exp Med, 1964, 120, 569

Zuckerman H, Sadowsky E, Diamant YZ, Polishuk WZ: Monitoring of leukocyte alkaline phosphatase activity in pregnancy. Isr J Med Sci, 1969, 5, 1159

Zukovskaya ES, Khramova NV: System of blood coagulation in patients with various forms of acute leukemia (in Russian). Probl Gematol, 1973, 18, 41–47

Żupańska B: Verification of biochemical studies on activity of catalase in leukocytes (in Polish). Acta Haematol Pol, 1970, 1, 191–198

Zurier RB: Prostaglandins, inflammation and asthma. Arch Intern Med, 1974, 133, 101

Zurier RB: Reduction of phagocytosis and lysosomal enzyme release from human leukocytes by serum from patients with systemic lupus. Arthritis Rheum, 1976, 19, 73–78

Zurier RB, Hoffstein S, Weissman G: Cytochalasin B: effect on lysosomal enzyme release from human leukocytes. Proc Natl Acad Sci, 1973, 70, 844–848

Zvaifler NJ: Immunoreactants in rheumatoid synovial effusions. J Exp Med, 1971, 134, 276–285

SUBJECT INDEX

alpha₂-Macroglobulin 100
Macrophages 242, 244
Macropolycytosis 32
Magnesium 47, 93, 104, 111
Magnesium-deficient diet 59, 60
Malnutrition 163
Malonic acid dehydrogenase 183
Mannosidase 55
May-Hegglin anomaly 28
McArdle's disease 203
Measles 233
Menstrual cycle 69
Metabolic diseases 199
Metamyelocytes 21
Methionine 182
Methotrexate 155
Methylaminocyclohexanocarboxylic acid 134
Micronucleoli 21
Microtubules 64
MIF 167
Migration of neutrophils 88–92
Mitochondria 20, 21
Mobilization of neutrophils 87–92, 150, 210
Monoblasts 24, 190
Monocytes 99
Muramidase 65
Myasthenia 36
Mycoses 242
Myeloblasts 20, 22, 24, 130, 134, 135, 141, 142, 150, 190
Myelomonocytic leukemia 193
Myeloperoxidase 32, 49, 50, 51, 175, 194, 202

N-acetyl-beta-glucosaminidase 55, 218–221
NADP 104, 109, 174
NADPH 104, 109, 110, 174
NADPH oxidase 18, 21–23, 173
NADPH₂ oxidase 51
Naphthol AS-D-chloroacetate 61
NBT—see Nitroblue tetrazolium reduction
Neonatal isoimmunization neutropenia 124
Neuraminidase, bacterial 52
Neurohormones 64
Neutropenia 153–161, 239
Neutrophilia 150–153
Neutrophilia promoting factor 87
Neutrophil immobilizing factor 100

Neutrophils 15, 39, 75, 97, 115, 129, 145, 179, 199, 209, 229
Nitroblue tetrazolium reduction 67, 68, 112, 119, 165, 167, 170, 171, 173, 176, 187, 190, 192, 193, 195, 214–216, 229, 235, 236, 244
Nuclear chromatin 20
Nucleoli 20, 21, 24
Nucleosidase 56
Nucleosomes 181
Nucleotidase 56
5-Nucleotidase 23, 56
Nucleotide synthesis in neutrophils 41

Oleinic acid 45
Oligosaccharases 62
Opsonization 100, 169
Orosomucoid 112
Orotidyl decarboxylase 41
Oxygen 108–110
Oxygen-dependent systems, antimicrobial 49
Oxygen-independent systems, antimicrobial 54
Ovarian insufficiency 69

Palmitinic acid 45
Papain 98, 99
Pappataci fever 71
Paracolon hornia 172
PAS reaction 24
Pasteur effect 43
Pelger-Huët anomaly 29, 30
Pentose cycle 43, 108, 109
Peptidase 23
Peroxidase 24, 32, 46
Phagocytic vacuole 102, 105, 172, 176
Phagocytosis 31, 95, 103, 163, 169, 172, 185, 186, 201, 208
Phagosome 36, 102, 105, 110
Pharyngitis 229
Ph₁ chromosome 34, 159, 181
Phocomelia 153
Phosphatase, acid—see Alkaline phosphatase
Phosphatase, alkaline—see Alkaline phosphatase
Phosphatidic acid 110
Phosphatidyl ethanolamine 44, 45
Phosphatidyl inositol 44, 110
Phosphatidyl serine 44, 45, 110